Learning Disabilities Sourcebook, 3rd Edition

Leukemia Sourcebook

Liver Disorders Sourcebook

Lung Disorders Sourcebook

Medical Tests Sourcebook, 3rd Edition

Men's Health Concerns Sourcebook, 2nd Edition

Mental Health Disorders Sourcebook, 4th Edition

Mental Retardation Sourcebook

Movement Disorders Sourcebook, 2nd Edition

Multiple Sclerosis Sourcebook

Muscular Dystrophy Sourcebook

Obesity Sourcebook

Osteoporosis S...

Pain Sourcebo...

Pediatric Canc...

Physical & Me...

Podiatry Sou...

Pregnancy &...

Prostate & U...

Prostate Can...

Reconstructi...

Rehabilitatio...

Respiratory...

Sexually Tra...
   3rd Editi...

Sleep Disord...

Smoking Co...

Sports Injuri...

Stress-Relate...

Stroke Sourc...

Surgery Sou...

Thyroid Dis...

Transplantati...

Traveler's H...

Urinary Trac...
   Sourcebo...

Vegetarian Sourcebook

Women's Health Concerns Sourcebook, 3rd Edition

Workplace Health & Safety Sourcebook

Worldwide Health Sourcebook

Teen Health Series

Abuse & Violence Information for Teens

Accident & Safety Information for Teens

Alcohol Information for Teens, 2nd Edition

Allergy Information for Teens

Asthma Information for Teens, 2nd Edition

...ens

...Edition

...Edition

...Teens,

...d

...n for

...ens,

...ens,

...s, 2nd

...eens,

...nd

Tobacco Information for Teens, 2nd Edition

Alcoholism
SOURCEBOOK

Third Edition

Health Reference Series

Third Edition

Alcoholism
SOURCEBOOK

Basic Consumer Health Information about Alcohol Use, Abuse, and Addiction, Including Facts about the Physical Consequences of Alcohol Abuse, Such as Brain Changes and Problems with Cognitive Functioning, Cirrhosis and Other Liver Diseases, Cardiovascular Disease, Pancreatitis, and Alcoholic Neuropathy, and the Effects of Alcohol on Reproductive Health and Fetal Development, Mental Health Problems Associated with Alcohol Abuse, and Alcohol's Impact on Families, Workplaces, and the Community

Along with Information about Underage Drinking, Alcohol Treatment and Recovery, a Glossary of Related Terms, and Directories of Resources for More Information

Edited by
Joyce Brennfleck Shannon

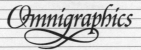

P.O. Box 31-1640, Detroit, MI 48231

Bibliographic Note
Because this page cannot legibly accommodate all the copyright notices, the Bibliographic
Note portion of the Preface constitutes an extension of the copyright notice.

Edited by Joyce Brennfleck Shannon

Health Reference Series

Karen Bellenir, *Managing Editor*
David A. Cooke, MD, FACP, *Medical Consultant*
Elizabeth Collins, *Research and Permissions Coordinator*
Cherry Edwards, *Permissions Assistant*
EdIndex, Services for Publishers, *Indexers*

* * *

Omnigraphics, Inc.
Matthew P. Barbour, *Senior Vice President*
Kevin M. Hayes, *Operations Manager*

* * *

Peter E. Ruffner, *Publisher*

Copyright © 2010 Omnigraphics, Inc.

ISBN 978-0-7808-1141-6

Library of Congress Cataloging-in-Publication Data

Alcoholism sourcebook : basic consumer health information about alcohol use, abuse, and addiction,
including facts about the physical consequences of alcohol abuse, such as brain changes and
problems with cognitive functioning, cirrhosis and other liver diseases, cardiovascular disease,
pancreatitis, and alcoholic neuropathy, and the effects of alcohol on reproductive health and fetal
development, mental health problems associated with alcohol abuse, and alcohol's impact on
families, workplaces, and the community; along with information about underage drinking, alcohol
treatment and recovery, a glossary of related terms, and directories of resources for more information
/ edited by Joyce Brennfleck Shannon. -- 3rd ed.
    p. cm. -- (Health reference series)
  Includes bibliographical references and index.
  Summary: "Provides basic consumer health information about alcohol abuse, addiction, and related
health effects, with facts about treatment and recovery. Includes index, glossary of related terms, and
other resources"--Provided by publisher.
  ISBN 978-0-7808-1141-6 (hardcover : alk. paper) 1. Alcoholism--Popular works. 2. Consumer
education. I. Shannon, Joyce Brennfleck.
  RC565.A4493 2010
  362.292'86--dc22
                                                                                        2010031843

Table of Contents

Visit www.healthreferenceseries.com to view *A Contents Guide to the Health Reference Series*, a listing of more than 15,000 topics and the volumes in which they are covered.

Part III: The Physical Effects and Consequences of Alcohol Abuse

Part VIII: Additional Help and Information

Preface

About This Book

Excessive alcohol use causes approximately 79,000 deaths each year, making it the third leading lifestyle-related cause of death in the United States. Alcohol affects every organ in the drinker's body. While moderate alcohol use can have some health benefits for adults, heavy alcohol use and binge drinking can harm the body, disrupt relationships, and lead to risky behaviors, injury, illness, or death. Furthermore, any alcohol use can cause permanent harm to underage drinkers and to the unborn children of pregnant women.

Alcoholism Sourcebook, Third Edition provides readers with updated information about alcohol use, abuse, and dependence. Physical alcohol-related effects on the brain, liver, pancreas, heart, lungs, nerves, and kidneys are described, and mental health issues that often accompany alcohol problems are discussed. A section on the problem of underage drinking looks at the causes and consequences of drinking among adolescents, and another section discusses the effects of alcohol use on reproductive and fetal health. Facts about alcohol's impact on families, workplaces, and communities are included, and guidance is provided for helping someone with an alcohol problem receive appropriate treatment and recovery services. The book concludes with a glossary of terms related to alcohol use and abuse and directories of resources for support and additional information.

How to Use This Book

This book is divided into parts and chapters. Parts focus on broad areas of interest. Chapters are devoted to single topics within a part.

Part I: Understanding Alcohol Use, Abuse, and Dependence reviews guidelines for the safe consumption of alcohol and offers facts about identifying when alcohol use transitions into abuse and may precipitate problems. It explains the course of alcohol dependence and discusses risk factors, including genetic links to addiction vulnerabilities.

Part II: The Problem of Underage Drinking describes drinking patterns and alcohol-related problems experienced by teens and college students. It discusses alcohol's impact on development, offers prevention strategies for families, schools, and communities, and explains the rationale behind laws establishing a minimum legal drinking age.

Part III: The Physical Effects and Consequences of Alcohol Abuse gives facts about alcohol impairment from various levels of blood alcohol concentration (BAC), alcohol poisoning, and alcohol hangover. It describes how alcohol changes the brain and affects the liver, cardiovascular system, kidneys, lungs, and bones. Information about alcohol interactions with other disorders and medications is also included.

Part IV: The Effects of Alcohol on Reproductive and Fetal Health describes how alcohol use impacts the reproductive organs and how it can lead to life-long impairments among children of women who drink during pregnancy. Detailed information about the effects of alcohol on a fetus is presented along with a discussion of fetal alcohol spectrum disorders (FASD).

Part V: Mental Health Problems Associated with Alcohol Abuse discusses the impact alcohol has on anxiety disorders, depression, post-traumatic stress disorder (PTSD), and attention deficit/hyperactivity disorder (ADHD). Separate chapters describe the connection of alcohol with other addiction disorders and suicide.

Part VI: Alcohol's Impact on Family, Work, and the Community includes information about children living with alcohol-abusing parents, interpersonal violence related to alcohol, the effects of alcohol-impaired driving, and problems associated with alcohol use in the workplace.

Part VII: Treatment and Recovery discusses helping strategies, programs, and support groups for families and individuals who decide to change their alcohol consumption habits. It describes alcohol addiction screening and explains the differences between brief interventions and long-term treatments. It also offers facts about the treatment process, including information on detoxification, withdrawal, pharmacological treatments, and integrated treatments for co-occurring disorders such as drug abuse or mental illness.

Part VIII: Additional Help and Information provides a glossary of terms related to alcohol use and abuse. Resource directories with listings of support groups for alcohol-related concerns, state agencies for substance abuse services, and organizations with additional information about alcohol use and abuse are also included.

Bibliographic Note

This volume contains documents and excerpts from publications issued by the following U.S. government agencies: Agency for Healthcare Research and Quality (AHRQ); Alcohol Policy Information System (APIS); Centers for Disease Prevention and Control (CDC); Federal Trade Commission (FTC); Higher Education Center for Alcohol and Other Drug Abuse and Violence Prevention; National Digestive Diseases Information Clearinghouse; National Institute of Diabetes and Digestive and Kidney Diseases (NIDDK); National Heart, Lung, and Blood Institute (NHLBI); National Highway Traffic Safety Administration (NHTSA); National Institute of Arthritis and Musculoskeletal and Skin Diseases (NIAMS); National Institute of Environmental Health Science (NIEHS); National Institute on Aging (NIA); National Institute on Alcohol Abuse and Alcoholism (NIAAA); National Institute on Drug Abuse (NIDA); National Institutes of Health (NIH); NIAAA College Drinking Changing the Culture; Substance Abuse and Mental Health Services Administration (SAMHSA); United States Coast Guard; United States Department of Agriculture (USDA); United States Department of Health and Human Services Administration (HHS); United States Department of Labor (DOL); United States Department of Veterans Affairs (VA); United States Fire Administration; and the VA National Center for Posttraumatic Stress Disorder.

In addition, this volume contains copyrighted documents from the following organizations and individuals: A.D.A.M., Inc.; American Diabetes Association; American Heart Association; American Institute for Cancer Research; American Liver Foundation; American Psychiatric Association; Anxiety Disorders Association of America; Go Ask Alice of Columbia University Health Education Program; HealthDay/Scout News LLC; International Center for Alcohol Policies; Marin Institute; Nemours Foundation; Steven M. Melemis, MD; and the World Health Organization.

, Full citation information is provided on the first page of each chapter or section. Every effort has been made to secure all necessary rights to reprint the copyrighted material. If any omissions have been made, please contact Omnigraphics to make corrections for future editions.

Acknowledgements

In addition to the listed organizations, agencies, and individuals who have contributed to this *Sourcebook*, special thanks go to managing editor Karen Bellenir, research and permissions coordinator Liz Collins, and document engineer Bruce Bellenir for their help and support.

About the Health Reference Series

The *Health Reference Series* is designed to provide basic medical information for patients, families, caregivers, and the general public. Each volume takes a particular topic and provides comprehensive coverage. This is especially important for people who may be dealing with a newly diagnosed disease or a chronic disorder in themselves or in a family member. People looking for preventive guidance, information about disease warning signs, medical statistics, and risk factors for health problems will also find answers to their questions in the *Health Reference Series*. The *Series*, however, is not intended to serve as a tool for diagnosing illness, in prescribing treatments, or as a substitute for the physician/patient relationship. All people concerned about medical symptoms or the possibility of disease are encouraged to seek professional care from an appropriate health care provider.

A Note about Spelling and Style

Health Reference Series editors use *Stedman's Medical Dictionary* as an authority for questions related to the spelling of medical terms and the *Chicago Manual of Style* for questions related to grammatical structures, punctuation, and other editorial concerns. Consistent adherence is not always possible, however, because the individual volumes within the *Series* include many documents from a wide variety of different producers and copyright holders, and the editor's primary goal is to present material from each source as accurately as is possible following the terms specified by each document's producer. This sometimes means that information in different chapters or sections may follow other guidelines and alternate spelling authorities. For example, occasionally a copyright holder may require that eponymous terms be shown in possessive forms (Crohn's disease *vs.* Crohn disease) or that British spelling norms be retained (leukaemia *vs.* leukemia).

Locating Information within the Health Reference Series

The *Health Reference Series* contains a wealth of information about a wide variety of medical topics. Ensuring easy access to all the fact sheets, research reports, in-depth discussions, and other material contained within the individual books of the *Series* remains one of our highest priorities. As the *Series* continues to grow in size and scope, however, locating the precise information needed by a reader may become more challenging.

A *Contents Guide to the Health Reference Series* was developed to direct readers to the specific volumes that address their concerns. It presents an extensive list of diseases, treatments, and other topics of general interest compiled from the Tables of Contents and major index headings. To access *A Contents Guide to the Health Reference Series*, visit www.healthreferenceseries.com.

Medical Consultant

Medical consultation services are provided to the *Health Reference Series* editors by David A. Cooke, MD, FACP. Dr. Cooke is a graduate of Brandeis University, and he received his MD degree from the University of Michigan. He completed residency training at the University of Wisconsin Hospital and Clinics. He is board-certified in Internal Medicine. Dr. Cooke currently works as part of the University of Michigan Health System and practices in Ann Arbor, MI. In his free time, he enjoys writing, science fiction, and spending time with his family.

Our Advisory Board

We would like to thank the following board members for providing guidance to the development of this *Series*:

- Dr. Lynda Baker, Associate Professor of Library and Information Science, Wayne State University, Detroit, MI

- Nancy Bulgarelli, William Beaumont Hospital Library, Royal Oak, MI

- Karen Imarisio, Bloomfield Township Public Library, Bloomfield Township, MI

- Karen Morgan, Mardigian Library, University of Michigan-Dearborn, Dearborn, MI

- Rosemary Orlando, St. Clair Shores Public Library, St. Clair Shores, MI

Health Reference Series *Update Policy*

The inaugural book in the *Health Reference Series* was the first edition of *Cancer Sourcebook* published in 1989. Since then, the *Series* has been enthusiastically received by librarians and in the medical community. In order to maintain the standard of providing high-quality health information for the layperson the editorial staff at Omnigraphics felt it was necessary to implement a policy of updating volumes when warranted.

Medical researchers have been making tremendous strides, and it is the purpose of the *Health Reference Series* to stay current with the most recent advances. Each decision to update a volume is made on an individual basis. Some of the considerations include how much new information is available and the feedback we receive from people who use the books. If there is a topic you would like to see added to the update list, or an area of medical concern you feel has not been adequately addressed, please write to:

Editor
Health Reference Series
Omnigraphics, Inc.
P.O. Box 31-1640
Detroit, MI 48231-1640
E-mail: editorial@omnigraphics.com

Part One

Understanding Alcohol Use, Abuse, and Dependence

Chapter 1

When Can Alcohol Be Used Safely?

Chapter Contents

3

Section 1.1

Drinking Alcohol: Low Risk Versus High Risk

This section is excerpted from "Rethinking Drinking: Alcohol and Your
Health," National Institute on Alcohol Abuse and Alcoholism (NIAAA),
NIH Publication No. 10–3770, revised April 2010.

Do you enjoy a drink now and then? Many of us do, often when so-
cializing with friends and family. Drinking can be beneficial or harmful,
depending on your age and health status, the situation, and of course,
how much you drink. Do you think you may drink too much at times?
Do you think everyone drinks a lot? Following are results from a nationwide survey of 43,000 adults by the National Institutes of Health
(NIH) on alcohol use and its consequences.

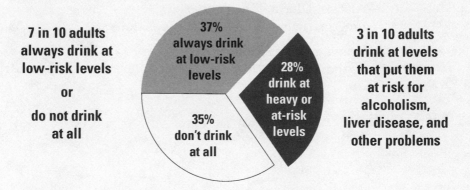

7 in 10 adults always drink at low-risk levels or **do not drink at all**

37% always drink at low-risk levels

28% drink at heavy or at-risk levels

35% don't drink at all

3 in 10 adults drink at levels that put them at risk for alcoholism, liver disease, and other problems

*Figure 1.1. Alcohol use by adults in the United States. (Although the mini-
mum legal drinking age in the U.S. is 21, this survey included people aged
18 or older.)*

Many heavy drinkers do not have alcohol-related problems yet
and can reduce their risk of harm by cutting back. For the nearly 18
million Americans who have alcoholism or related problems, however,
it's safest to quit.

What counts as a drink?

Many people are surprised to learn what counts as a drink. In the United States, a standard drink is any drink that contains about 0.6 fluid ounces or 14 grams of pure alcohol. Although the drinks pictured in Figure 1.2 are different sizes, each contains approximately the same amount of alcohol and counts as a single drink.

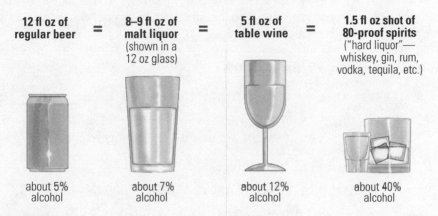

| **12 fl oz of regular beer** | = | **8–9 fl oz of malt liquor** (shown in a 12 oz glass) | = | **5 fl oz of table wine** | = | **1.5 fl oz shot of 80-proof spirits** ("hard liquor"—whiskey, gin, rum, vodka, tequila, etc.) |

about 5% alcohol   about 7% alcohol   about 12% alcohol   about 40% alcohol

Figure 1.2. *Standard Drinks. The percent of "pure" alcohol, expressed here as alcohol by volume (alc/vol), varies by beverage.*

How many drinks are in common containers?

Table 1.1. Approximate Number of Standard Drinks in Different Sized Containers

regular beer (fluid ounces [fl oz])	malt liquor	table wine (milliliter [ml])	80-proof spirits or hard liquor
12 fl oz = 1	12 fl oz = 1.5	750 ml (a regular wine bottle) = 5	a shot (1.5 oz glass/50 ml bottle) = 1
16 fl oz = 1.3	16 fl oz = 2		a mixed drink or cocktail = 1 or more
22 fl oz = 2	22 fl oz = 2.5		200 ml (a half pint) = 4.5
40 fl oz = 3.3	40 fl oz = 4.5		375 ml (a pint or half bottle) = 8.5
			750 ml (a fifth) = 17

The examples shown serve as a starting point for comparison. For different types of beer, wine, or malt liquor, the alcohol content can vary greatly. Some differences are smaller than you might expect, however. Many light beers, for example, have almost as much alcohol as regular beer—about 85% as much, or 4.2% versus 5.0% alcohol by volume (alc/vol), on average.

Although the standard drink sizes are helpful for following health guidelines, they may not reflect customary serving sizes. A mixed drink, for example, can contain one, two, or more standard drinks, depending on the type of spirits and the recipe.

What's your drinking pattern?

Using the drink sizes, answer the following questions:

1. On any day in the past year, have you ever had more than four drinks (men), or more than three drinks (women)?

2. Think about your typical week:

   a. on average, how many days a week do you drink alcohol?

   b. on a typical drinking day, how many drinks do you have?

To learn your weekly average, multiply a by b.

Sometimes even a little is too much: Even moderate levels of drinking (up to two drinks per day for men or one for women) can be too much in some circumstances. It's safest to avoid alcohol if you are: planning to drive a vehicle or operate machinery; taking medications that interact with alcohol; managing a medical condition that can be made worse by drinking; or pregnant or trying to become pregnant.

Can you hold your liquor?

If so, you may be at greater risk. For some people, it takes quite a few drinks to get a buzz or feel relaxed. Often they are unaware that being able to hold your liquor isn't protection from alcohol problems, but instead a reason for caution. They tend to drink more, socialize with people who drink a lot, and develop a tolerance to alcohol. As a result, they have an increased risk for developing alcoholism. The higher alcohol levels can also cause liver, heart, and brain damage that can go unnoticed until it's too late. And all drinkers need to be aware that even moderate amounts of alcohol can significantly impair driving performance, even when they don't feel a buzz from drinking.

What's low-risk drinking?

A major nationwide survey of 43,000 U.S. adults by the National Institutes of Health shows that only about two in 100 people who drink within both the single-day and weekly limits shown in Figure 1.3 have alcoholism or alcohol abuse. How do these low-risk levels compare with your drinking pattern?

Low risk is not no risk. Even within these limits, drinkers can have problems if they drink too quickly, have health problems, or are older (both men and women over 65 are generally advised to have no more than three drinks on any day and seven per week). Based on your health and how alcohol affects you, you may need to drink less or not at all.

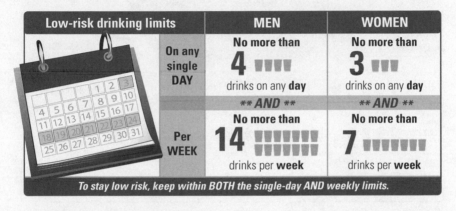

Figure 1.3. Low-Risk Drinking Limits

What's heavy or at-risk drinking?

For healthy adults in general, drinking more than the single-day or weekly amounts shown is considered at-risk or heavy drinking. About one in four people who drink this much already has alcoholism or is abusing alcohol, and the rest are at greater risk for developing these and other problems.

It makes a difference both how much you drink on any day and how often you have a heavy drinking day—that is, more than four drinks in a day for men or more than three drinks for women. The more drinks in a day and the more heavy drinking days over time, the greater the chances for problems.

Why are women's low-risk limits different from men's?

Research shows that women start to have alcohol-related problems at lower drinking levels than men do. One reason is that, on average, women weigh less than men. In addition, alcohol disperses in body water, and pound for pound, women have less water in their bodies than men do. So after a man and woman of the same weight drink the same amount of alcohol, the woman's blood alcohol concentration will tend to be higher, putting her at greater risk for harm.

How much do U.S. adults drink?

The majority—seven out of ten—either abstain or always drink within low-risk limits.

Drinking patterns in U.S. adults		
9 %	drink more than *both* the single-day limits **and** the weekly limits	**Highest risk**
19 %	drink more than *either* the single-day limits **or** the weekly limits	**Increased risk**
37 %	**always** drink **within** low-risk limits	**Low risk**
35 %	**never** drink alcohol	—

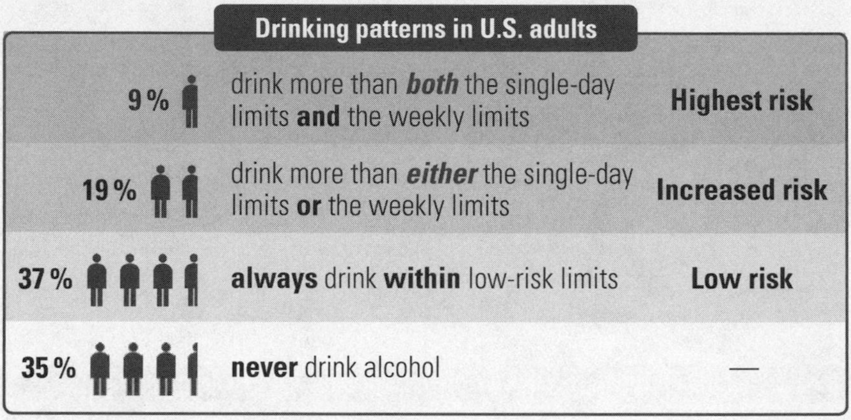

Figure 1.4. Patterns of Drinking

What's the harm?

Not all drinking is harmful. You may have heard that regular light to moderate drinking (from half of a drink a day up to one drink a day for women and two for men) can even be good for the heart. With at-risk or heavy drinking, however, any potential benefits are outweighed by greater risks.

Injuries: Drinking too much increases your chances of being injured or even killed. Alcohol is a factor, for example, in about 60% of fatal burn injuries, drowning, and homicides; 50% of severe trauma injuries and sexual assaults; and 40% of fatal motor vehicle crashes, suicides, and fatal falls.

Health problems: Heavy drinkers have a greater risk of liver disease, heart disease, sleep disorders, depression, stroke, bleeding from the stomach, sexually transmitted infections from unsafe sex, and several types of cancer. They may also have problems managing diabetes, high blood pressure, and other conditions.

Birth defects: Drinking during pregnancy can cause brain damage and other serious problems in the baby. Because it is not yet known whether any amount of alcohol is safe for a developing baby, women who are pregnant or may become pregnant should not drink.

Alcohol use disorders: Generally known as alcoholism and alcohol abuse, alcohol use disorders are medical conditions that doctors can diagnose when a patient's drinking causes distress or harm. In the United States, about 18 million people have an alcohol use disorder.

Section 1.2

Alcohol Dietary Guidelines for Americans

This section includes an excerpt from "Dietary Guidelines for Americans 2005," United States Department of Agriculture (USDA), updated July 9, 2008; and "Alcohol Calorie Calculator," National Institute on Alcohol Abuse and Alcoholism (NIAAA), July 11, 2007.

Alcoholic beverages supply calories but few essential nutrients. As a result, excessive alcohol consumption makes it difficult to ingest sufficient nutrients within an individual's daily calorie allotment and to maintain a healthy weight. Although the consumption of one to two alcoholic beverages per day is not associated with macronutrient or micronutrient deficiencies or with overall dietary quality, heavy drinkers may be at risk of malnutrition if the calories derived from alcohol are substituted for those in nutritious foods.

Alcohol Calorie Calculation

Find out the number of beer and hard alcohol calories you are consuming. Multiply the number of calories by the number of each drink you have in an average week and add the totals to see the number of alcohol calories you average in a week.

Table 1.2. Calories in Alcoholic Beverages

Beverage	Serving Amount (ounce)	Calories
Beer		
Regular	12	149
Light	12	110
Distilled (80 proof)		
Gin, rum, vodka, whisky, tequila	1.0	65
Brandy, cognac	1.0	65
Liqueurs (Drambuie, Cointreau, Kahlua)	1.5	188
Wine		
Red	4	80
Dry white	4	75
Sweet	4	105
Sherry	2	75
Port	2	90
Champagne	4	84
Vermouth, sweet	3	140
Vermouth, dry	3	105
Cocktails		
Martini	3.5	140
Manhattan	3.5	164
Daiquiri	4	122
Whiskey sour	3	122
Margarita cocktail	4	168
Coolers	6	150

Table 1.3. Nutrient Intakes from Food: Percentages of Calories from Protein, Carbohydrate, Fat, and Alcohol, One Day, 2005–2006

Gender and age (years)	Food energy (% kcal)	Protein (% kcal)	Carbohydrate (% kcal)	Total fat (% kcal)	Saturated fat (%kcal)	Monoun-saturated fat (% kcal)	Poly-unsaturated fat (% kcal)	Alcohol (% kcal)
Males:								
2–5	1641	13.9	55.9	31.4	11.5	11.5	5.8	#*
6–11	2092	13.8	53.7	33.8	12.1	12.4	6.5	#*
12–19	2707	14.6	52.7	33.1	11.6	12.3	6.2	0.5
20–29	2821	15.4	49.0	31.7	10.7	11.9	6.4	4.6

30–39	2978	16.0	46.8	34.0	11.4	12.7	7.0	4.1
40–49	2753	16.0	45.6	34.0	11.2	12.7	7.1	5.5
50–59	2597	15.2	47.7	34.6	11.3	12.9	7.5	3.8
60–69	2202	16.4	47.2	33.7	11.2	12.3	7.1	4.1
70 and over	1984	15.9	48.7	34.5	11.5	12.7	7.3	2.6
20 and over	2638	15.8	47.4	33.7	11.2	12.5	7.0	4.3
Females:								
2–5	1486	14.3	56.0	31.1	11.3	11.2	6.0	#*
6–11	1879	13.5	53.8	33.9	12.0	12.5	6.6	#*
12–19	1906	13.7	53.6	33.4	11.5	12.1	7.0	#0.4
20–29	1959	15.1	51.0	33.1	11.3	12.0	6.9	2.0
30–39	1923	16.1	49.0	34.2	11.1	12.6	7.5	2.1
40–49	1873	16.5	47.9	33.6	11.4	11.9	7.3	3.3
50–59	1718	16.7	48.3	34.5	11.8	12.4	7.3	1.8
60–69	1598	16.0	49.2	34.8	11.6	12.6	7.6	1.7
70 and over	1495	15.6	51.9	33.0	11.2	11.7	7.3	1.3
20 and over	1785	16.0	49.4	33.8	11.4	12.2	7.3	2.1
Males and females:								
2 and over	2157	15.4	49.9	33.6	11.4	12.3	7.0	2.4

# indicates an estimate with a relative standard error greater than 30%.
* indicates a non-zero value too small to print.
Source: U.S. Department of Agriculture, Agricultural Research Service. 2008. Available: http://www.ars.usda.gov/ba/bhnrc/fsrg.

Section 1.3

Prevalence of Alcohol Use in the United States

Text in this section is excerpted from "Results from the 2008 National Survey on Drug Use and Health: National Findings," Substance Abuse and Mental Health Services Administration (SAMHSA), HHS Publication No. SMA 09–4434, 2009.

The National Survey on Drug Use and Health (NSDUH) includes questions about the recency and frequency of consumption of alcoholic beverages, such as beer, wine, whiskey, brandy, and mixed drinks. An extensive list of examples of the kinds of beverages covered is given to respondents prior to the question administration. A drink is defined as a can or bottle of beer, a glass of wine or a wine cooler, a shot of liquor, or a mixed drink with liquor in it. Times when the respondent only had a sip or two from a drink are not considered to be consumption. For this report, estimates for the prevalence of alcohol use are reported primarily at three levels defined for both males and females and for all ages as follows:

Current (past month) use: At least one drink in the past 30 days.

Binge use: Five or more drinks on the same occasion (for example, at the same time or within a couple of hours of each other) on at least one day in the past 30 days.

Heavy use: Five or more drinks on the same occasion on each of five or more days in the past 30 days.

These levels are not mutually exclusive categories of use; heavy use is included in estimates of binge and current use, and binge use is included in estimates of current use.

Alcohol Use among Persons Aged 12 or Older

- Slightly more than half of Americans aged 12 or older reported being current drinkers of alcohol in the 2008 survey (51.6%). This translates to an estimated 129.0 million people, which is similar to the 2007 estimate of 126.8 million people (51.1%).

- More than one-fifth (23.3%) of persons aged 12 or older partici-pated in binge drinking at least once in the 30 days prior to the survey in 2008. This translates to about 58.1 million people. The rate in 2008 is the same as the rate in 2007 (23.3%).

- In 2008, heavy drinking was reported by 6.9% of the population aged 12 or older, or 17.3 million people. This percentage is the same as the rate of heavy drinking in 2007 (6.9%).

Age

- In 2008, rates of current alcohol use were 3.4% among persons aged 12 or 13, 13.1% of persons aged 14 or 15, 26.2% of 16- or 17-year-olds, 48.7% of those aged 18 to 20, and 69.5% of 21- to 25-year-olds. These estimates showed significant declines from 2007 for the 14- or 15-year-olds (from 14.7 to 13.1%) and for the 16- or 17-year-olds (from 29.0 to 26.2%).

- Among older age groups, the prevalence of current alcohol use decreased with increasing age, from 67.4% among 26- to 29-year-olds to 50.3% among 60- to 64-year-olds and 39.7% among people aged 65 or older.

- Rates of binge alcohol use in 2008 were 1.5% among 12- or 13-year-olds, 6.9% among 14- or 15-year-olds, 17.2% among 16- or 17-year olds, 33.7% among persons aged 18 to 20, and peaked among those aged 21 to 25 at 46.0%. The 2008 binge drinking rate for 16- or 17-year-olds showed a decrease from 2007 when it was 19.4%.

- The binge drinking rate decreased beyond young adulthood from 36.4% of 26- to 34-year-olds to 18.8% of persons aged 35 or older.

- The rate of binge drinking was 41.0% for young adults aged 18 to 25. Heavy alcohol use was reported by 14.5% of persons aged 18 to 25. These rates are similar to the rates in 2007 (41.8% and 14.7% respectively).

- Persons aged 65 or older had lower rates of binge drinking (8.2%) than adults in other age groups. The rate of heavy drink-ing among persons aged 65 or older was 2.2%.

- The rate of current alcohol use among youths aged 12 to 17 was 14.6% in 2008, which is lower than it was in 2007, when it was 15.9%. Youth binge and heavy drinking rates were 8.8% and 2.0% respectively. The 2008 rate for youth binge drinking is also lower than the 2007 rate which was 9.7%.

Gender

- In 2008, 57.7% of males aged 12 or older were current drinkers, higher than the rate for females (45.9%). However, among youths aged 12 to 17, the percentage of males who were current drinkers (14.2%) was similar to the rate for females (15.0%).

- Among adults aged 18 to 25, an estimated 58.0% of females and 64.3% of males reported current drinking in 2008. These rates are similar to those reported in 2007 (57.1% and 65.3% respectively).

Pregnant Women

- Among pregnant women aged 15 to 44, an estimated 10.6% reported current alcohol use, 4.5% reported binge drinking, and 0.8% reported heavy drinking. These rates were significantly lower than the rates for non-pregnant women in the same age group (54.0%, 24.2%, and 5.5% respectively). Binge drinking during the first trimester of pregnancy was reported by 10.3% of pregnant women aged 15 to 44. All of these estimates by pregnancy status are based on data averaged over 2007 and 2008. The 2007–2008 estimate for first-trimester binge drinking is higher than in 2005–2006, when it was 4.6%.

Race/Ethnicity

- Among persons aged 12 or older, Whites in 2008 were more likely than other racial/ethnic groups to report current use of alcohol (56.2%). The rates were 47.5% for persons reporting two or more races, 43.3% for American Indians or Alaska Natives, 43.2% for Hispanics, 41.9% for Blacks, and 37.0% for Asians.

- The rate of binge alcohol use was lowest among Asians (11.9%). Rates for other racial/ethnic groups were 20.4% for Blacks, 22.0% for persons reporting two or more races, 24.0% for Whites, 24.4% for American Indians or Alaska Natives, and 25.6% for Hispanics.

- Among youths aged 12 to 17 in 2008, Asians had lower rates of current alcohol use than any other racial/ethnic group (5.7%), while 10.1% of Black youths, 13.6% of those reporting two or more races, 14.8% of Hispanic youths, and 16.3% of White youths were current drinkers.

Education

- Among adults aged 18 or older, the rate of past month alcohol use increased with increasing levels of education. Among adults with less than a high school education, 36.8% were current drinkers in 2008, significantly lower than the 67.9% of college graduates who were current drinkers. However, among adults aged 26 or older, binge and heavy alcohol use rates were lower among college graduates (19.5% and 4.6% respectively) than among those who had not completed college (23.2% versus 7.0% respectively).

College Students

- Young adults aged 18 to 22 enrolled full time in college were more likely than their peers not enrolled full time (for example, part-time college students and persons not currently enrolled in college) to use alcohol in the past month, binge drink, and drink heavily. Among full-time college students in 2008, 61.0% were current drinkers, 40.5% binge drank, and 16.3% were heavy drinkers. Among those not enrolled full time in college, these rates were 54.2%, 38.1%, and 13.0%, respectively. Rates of current alcohol use and binge use for full-time college students decreased from 2007, when they were 63.7% and 43.6% respectively.

- The pattern of higher rates of current alcohol use, binge alcohol use, and heavy alcohol use among full-time college students compared with rates for others aged 18 to 22 has remained consistent since 2002.

Employment

- The rate of current alcohol use was 63.0% for full-time employed adults aged 18 or older in 2008, higher than the rate for unemployed adults (55.5%). However, the rate of heavy use for unemployed persons was 12.8%, which was higher than the rate of 8.8% for full-time employed persons. There was no significant difference in binge alcohol use rates between full-time employed adults (30.3%) and unemployed adults (33.4%).

- Most binge and heavy alcohol users were employed in 2008. Among 55.9 million adult binge drinkers, 44.6 million (79.7%) were employed either full or part time. Among 16.8 million heavy drinkers, 13.1 million (78.0%) were employed.

- Rates of binge and heavy alcohol use did not change significantly between 2007 and 2008 for full-time employed or unemployed adults. However, the number of unemployed binge and heavy drinkers did increase (from 2.3 million to 3.0 million for binge use and from 851,000 to 1.2 million for heavy use).

Geographic Area

- The rate of past month alcohol use for people aged 12 or older in 2008 was lower in the South (47.3%) than in the Northeast (56.8%), Midwest (54.2%), or West (51.8%).

- Among people aged 12 or older, the rate of past month alcohol use in large metropolitan areas (53.6%) was higher than the 51.3% in small metropolitan areas and 45.8% in nonmetropolitan areas. Binge drinking was equally prevalent in small metropolitan areas (22.5%), large metropolitan areas (23.9%), and nonmetropolitan areas (22.8%).

- The rates of binge alcohol use among youths aged 12 to 17 were 9.8% in nonmetropolitan areas, 9.0% in small metropolitan areas, and 8.4% in large metropolitan areas.

Chapter 2

Ethnicity, Culture, and Alcohol

Alcohol Consumption and Drinking Patterns across Groups within the United States

Alcohol consumption trends and patterns vary markedly across various groups within the United States (U.S.) Recognition of diversity in alcohol-related problems is an important aspect of developing tailored and targeted intervention and prevention responses. Most research into this issue is centered on the study of four main groups, often in comparison or contrast to White/Caucasian Americans. The four groups include: African Americans, Hispanics, Asian Americans/Pacific Islanders, and American Indians/Alaska Natives. Note that these categories include hundreds of distinct ethnic or racial populations which differ markedly in cultural characteristics and drinking behavior. The problem with aggregate data is that it masks very important differences across subgroups within an ethnic or cultural category.

This chapter includes excerpts from "Module 10H: Ethnicity, Culture and Alcohol," National Institute on Alcohol Abuse and Alcoholism (NIAAA), 2005. Reviewed in May 2010 by Dr. David A. Cooke, MD, FACP, Diplomate, American Board of Internal Medicine. The complete module is available at http://pubs.niaaa .nih.gov/publications/Social/Module10HEthnicity&Culture/Module10H.html. Also included are an excerpt from "Prevalence of Alcohol Use among Racial and Ethnic Subgroups in the U.S.," Substance Abuse and Mental Health Services Administration (SAMHSA), 2008; and, an excerpt from "Substance Use and Substance Use Disorders among American Indians and Alaska Natives," SAMHSA, January 19, 2007.

17

In addition, the results of ethnic group comparisons may not be consistent across the life cycle. For example, in 2000, Muthen and Muthen observed that gender and ethnicity effects related to alcohol consumption patterns among individuals in their twenties did not follow the same trajectory as for individuals in their thirties. Furthermore, American Indian experiences may vary tremendously depending on where they reside during different periods of their lives—in large urban centers, rural areas, within reservation areas, or as youths living in boarding schools.

Impact of Alcohol on Ethnic and Cultural Groups

In addition to differences in drinking patterns, differences in the consequences of alcohol use may exist among various ethnic and cultural groups. The differential consequences may, in part, be a function of different vulnerabilities and resiliencies conferred by biological and genetic factors. Or, differences in outcomes and impacts may be related to disparities in the timing and types of services experienced by individuals from various ethnic and cultural groups.

As the U.S. Surgeon General, Dr. David Satcher issued a statement concerning health disparities and service inequities that exist across our nation. His position is that some communities, defined by race and ethnicity, disproportionately bear the burden of disability from under- or poorly-treated mental health problems. For example, Hispanics in the U.S. are approximately twice as likely as Whites to die from cirrhosis of the liver, despite lower drinking and heavy drinking prevalence. This is possibly attributable to higher cumulative doses per drinking occasion, the prevalence of hepatitis C which enhances risks to the liver from heavy drinking, and differences in access to early, effective treatment. With regard to mental health services, Satcher stated that culture counts in critical ways, and that the nation's diversity has to be addressed in the conduct of basic and applied research, in service delivery, and in the ways that future generations of service providers are educated.

Ethnic and Cultural Influences on Drinking Patterns

Alcohol consumption is governed, in large part, by the social rules, norms, customs, and traditions acquired through an individual's cultural and ethnic contextual experiences, including immediate family, extended kin, peers, and teachings. Ignoring these influences can lead to misguided judgments about the appropriateness and inappropriateness of alcohol consumption and concomitant behaviors.

18

Many interventions are based on assumptions that do not recognize the importance of these norms, practices, and influences on alcohol consumption and abuse. Such a lack of cultural relativity may result in a misinterpretation of intervention outcomes. Researchers need to be alert to implicit assumptions about relationships between ethnicity and addiction, particularly in reference to differences in prevalence rates, associated problems, and use-related attitudes.

Cultural Norms and Values

Ethnic and cultural group norms, values, and expectations concerning alcohol vary markedly, as do cultural strengths and resiliency factors. Members of different ethnic and cultural groups show preferences for different types of alcoholic beverages which may in turn affect access and relative alcohol content and exposure. Individuals that drink in social groups and in situations where there are linked activities, adjust their consumption rates and rhythms to others in the group and to the linked activities rather than follow an individually-determined pattern of consumption. Some cultures abhor any alcohol use. Unfortunately, this does not guarantee an absence of alcohol-related problems, and when alcohol is a problem, these cultural norms may lead to hiding, minimizing, denial, or exclusion. In cultures that accept some alcohol consumption, norms govern what types are consumed. There are also norms concerning how much is consumed, and what are acceptable forms of intoxicated behavior. Any specific type of substance use could be differentially viewed as normative, deviant to some degree, or quite deviant behavior, depending on the cultural context. Culture has a powerful influence on alcohol-related behaviors, as well as on belief systems about alcohol among users and among members of the users' support systems.

Socialization theory explains how specific drinking customs and rituals are transmitted across generations and from one individual to another within a family, ethnic, or cultural group. The degree to which cultural norms influence an individual's drinking behavior is determined, in part, by the extent of that person's identification with the group, the degree of consistency in the group's norms, and the presence of confounding or complementary forces, such as gender and age norms. Drinking and other drug use behavior are also associated with the perception of risk associated with consumption, and the risk perception may differ among ethnic and cultural groups. White individuals in a general population survey are the least likely to perceive risks for alcohol use (compared to Black and Hispanic respondents), and have the highest prevalence of past month use.

The Hispanic community has strong cultural prohibitions about women drinking. This may account for the high number of Hispanic women (70%) who have less than one drink per month, if they drink at all. These community injunctions do not exist for Hispanic men—a fact that is offered as a potential explanation for their significantly higher drinking rates when compared to Hispanic women.

Similarly, the influence of the Confucian and Taoist philosophies has been considered as an explanation for the low rate of alcohol consumption among Asian Americans. The emphasis on peace, congruence, and harmony may serve to moderate alcohol consumption. The degree of acculturation to American cultural patterns may also serve as a means of explaining differences in drinking behavior across Asian and Pacific Islander groups. Studies of youth and young adults generally associate higher degrees of assimilation with higher levels of drinking, particularly among men. Risk factors that have been identified through key informant surveys among Asian American groups include: drinking as an intrinsic part of business transactions (Chinese and Japanese men), waitresses and hostesses encouraged to drink with clients (Korean women), isolated elders (Japanese and Filipino men), recent immigrants experiencing posttraumatic stress (Southeast Asians), young men who engage in pack social behaviors, and increasing numbers of young women whose group behaviors reflect their male counterparts. Alcohol problems among Asian Americans are often related to struggles with the transition to Western culture. The transition process creates stress, disrupts traditional family structures and the extensive support system provided by extended family members, and can hinder self-identity development. Some individuals use alcohol to cope with the stress associated with these difficulties.

Historically, African Americans who drank did so primarily on weekends or as part of celebrations and holidays. West African traditions involved alcohol as an integral part of medicine, religion, and special celebrations, but placed high value on moderate drinking and disapproved of drunken behavior. Slavery, emancipation, abolition, and civil rights have since intervened, and one contemporary result is a tremendous degree of variability and ambiguity in attitudes, meanings, norms, and behaviors related to alcohol consumption. A large segment of the African American community is characterized by abstinence. Many of the African Americans who do drink tend to follow a pattern of group or weekend drinking. The cultural-specific approach to understanding alcohol use disorders leads to an awareness of where people seek and receive help with their problems. African Americans very often rely on the church as a critical resource for addressing substance use problems.

It is important to note that the research concerning drinking patterns among African Americans does not tend to employ ethnographic approaches or to address cultural theories, and therefore is limited in its usefulness for within group comparisons.

Alcohol Use by Race or Ethnicity

* Among persons aged 12 or older, Whites in 2008 were more likely than other racial or ethnic groups to report current use of alcohol (56.2%). The rates were 47.5% for persons reporting two or more races, 43.3% for American Indians or Alaska Natives, 43.2% for Hispanics, 41.9% for Blacks, and 37.0% for Asians.

* The rate of binge alcohol use was lowest among Asians (11.9%). Rates for other racial or ethnic groups were 20.4% for Blacks, 22.0% for persons reporting two or more races, 24.0% for Whites, 24.4% for American Indians or Alaska Natives, and 25.6% for Hispanics.

* Among youths aged 12 to 17 in 2008, Asians had lower rates of current alcohol use than any other racial or ethnic group (5.7%), while 10.1% of Black youths, 13.6% of those reporting two or more races, 14.8% of Hispanic youths, and 16.3% of White youths were current drinkers.

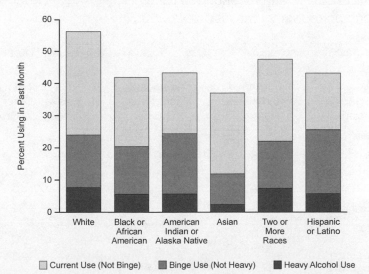

Figure 2.1. Current, Binge, and Heavy Alcohol Use among Persons Aged 12 or Older, by Race/Ethnicity: 2008. Note: Due to low precision, estimates for Native Hawaiians or Other Pacific Islanders are not shown.

Substance Use and Substance Use Disorders among American Indians and Alaska Natives

* In 2002–2005, American Indians and Alaska Natives aged 12 or older were less likely to have used alcohol at least once in the past year than were members of other racial groups (60.8% versus 65.8%), but they were more likely than members of other racial groups to have a past year alcohol use disorder (10.7% versus 7.6%). Additionally, generally consistent patterns were found within gender and age groups. For example, American Indian and Alaska Native males aged 12 or older were less likely to have used alcohol in the past year than males in other racial groups (65.5% versus 70.2%), but they more likely to have a past year alcohol use disorder (13.6% versus 10.5%). One exception was that American Indians and Alaska Natives aged 12 to 17 were equally likely as same-aged youths in other racial groups to report past year alcohol use, but they nevertheless were more likely than youths in other racial groups to have a past year alcohol use disorder (8.5% versus 5.8%).

Table 2.1. Percentages of Persons Aged 12 or Older Reporting Past Year Alcohol Use and Alcohol Use Disorder, by Racial Group and Demographic Characteristics: 2002–2005

| | Past Year Alcohol Use | | Past Year Alcohol Use Disorder | |
Demographic Characteristics	American Indians and Alaska Natives	Members of Other Racial Groups	American Indians and Alaska Natives	Members of Other Racial Groups
Gender				
Male	65.5	70.2	13.6	10.5
Female	56.4	61.6	7.9	4.9
Age Group				
12 to 17	35.2	34.0	8.5	5.8
18 to 25	72.9	78.1	20.8	17.4
26 or Older	62.8	68.0	9.1	6.1

Source: SAMHSA, 2002–2005 National Survey on Drug Use and Health (NSDUH).

Chapter 3

Binge Drinking

Quick Stats on Binge Drinking

Binge drinking is a common pattern of excessive alcohol use in the United States (U.S.). The National Institute of Alcohol Abuse and Alcoholism defines binge drinking as a pattern of drinking that brings a person's blood alcohol concentration (BAC) to 0.08% or above. This typically happens when men consume five or more drinks, and when women consume four or more drinks, in about two hours. Most people who binge drink are not alcohol dependent.

According to national surveys:

- Approximately 92% of U.S. adults who drink excessively report binge drinking in the past 30 days.

- Although college students commonly binge drink, 70% of binge drinking episodes involve adults over age 25 years.

- The prevalence of binge drinking among men is two times the prevalence among women.

- Binge drinkers are 14 times more likely to report alcohol-impaired driving than non-binge drinkers.

- About 90% of the alcohol consumed by youth under the age of 21 years in the United States is in the form of binge drinks.

This chapter is excerpted from "Quick Stats: Binge Drinking," Centers for Disease Control and Prevention (CDC), August 6, 2008; and includes excerpts from "2008 National Health Interview Survey," CDC, 2009.

- About 75% of the alcohol consumed by adults in the United States is in the form of binge drinks.
- The proportion of current drinkers that binge is highest in the 18- to 20-year-old group (51%).

Binge drinking is associated with many health problems, including but not limited to the following:

- Unintentional injuries (for example: car crashes, falls, burns, drowning)
- Intentional injuries (such as firearm injuries, sexual assault, domestic violence)
- Alcohol poisoning
- Sexually transmitted diseases
- Unintended pregnancy
- Children born with fetal alcohol spectrum disorders (FASD)
- High blood pressure, stroke, and other cardiovascular diseases
- Liver disease
- Neurological damage
- Sexual dysfunction
- Poor control of diabetes

Evidence-based interventions to prevent binge drinking and related harms include the following:

- Increasing alcoholic beverage costs and excise taxes
- Limiting the number of retail alcohol outlets that sell alcoholic beverages in a given area
- Consistent enforcement of laws against underage drinking and alcohol-impaired driving
- Screening and counseling for alcohol misuse

Alcohol Consumption Information from the National Health Interview Survey

- The percentage of adults who had five or more drinks in one day at least once in 2008 was similar for men aged 18–24 years and 25–44 years and lower among men in older age groups. The percentage of adult women who had five or more drinks in one day at least once in 2008 decreased with age.

Table 3.1. Percentage of adults who reported binge drinking by state and gender in 2008, Behavioral Risk Factor Surveillance System (BRFSS), 2008

State	Total	Men	Women
Alaska	16.0	21.9	9.9
Arizona	15.7	21.1	10.4
Arkansas	1.6	18.5	7.2
California	15.6	22.1	9.2
Colorado	16.1	21.7	10.5
Connecticut	16.8	23.1	11.0
District of Columbia	18.1	22.5	14.4
Florida	13.1	18.4	8.1
Georgia	14.1	19.7	8.9
Hawaii	17.6	25.5	9.9
Idaho	13.2	17.0	9.3
Illinois	19.5	25.9	13.4
Indiana	16.2	23.8	8.9
Iowa	20.3	26.9	14.0
Kansas	13.8	19.6	8.2
Kentucky	11.4	16.8	6.4

State	Total	Men	Women
Louisiana	13.6	20.0	8.0
Maine	15.8	20.8	11.1
Maryland	13.8	18.0	10.1
Massachusetts	17.7	23.0	13.0
Michigan	17.9	23.4	12.7
Minnesota	19.8	26.8	13.1
Mississippi	10.8	16.4	5.8
Missouri	15.4	20.8	10.4
Montana	17.8	23.6	12.1
Nebraska	19.2	26.0	12.7
Nevada	19.0	24.8	13.0
New Hampshire	16.5	24.9	8.6
New Jersey	14.2	18.2	10.4
New Mexico	11.4	16.5	6.6
New York	14.7	21.0	9.0
North Carolina	12.9	18.6	7.7
North Dakota	21.6	29.3	14.1

State	Total	Men	Women
Ohio	15.9	22.0	10.4
Oklahoma	12.2	17.3	7.5
Oregon	12.9	17.2	8.9
Pennsylvania	16.8	22.7	11.4
Rhode Island	17.6	24.2	11.6
South Carolina	12.3	17.4	7.7
South Dakota	17.9	24.1	11.8
Tennessee	10.5	15.7	5.7
Texas	14.9	21.6	8.5
Utah	8.2	11.3	5.2
Vermont	17.5	24.3	11.0
Virginia	13.8	17.8	10.0
Washington	15.2	19.9	10.7
West Virginia	8.8	14.0	3.9
Wisconsin	22.9	28.5	17.4
Wyoming	15.5	20.6	10.2
Puerto Rico	10.9	17.6	5.1
Guam	20.2	34.5	5.9
Virgin Islands	12.3	19.6	6.0

Source: National Institute on Alcohol Abuse and Alcoholism (NIAAA), September 2009.

- In all four age groups, men were considerably more likely than women to have had five or more drinks in one day at least once in 2008.

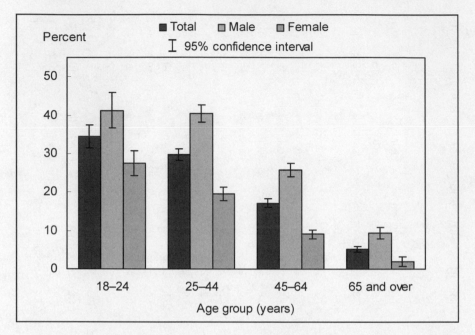

Figure 3.1. *Percentage of adults aged 18 years and over who had five or more drinks in one day at least once in the past year, by age group and sex: United States, 2008 (Note: The analyses excluded 359 adults (1.6%) with unknown alcohol consumption. Data Source: Based on data collected in the Sample Adult Core component of the 2008 National Health Interview Survey. Data are based on household interviews of a sample of the civilian non-institutionalized population.)*

Table 3.2. Age-sex-adjusted percentage of adults aged 18 years and older who had five or more drinks in one day at least once in the past year by race/ethnicity: United States, 2008

Race/ethnicity	Percent[1]
Hispanic or Latino	18.3
Not Hispanic or Latino, single race, White	26.2
Not Hispanic or Latino, single race, Black	13.9

[1]Estimates are age-sex adjusted using the projected 2000 U.S. population as the standard population and using four age groups: 18–24 years, 25–44 years, 45–64 years, and 65 years and over.

Chapter 4

Facts about Alcoholism

Chapter Contents

Section 4.1

What Does Alcoholism Look Like?

Excerpted from "Alcoholism Isn't What It Used to Be," National Institute
on Alcohol Abuse and Alcoholism (NIAAA), 2009.

The realization dawned gradually as researchers analyzed data
from the National Institute on Alcohol Abuse and Alcoholism (NIAAA)
2001–2002 National Epidemiologic Survey on Alcohol and Related
Conditions (NESARC). In most persons affected, alcohol dependence
(commonly known as alcoholism) looks less like Nicolas Cage in *Leaving Las Vegas* than it does your party-hardy college roommate or that
hard-driving colleague in the next cubicle.

"We knew from the 1991–1992 National Longitudinal Alcohol Epidemiologic Study that alcohol dependence is most prevalent among
younger adults aged 18 to 29," says Bridget Grant, PhD, chief of
NIAAA's Laboratory Epidemiology and Biometry. "However, it was
not until we examined the NESARC data that we pinpointed age 22
as the mean age of alcohol dependence onset." Subsequent analysis by
Ralph Hingson, Doctor of Science (ScD), director, Division of Epidemiology and Prevention Research, showed that nearly half of people who
become alcohol dependent do so by age 21 and two-thirds by age 25.

The NESARC surveyed more than 43,000 individuals representative
of the United States (U.S.) adult population using questions based on
criteria in the *Diagnostic and Statistical Manual of Mental Disorders,
Fourth Edition* (*DSM-IV*) of the American Psychiatric Association (APA).
Published in 1994, *DSM-IV* recognizes alcohol dependence by preoccupation with drinking, impaired control over drinking, compulsive drinking,
drinking despite physical or psychological problems caused or made
worse by drinking, and tolerance and/or withdrawal symptoms.

Meanwhile, findings continue to accumulate to challenge past
perceptions of the nature, course, and outcome of alcoholism. Among
those findings:

- Many heavy drinkers do not have alcohol dependence. For example, even in people who have five or more drinks a day (the
equivalent of a bottle of wine) the rate of developing dependence
is less than 7% per year.

- Most persons who develop alcohol dependence have mild to moderate disorder, in which they primarily experience impaired control. For example, they set limits and go over them or find it difficult to quit or cut down. In general, these people do not have severe alcohol-related relationship, health, vocational, or legal problems.

- About 70% of affected persons have a single episode of less than four years. The other 30% of affected persons experience an average of five episodes. Thus, it appears that there are two forms of alcohol dependence—time-limited, and recurrent or chronic.

- Although 22 is the average age when alcohol dependence begins, the onset varies from the mid-teens to middle age.

- Twenty years after onset of alcohol dependence, about three-fourths of individuals are in full recovery; more than half of those who have fully recovered drink at low-risk levels without symptoms of alcohol dependence.

- About 75% of persons who recover from alcohol dependence do so without seeking any kind of help, including specialty alcohol (rehab) programs and Alcoholics Anonymous (AA). Only 13% of people with alcohol dependence ever receive specialty alcohol treatment.

"These and other recent findings turn on its head much of what we thought we knew about alcoholism," according to Mark Willenbring, MD, director of NIAAA's Division of Treatment and Recovery Research. "As is so often true in medicine, researchers have studied the patients seen in hospitals and clinics most intensively. This can greatly skew understanding of a disorder, especially in the alcohol field where most people neither seek nor receive treatment, and those who seek it do so well into the course of disease. Longitudinal, general population studies such as the NESARC permit us to see the entire disease continuum from before onset to late-stage disease."

To Willenbring, these realizations call for a public health approach that targets at-risk drinkers and persons with mild alcohol disorder to prevent or arrest problems before they progress. NIAAA is addressing this need with tools to expand risk awareness (http://rethinkingdrinking.niaaa.nih.gov) and inform secondary prevention and primary care screening (http://www.niaaa.nih.gov/guide).

"NIAAA's goal now and for the foreseeable future is to develop and disseminate research-based resources for each stage of the alcohol use disorder continuum, from primary prevention to disease management," according to acting NIAAA director Ken Warren, PhD.

Section 4.2

Questions and Answers about Alcoholism

Text in this section is from "FAQs for the General Public: Alcoholism," National Institute on Alcohol Abuse and Alcoholism (NIAAA), February, 2007.

What is alcoholism?

Alcoholism, also known as alcohol dependence, is a disease that includes the following four symptoms:

- **Craving:** A strong need, or urge, to drink

- **Loss of control:** Not being able to stop drinking once drinking has begun

- **Physical dependence:** Withdrawal symptoms, such as nausea, sweating, shakiness, and anxiety after stopping drinking

- **Tolerance:** The need to drink greater amounts of alcohol to get high

For clinical and research purposes, formal diagnostic criteria for alcoholism also have been developed. Such criteria are included in the *Diagnostic and Statistical Manual of Mental Disorders, Fourth Edition*, published by the American Psychiatric Association, as well as in the *International Classification Diseases*, published by the World Health Organization.

Is alcoholism a disease?

Yes, alcoholism is a disease. The craving that an alcoholic feels for alcohol can be as strong as the need for food or water. An alcoholic will continue to drink despite serious family, health, or legal problems. Like many other diseases, alcoholism is chronic, meaning that it lasts a person's lifetime; it usually follows a predictable course; and it has symptoms. The risk for developing alcoholism is influenced both by a person's genes and by his or her lifestyle.

Is alcoholism inherited?

Research shows that the risk for developing alcoholism does indeed run in families. The genes a person inherits partially explain this—pattern, but lifestyle is also a factor. Currently, researchers are working to discover the actual genes that put people at risk for alcoholism. Your friends, the amount of stress in your life, and how readily available alcohol is also are factors that may increase your risk for alcoholism.

But remember: Risk is not destiny. Just because alcoholism tends to run in families doesn't mean that a child of an alcoholic parent will automatically become an alcoholic. Some people develop alcoholism even though no one in their family has a drinking problem. By the same token, not all children of alcoholic families get into trouble with alcohol. Knowing you are at risk is important, though, because then you can take steps to protect yourself from developing problems with alcohol.

Can alcoholism be cured?

No, alcoholism cannot be cured at this time. Even if an alcoholic hasn't been drinking for a long time, he or she can still suffer a relapse. Not drinking is the safest course for most people with alcoholism.

Can alcoholism be treated?

Yes, alcoholism can be treated. Alcoholism treatment programs use both counseling and medications to help a person stop drinking. Treatment has helped many people stop drinking and rebuild their lives.

Does alcoholism treatment work?

Alcoholism treatment works for many people. But like other chronic illnesses, such as diabetes, high blood pressure, and asthma, success varies when it comes to treatment. Some people stop drinking and remain sober. Others have long periods of sobriety with bouts of relapse. And still others cannot stop drinking for any length of time. With treatment, one thing is clear, the longer a person abstains from alcohol, the more likely he or she will be able to stay sober.

Do you have to be an alcoholic to experience alcohol-related problems?

No. Alcoholism is only one type of an alcohol problem. Alcohol abuse can be just as harmful. A person can abuse alcohol without actually being an alcoholic—that is, he or she may drink too much and too often but still not be dependent on alcohol. Some of the problems linked to alcohol abuse include not being able to meet work, school, or family responsibilities; drunk-driving arrests and car crashes; and drinking-related medical conditions. Under some circumstances, even social or moderate drinking is dangerous such as when driving, during pregnancy, or when taking certain medications.

Are specific groups of people more likely to have alcohol-related problems?

Alcohol abuse and alcoholism cut across gender, race, and nationality. In the United States, 17.6 million people—about one in every 12 adults—abuse alcohol or are alcohol dependent. In general, more men than women are alcohol dependent or have alcohol problems. And alcohol problems are highest among young adults ages 18–29 and lowest among adults ages 65 and older. We also know that people who start drinking at an early age—for example, at age 14 or younger—are at much higher risk of developing alcohol problems at some point in their lives compared to someone who starts drinking at age 21 or after.

How can you tell if someone has a problem?

Answering the following four questions can help you find out if you or a loved one has a drinking problem:

- Have you ever felt you should cut down on your drinking?
- Have people annoyed you by criticizing your drinking?
- Have you ever felt bad or guilty about your drinking?
- Have you ever had a drink first thing in the morning to steady your nerves or to get rid of a hangover?

One "yes" answer suggests a possible alcohol problem. More than one "yes" answer means it is highly likely that a problem exists. If you think that you or someone you know might have an alcohol problem, it is important to see a doctor or other health care provider right away. They can help you determine if a drinking problem exists and plan the best course of action.

Section 4.3

Researchers Identify Alcoholism Subtypes

NIH News, National Institute on Alcohol Abuse and Alcoholism (NIAAA), June 28, 2007.

Analyses of a national sample of individuals with alcohol dependence (alcoholism) reveal five distinct subtypes of the disease, according to a new study by scientists at the National Institute on Alcohol Abuse and Alcoholism (NIAAA), part of the National Institutes of Health (NIH).

"Our findings should help dispel the popular notion of the typical alcoholic," notes first author Howard B. Moss, MD, NIAAA Associate Director for Clinical and Translational Research. "We find that young adults comprise the largest group of alcoholics in this country, and nearly 20% of alcoholics are highly functional and well-educated with good incomes. More than half of the alcoholics in the United States have no multigenerational family history of the disease, suggesting that their form of alcoholism was unlikely to have genetic causes."

"Clinicians have long recognized diverse manifestations of alcoholism," adds NIAAA Director Ting-Kai Li, MD, "and researchers have tried to understand why some alcoholics improve with specific medications and psychotherapies while others do not. The classification system described in this study will have broad application in both clinical and research settings." A report of the study is available online in the journal *Drug and Alcohol Dependence*.

Previous efforts to identify alcoholism subtypes focused primarily on individuals who were hospitalized or otherwise receiving treatment for their alcoholism. However, reports from NIAAA's National Epidemiologic Survey on Alcohol and Related Conditions (NESARC), a nationally representative epidemiological study of alcohol, drug, and mental disorders in the United States, suggest that only about one-fourth of individuals with alcoholism have ever received treatment. Thus, a substantial proportion of people with alcoholism were not represented in the samples previously used to define subtypes of this disease.

In the current study, Dr. Moss and colleagues applied advanced statistical methods to data from the NESARC. Their analyses focused on the 1,484 NESARC survey respondents who met diagnostic criteria for alcohol dependence, and included individuals in treatment as well as those not seeking treatment. The researchers identified unique subtypes of alcoholism based on respondents' family history of alcoholism, age of onset of regular drinking and alcohol problems, symptom patterns of alcohol dependence and abuse, and the presence of additional substance abuse and mental disorders:

Young adult subtype: 31.5% of United States (U.S.) alcoholics. Young adult drinkers, with relatively low rates of co-occurring substance abuse and other mental disorders, a low rate of family alcoholism, and who rarely seek any kind of help for their drinking.

Young antisocial subtype: 21% of U.S. alcoholics. Individuals tend to be in their mid-twenties, had early onset of regular drinking, and alcohol problems. More than half come from families with alcoholism, and about half have a psychiatric diagnosis of antisocial personality disorder. Many have major depression, bipolar disorder, and anxiety problems. More than 75% smoked cigarettes and marijuana, and many also had cocaine and opiate addictions. More than one-third of these alcoholics seek help for their drinking.

Functional subtype: 19.5% of U.S. alcoholics. These individuals are typically middle-aged, well-educated, with stable jobs and families. About one-third have a multigenerational family history of alcoholism, about one-quarter had major depressive illness sometime in their lives, and nearly 50% were smokers.

Intermediate familial subtype: 19% of U.S. alcoholics. These individuals are middle-aged with about 50% from families with multigenerational alcoholism. Almost half have had clinical depression, and 20% have had bipolar disorder. Most of these individuals smoked cigarettes, and nearly one in five had problems with cocaine and marijuana use. Only 25% ever sought treatment for their problem drinking.

Chronic severe subtype: 9% of U.S. alcoholics. This group is comprised mostly of middle-aged individuals who had early onset of drinking and alcohol problems with high rates of antisocial personality disorder and criminality. Almost 80% come from families with multigenerational alcoholism. They have the highest rates of other psychiatric disorders including depression, bipolar disorder, and anxiety disorders as well as high rates of smoking, and marijuana, cocaine, and opiate dependence. Two-thirds of these alcoholics seek help for their drinking problems, making them the most prevalent type of alcoholic in treatment.

The authors also report that co-occurring psychiatric and other substance abuse problems are associated with severity of alcoholism and entering into treatment. Attending Alcoholics Anonymous (AA) and other 12-step programs is the most common form of help-seeking for drinking problems, but help-seeking remains relatively rare.

Chapter 5

Alcohol-Related Problems: Are You at Risk?

Chapter Contents

Section 5.1

Risk Factors for Alcohol-Related Problems across the Lifespan

Excerpted from "Alcohol Research: A Lifespan Perspective," National Institute on Alcohol Abuse and Alcoholism (NIAAA), January, 2008. The complete document with references is available at http://pubs.niaaa.nih.gov/publications/AA74/AA74.pdf.

Alcohol use and the risk for alcohol-related problems change over the lifespan. College students and young adults, who often drink large quantities of alcohol at one time, are more likely to experience problems such as alcohol poisoning, drunk-driving crashes, and assaults; whereas, older individuals who drink even moderately while taking certain medications run the risk of harmful drug interactions. Also, patterns of alcohol use may differ across the human lifespan—adolescents who begin drinking prior to age 14 are more likely to develop a serious problem with alcohol later in life. Understanding how alcohol influences people across different life stages is important, especially when designing effective approaches for diagnosing, treating, and preventing alcohol abuse and dependence and their related problems.

The Embryo and Fetus

Alcohol is a leading preventable cause of birth defects with mental deficiency. Prenatal alcohol exposure can cause a variety of problems known collectively as fetal alcohol spectrum disorder (FASD). The most severe form of FASD, fetal alcohol syndrome (FAS), often is characterized by certain physical traits, such as a flattened mid-face, wide-set eyes and slow growth, nervous system impairments, and a range of learning and behavioral problems. Additionally, people exposed to alcohol prenatally are at higher risk of developing an alcohol and other drug use disorder later in life.

It has been reported that up to one in 100 children in the United States are born with FASD. Also, 0.5 to 3.0 children out of 1,000 are diagnosed with FAS. Research suggests that other factors, such as the mother's hormone status, nutrition, age, the number of children she has had previously, and the length of time she has been drinking, as well as genetic factors including those affecting the way the body breaks down alcohol, also may contribute to the development of FASD.

Youth and Adolescence

Adolescence is the period between 12 and 17 years of age. This is a time of dramatic physical, psychological, and social change. The brain continues to develop and mature throughout adolescence and into the mid-20s, and studies suggest that consuming alcohol during this time may have lasting effects on brain development. For example, a region of the brain involved in learning and memory, the hippocampus, is smaller in adolescents who begin drinking at an early age. In addition, studies of adolescents who were receiving treatment for alcohol withdrawal showed that they were more likely to have memory problems than adolescents who did not drink.

Adolescents tend to drink differently than adults. They are more likely to engage in risky behaviors such as heavy episodic (or binge) drinking. Researchers believe these risky behaviors are the result of certain social factors, such as a greater independence and pressure from peers, as well as biological factors. Adolescents tend to be less sensitive to negative effects of alcohol, such as increased sleepiness and lack of coordination. This may explain why they are able to drink so much alcohol at one time. On the other hand, adolescents are more likely to have trouble with complex tasks, such as driving a motor vehicle, making adolescent alcohol use especially dangerous.

Young Adults

Young adulthood is the period between the ages of 18 and 29 years. During this period many young people pursue postsecondary education, enlist in the military, or enter the workforce. This is a time of transition and of increased risk for problems with alcohol. The youngest segment of this population—young adults ages 18–24 years—are most at risk for alcohol problems, compared with other age groups. This group is most likely to drink heavily, regardless of their gender, ethnicity, and school or work status—that is, whether they attend college or are employed full time. Despite increased attention in recent years, the problem of young adult drinking continues to escalate: alcohol-related deaths rose 5% for 18- to 24-year-olds between 1998 and 2001.

Nonstudent, nonmilitary personnel may be more likely to continue dangerous drinking patterns into adulthood. This population does not have access to institutionally based programs that typically serve college students and military personnel. Additionally, this population may not have access to mental health services, making them vulnerable to psychiatric conditions, such as depression and anxiety, often associated with dangerous drinking patterns.

Although most young adults drink less as they transition into midlife, some continue to drink heavily. Research continues to explore the risk factors associated with continued drinking into midlife.

Alcohol and Human Immunodeficiency Virus (HIV) and Acquired Immunodeficiency Virus (AIDS)

HIV, the virus that causes AIDS, is epidemic in the United States. As many as 950,000 people in the United States may be infected with the HIV virus, and more than 500,000 people have died from the infection. Eighty percent of people infected with HIV drink alcohol, and between 30% and 60% have been diagnosed with an alcohol use disorder.

The relationship between HIV and alcohol is complex and needs further study. Drinking might make it easier for the HIV virus to establish an infection; additionally, alcohol use might actually accelerate the course of the disease. Alcohol also may change the way the body breaks down HIV medications, interfering with their effectiveness. In addition, it has been shown that people who drink are less likely to get tested for HIV. When they do test positive they are less likely to seek treatment and are less compliant with treatment. Drinking also is associated with risk-taking behaviors that might put people at increased risk for contracting HIV.

Midlife

Midlife is considered here as spanning the ages of 30–59. During this period the consequences of heavy drinking often become evident. Alcoholic liver disease, alcohol pancreatitis, several types of cancer, disorders of the heart and circulatory system, alcohol-related brain disorders, and other adverse effects upon the endocrine and immune system are most likely to emerge during this time. For people in midlife, research often has focused on how alcohol damages body tissues, as well as methods for better tailoring treatments and interventions to this segment of the population. Individuals in midlife are more likely to seek treatment for alcohol dependence. Research shows that a variety of factors—both biological and social—influence an individual's response to therapy.

Senior Adults and Alcohol

Senior adults tend to drink less than other age groups; however, research suggests that alcohol problems in older adults soon may become a national health issue. Senior adult drinking is on the rise; as people live longer, the number of people who drink will increase. Research also shows that people born in recent years tend to drink more than older generations, suggesting that as the current population ages, these individuals will continue to drink more.

Older adults are at particular risk for alcohol-related problems. As individuals age they metabolize alcohol more slowly; as a result, alcohol remains in the body longer. Older adults are more likely to have health conditions that can be exacerbated by alcohol, including stroke, hypertension, neurological degeneration, memory loss, mood disorders, and cognitive or emotional problems. Additionally, older adults are more likely than younger people to take medications, putting them at risk for interactions that can be dangerous or even life-threatening. Alcohol also may decrease effectiveness of some medications.

According to the current literature, the most beneficial treatment for alcohol use disorders in older adults may be education; many seniors lack information on the dangers of alcohol use. The age at which they begin drinking also is important. Older adults who began problem drinking earlier in life tend to have worse treatment outcomes than those who began drinking later in life.

Section 5.2

Alcohol and Women's Health Issues

Text in this section is excerpted from "Alcohol: A Woman's Health Issue,"
National Institute on Alcohol Abuse and Alcoholism (NIAAA), 2008.

Alcohol presents yet another health challenge for women. Even in
small amounts, alcohol affects women differently than men. In some
ways, heavy drinking is much more risky for women than it is for
men. With any health issue, accurate information is key. There are
times and ways to drink that are safer than others. Every woman is
different. No amount of drinking is 100% safe, 100% of the time, for
every woman. With this in mind, it's important to know how alcohol
can affect a woman's health and safety.

How much is too much?

In the United States (U.S.), 60% of women have at least one drink
a year. Among women who drink, 13% have more than seven drinks
per week. For women, this level of drinking is above the recommended limits published in the Dietary Guidelines for Americans,
which are issued jointly by the U.S. Department of Agriculture and
the U.S. Department of Health and Human Services. The Dietary
Guidelines define moderate drinking as no more than one drink a
day for women and no more than two drinks a day for men. The
Dietary Guidelines point out that drinking more than one drink
per day for women can increase the risk for motor vehicle crashes,
other injuries, high blood pressure, stroke, violence, suicide, and
certain types of cancer.

Some people should not drink at all, including the following:

- Anyone under age 21
- People of any age who are unable to restrict their drinking to
  moderate levels
- Women who may become pregnant or who are pregnant
- People who plan to drive, operate machinery, or take part in
  other activities that require attention, skill, or coordination

- People taking prescription or over-the-counter medications that can interact with alcohol

Why are lower levels of drinking recommended for women than for men? Lower levels of drinking are recommended because women are at greater risk than men for developing alcohol-related problems. Alcohol passes through the digestive tract and is dispersed in the water in the body. The more water available, the more diluted the alcohol. As a rule, men weigh more than women, and pound for pound, women have less water in their bodies than men. Therefore, a woman's brain and other organs are exposed to more alcohol and to more of the toxic byproducts that result when the body breaks down and eliminates alcohol.

Moderate Drinking: Benefits and Risks

Benefits

Heart disease: Once thought of as a threat mainly to men, heart disease also is the leading killer of women in the United States. Drinking moderately may lower the risk for coronary heart disease, mainly among women over age 55. However, there are other factors that reduce the risk of heart disease, including a healthy diet, exercise, not smoking, and keeping a healthy weight. Moderate drinking provides little, if any, net health benefit for younger people. (Heavy drinking can actually damage the heart.)

Risks

Drinking and driving: It doesn't take much alcohol to impair a person's ability to drive. The chances of being killed in a single-vehicle crash are increased at a blood alcohol level that a 140-pound woman would reach after having one drink on an empty stomach.

Medication interactions: Alcohol can interact with a wide variety of medicines, both prescription and over-the-counter. Alcohol can reduce the effectiveness of some medications, and it can combine with other medications to cause or increase side effects. Alcohol can interact with medicines used to treat conditions as varied as heart and blood vessel disease, digestive problems, and diabetes. In particular, alcohol can increase the sedative effects of any medication that causes drowsiness, including cough and cold medicines and drugs for anxiety and depression. When taking any medication, read package labels and warnings carefully.

Breast cancer: Research suggests that as little as one drink per day can slightly raise the risk of breast cancer in some women, especially those who are postmenopausal or have a family history of breast cancer. It is not possible, however, to predict how alcohol will affect the risk for breast cancer in any one woman.

Fetal alcohol syndrome (FAS): Drinking by a pregnant woman can harm her unborn baby, and may result in a set of birth defects called fetal alcohol syndrome (FAS).

Alcohol dependence: Another risk of drinking is that a woman may at some point abuse alcohol or become alcoholic (alcohol dependent). Drinking four or more drinks on any given day, or drinking eight or more drinks in a typical week increases a woman's risk of developing alcohol abuse or dependence. The ability to drink a man—or anyone—under the table is not a plus: it is a red flag. Research has shown that drinkers who are able to handle a lot of alcohol all at once are at higher—not lower—risk of developing problems, such as dependence on alcohol.

Heavy Drinking

An estimated 5.3 million women in the United States drink in a way that threatens their health, safety, and general well-being. A strong case can be made that heavy drinking is more risky for women than men:

- Heavy drinking increases a woman's risk of becoming a victim of violence and sexual assault.

- Drinking over the long term is more likely to damage a woman's health than a man's, even if the woman has been drinking less alcohol or for a shorter length of time than the man.

The health effects of alcohol abuse and alcoholism are serious. Some specific health problems include the following:

- **Alcoholic liver disease:** Women are more likely than men to develop alcoholic hepatitis (liver inflammation) and to die from cirrhosis.

- **Brain disease:** Most alcoholics have some loss of mental function, reduced brain size, and changes in the function of brain cells. Research suggests that women are more vulnerable than men to alcohol-induced brain damage.

- **Cancer:** Many studies report that heavy drinking increases the risk of breast cancer. Alcohol also is linked to cancers of the digestive tract and of the head and neck (the risk is especially high in smokers who also drink heavily).

- **Heart disease:** Chronic heavy drinking is a leading cause of cardiovascular disease. Among heavy drinkers, women are more susceptible to alcohol-related heart disease, even though women drink less alcohol over a lifetime than men.

- **Smoking effects:** Many alcoholics smoke; smoking in itself can cause serious long-term health consequences.

Alcohol in Women's Lives: Safe Drinking over a Lifetime

The pressures to drink more than what is safe—and the consequences—change as the roles that mark a woman's lifespan change. Knowing the signs that drinking may be a problem instead of a pleasure can help women who choose to drink do so without harm to themselves or others.

Adolescence: Despite the fact that drinking is illegal for anyone under the age of 21, the reality is that many adolescent girls drink. Research shows that about 37% of 9th grade girls—usually about 14 years old—report drinking in the past month. (This rate is slightly more than that for 9th grade boys.) Even more alarming is the fact that about 17% of these same young girls report having had five or more drinks on a single occasion during the previous month.

Consequences of unsafe underage drinking include the following:

- Drinking under age 21 is illegal in every state.

- Drunk driving is one of the leading causes of teen death.

- Drinking makes young women more vulnerable to sexual assault and unsafe and unplanned sex. On college campuses, assaults, unwanted sexual advances, and unplanned and unsafe sex are all more likely among students who drink heavily on occasion— for men, five drinks in a row, for women, four. In general, when a woman drinks to excess she is more likely to be a target of violence or sexual assault.

- Young people who begin drinking before age 15 have a 40% higher risk of developing alcohol abuse or alcoholism some time in their lives than those who wait until age 21 to begin drinking. This increased risk is the same for young girls as it is for boys.

Women in young and middle adulthood: Young women in their twenties and early thirties are more likely to drink than older women.

45

No one factor predicts whether a woman will have problems with alcohol, or at what age she is most at risk. However, there are some life experiences that seem to make it more likely that women will have drinking problems.

Heavy drinking and drinking problems among White women are most common in younger age groups. Among African American women, however, drinking problems are more common in middle age than youth. A woman's ethnic origins—and the extent to which she adopts the attitudes of mainstream versus her native culture—influence how and when she will drink. Hispanic women who are more mainstream are more likely to drink and to drink heavily (that is, to drink at least once a week and to have five or more drinks at one time).

Research suggests that women who have trouble with their closest relationships tend to drink more than other women. Heavy drinking is more common among women who have never married, are living unmarried with a partner, or are divorced or separated. (The effect of divorce on a woman's later drinking may depend on whether she is already drinking heavily in her marriage.) A woman whose husband drinks heavily is more likely than other women to drink too much.

Many studies have found that women who suffered childhood sexual abuse are more likely to have drinking problems. Also, depression is closely linked to heavy drinking in women, and women who drink at home alone are more likely than others to have later drinking problems.

Stress and drinking: Stress is a common theme in women's lives. Research confirms that one of the reasons people drink is to help them cope with stress. However, it is not clear just how stress may lead to problem drinking. Heavy drinking by itself causes stress in a job and family. Many factors, including family history, shape how much a woman will use alcohol to cope with stress. A woman's past and usual drinking habits are important. Different people have different expectations about the effect of alcohol on stress. How a woman handles stress, and the support she has to manage it, also may affect whether she uses alcohol in response to stress.

Consequences of unsafe drinking for young and middle-age women include the following:

- The number of female drivers involved in alcohol-related fatal traffic crashes is going up, even as the number of male drivers involved in such crashes has decreased. This trend may reflect the increasing number of women who drive themselves, even after drinking, as opposed to riding as a passenger.

- Long-term health problems from heavy drinking include liver, heart, and brain disease; suppression of the immune system; and cancer.

- Because women are more likely to become pregnant in their twenties and thirties, this age group faces the greatest risk of having babies with the growth and mental impairments of fetal alcohol syndrome which is caused by drinking during pregnancy.

Older women: As they grow older, fewer women drink. At the same time, research suggests that people born in recent decades are more likely to drink—throughout life—than people born in the early 1900s. Elderly patients are admitted to hospitals about as often for alcohol-related causes as for heart attacks. Older women may be especially sensitive to the stigma of being alcoholic, and therefore hesitate to admit if they have a drinking problem.

Consequences of unsafe drinking for older women include the following:

- Older women, more than any other group, use medications that can affect mood and thought, such as those for anxiety and depression. These psychoactive medications can interact with alcohol in harmful ways.

- Research suggests that women may be more likely to develop or to show alcohol problems later in life when compared with men.

- Older adults reach higher blood levels of alcohol even when drinking the same amount as younger people. This is because, with aging, the amount of water in the body is reduced and alcohol becomes more concentrated. But even at the same blood alcohol level, older adults may feel some of the effects of alcohol more strongly than younger people.

- Alcohol problems among older people often are mistaken for other aging-related conditions. As a result, alcohol problems may be missed and untreated by health care providers, especially in older women.

Women and Problem Drinking

Fewer women than men drink. However, among the heaviest drinkers, women equal or surpass men in the number of problems that result from their drinking. For example, female alcoholics have death rates 50%–100% higher than those of male alcoholics, including deaths from suicides, alcohol-related accidents, heart disease and stroke, and liver cirrhosis.

An Individual Decision

A woman's genetic makeup shapes how quickly she feels the effects of alcohol, how pleasant drinking is for her, and how drinking alcohol over the long term will affect her health, even the chances that she could have problems with alcohol. A family history of alcohol problems, a woman's risk of illnesses like heart disease and breast cancer, medications she is taking, and age are among the factors for each woman to weigh in deciding when, how much, and how often to drink.

What are alcohol abuse and alcoholism?

Alcohol abuse is a pattern of drinking that is harmful to the drinker or others. The following situations, occurring repeatedly in a 12-month period, would be indicators of alcohol abuse:

- Missing work or skipping child care responsibilities because of drinking

- Drinking in situations that are dangerous, such as before or while driving

- Being arrested for driving under the influence of alcohol or for hurting someone while drunk

- Continuing to drink even though there are ongoing alcohol-related tensions with friends and family

Research suggests that a woman is more likely to drink excessively if she has any of the following:

- Parents and siblings (or other blood relatives) with alcohol problems

- A partner who drinks heavily

- The ability to hold her liquor more than others

- A history of depression

- A history of childhood physical or sexual abuse

The presence of any of these factors is a good reason to be especially careful with drinking.

Section 5.3

Men's Health Risks from Excessive Alcohol Use

This section includes text excerpted from "Excessive Alcohol Use and Risks to Men's Health," Centers for Disease Control and Prevention (CDC), August 6, 2008; and excerpts from "Gender Differences in Alcohol Use and Alcohol Dependence or Abuse 2004 and 2005," Substance Abuse and Mental Health Services Administration (SAMHSA), August 2, 2007.

Excessive Alcohol Use and Risks to Men's Health

Men are more likely than women to drink excessively. Excessive drinking is associated with significant increases in short-term risks to health and safety, and the risk increases as the amount of drinking increases. Men are also more likely than women to take other risks (for example, drive fast or without a safety belt), when combined with excessive drinking, further increasing their risk of injury or death.

Drinking levels for men:

- Approximately 62% of adult men reported drinking alcohol in the last 30 days and were two times more likely to binge drink than women during the same time period.

- Men average about 12.5 binge drinking episodes per person per year, while women average about 2.7 binge drinking episodes per year.

- Most people who binge drink are not alcoholics or alcohol dependent.

- It is estimated that about 17% of men and about 8% of women will meet criteria for alcohol dependence at some point in their lives.

Injuries and deaths as a result of excessive alcohol use:

- Men consistently have higher rates of alcohol-related deaths and hospitalizations than women.

49

- Among drivers in fatal motor-vehicle traffic crashes, men are almost twice as likely as women to have been intoxicated (a blood alcohol concentration of 0.08% or greater).

- Excessive alcohol consumption increases aggression and, as a result, can increase the risk of physically assaulting another person.

- Men are more likely than women to commit suicide, and more likely to have been drinking prior to committing suicide.

Reproductive health and sexual function: Excessive alcohol use can interfere with testicular function and male hormone production, resulting in impotence, infertility, and reduction of male secondary sex characteristics such as facial and chest hair.

Excessive alcohol use is commonly involved in sexual assault. Impaired judgment caused by alcohol may worsen the tendency of some men to mistake a women's friendly behavior for sexual interest and misjudge their use of force. Also, alcohol use by men increases the chances of engaging in risky sexual activity including, unprotected sex, sex with multiple partners, or sex with a partner at risk for sexually transmitted diseases.

Cancer: Alcohol consumption increases the risk of cancer of the mouth, throat, esophagus, liver, and colon in men.

Gender Differences in Alcohol Use and Alcohol Dependence or Abuse: 2004 and 2005

Research indicates that rates of alcohol use and alcohol dependence or abuse are higher among males than females, and males account for more treatment admissions for alcohol abuse than do females, according to the Treatment Episode Data Set. Prior research has attempted to determine the extent to which higher rates of dependence reflect higher rates of use versus differences in the vulnerability to dependence among users.

The National Survey on Drug Use and Health (NSDUH) asks persons aged 12 or older to report on their frequency and quantity of alcohol use during the 30 days prior to the survey. NSDUH defines binge alcohol use as drinking five or more drinks on the same occasion (at the same time or within a couple of hours of each other) on at least one day in the past 30 days. Heavy alcohol use is defined as drinking five or more drinks on the same occasion on each of five or more days in the past 30 days. (All heavy alcohol users are also binge alcohol users.) NSDUH also asks questions to assess symptoms of alcohol dependence or abuse during the past year. NSDUH defines dependence on or abuse of alcohol using criteria specified in the *Diagnostic and Statistical Manual of Mental Disorders (DSM-IV)*. Alcohol dependence or abuse includes such symptoms as withdrawal, tolerance, use in dangerous situations, trouble with the law, and interference in major obligations at work, school, or home during the past year.

This report examines gender differences in past month alcohol use and past year alcohol dependence or abuse. All findings presented in this report are annual averages based on combined 2004 and 2005 NSDUH data.

Past Month Alcohol Use, by Gender

Combined data from 2004 and 2005 indicate that in the past month, 51.1% of persons aged 12 or older used alcohol, 22.7% reported binge alcohol use, and 6.8% indicated heavy alcohol use. Males were more likely than females to report past month alcohol use, binge alcohol use, and heavy alcohol use. These gender differences were generally consistent across demographic characteristics (age group, race/ethnicity, and family income).

Table 5.1. Percentages of Past Month Alcohol Use among Persons Aged 12 or Older, by Gender: 2004 and 2005

	Male	Female
Past month alcohol use	57.5%	45.0%
Binge alcohol use*	30.8%	15.1%
Heavy alcohol use*	10.5%	3.3%

Source: SAMHSA, 2004 and 2005 NSDUHs.

*NSDUH defines binge alcohol use as drinking five or more drinks on the same occasion (at the same time or within a couple of hours of each other) on at least one day in the past 30 days. Heavy alcohol use id defined as drinking five or more drinks on the same occasion on each of five or more days in the past 30 days. All heavy alcohol users are also binge alcohol users.

Alcohol Dependence or Abuse, by Gender

Combined data from 2004 and 2005 indicate that 7.7% of persons aged 12 or older (an estimated 18.7 million annually) were dependent on or abused alcohol in the past year. Males were twice as likely as females to have met the criteria for alcohol dependence or abuse in the past year (10.5% versus 5.1%). Although gender differences in alcohol dependence or abuse were generally consistent across demographic groups, there were some exceptions, for example, females aged 12 to 17 were equally likely to have met the criteria for alcohol dependence or abuse as their male counterparts (6.0% and 5.5% respectively).

Alcohol Dependence or Abuse, by Gender and Level of Alcohol Use

The rate of past year alcohol dependence or abuse varied by level of alcohol use. Nearly half of the past month heavy alcohol users aged 12 or older (44.7%) met the criteria for past year alcohol dependence or abuse, compared with 18.5% of those who were binge drinkers but not heavy alcohol users, 3.8% who were past month alcohol users but not binge drinkers, and 1.3% who were not past month alcohol users.

As noted, males aged 12 or older were more likely than their female counterparts to be heavy drinkers; however, among past month heavy alcohol users, there was no difference in the rate of past year alcohol dependence or abuse between males and females (Table 5.2). For all other levels of past month alcohol use, males were more likely to have met the criteria for past year alcohol dependence or abuse than females. For example, 19.2% of males who were binge drinkers but not heavy alcohol users met the criteria for past year alcohol dependence or abuse compared with 17.5% of females.

Table 5.2. Percentages Reporting Past Year Alcohol Dependence or Abuse among Persons Aged 12 or Older, by Gender and Level of Current Alcohol Use: 2004 and 2005

	Male	Female
No past month alcohol use	1.9%	0.9%
Past month alcohol use, but not binge use*	4.3%	3.5%
Binge but not heavy alcohol use*	19.2%	17.5%
Heavy alcohol use*	44.6%	44.9%

Source: SAMHSA, 2004 and 2005 NSDUHs.

*NSDUH defines binge alcohol use as drinking five or more drinks on the same occasion (at the same time or within a couple of hours of each other) on at least one day in the past 30 days. Heavy alcohol use id defined as drinking five or more drinks on the same occasion on each of five or more days in the past 30 days. All heavy alcohol users are also binge alcohol users.

Section 5.4

Alcohol Use in Older People

Text in this section is excerpted from "Alcohol Use In Older People,"
National Institute on Aging (NIA), May 2009.

Anyone at any age can have a drinking problem. Uncle George always liked his liquor, so his family may not see that his drinking is getting worse as he gets older. Grandma Betty was a teetotaler all her life—she started having a drink each night to help her get to sleep after her husband died. Now, no one realizes that she needs a couple of drinks to get through each day.

These are common stories. The fact is that families, friends, and health-care workers often overlook their concerns about older people drinking. Sometimes trouble with alcohol in older people is mistaken for other conditions related to aging. But, how the body handles alcohol can change with age. You may have the same drinking habits, but your body has changed.

Alcohol may act differently in older people than in younger people. Some older people can feel high without increasing the amount of alcohol they drink. This high can make them more likely to have accidents, including falls and fractures and car crashes.

Drinking too much alcohol over a long time can:

- lead to some kinds of cancer, liver damage, immune system disorders, and brain damage;

- worsen some health conditions like osteoporosis, diabetes, high blood pressure, and ulcers;

- make some medical problems hard for doctors to find and treat (for example, alcohol causes changes in the heart and blood vessels; these changes can dull pain that might be a warning sign of a heart attack); and

- cause some older people to be forgetful and confused—these symptoms could be mistaken for signs of Alzheimer disease.

Alcohol and Medicines

Many medicines—prescription, over-the-counter, or herbal remedies—can be dangerous or even deadly when mixed with alcohol. Many

53

older people take medications every day, making this a special worry. Before taking any medicine, ask your doctor or pharmacist if you can safely drink alcohol. Following are some examples of problems caused by mixing alcohol with some medicines:

- If you take aspirin and drink, your risk of stomach or intestinal bleeding is increased.

- When combined with alcohol, cold and allergy medicines (the label will say antihistamines) may make you feel very sleepy.

- Alcohol used with large doses of acetaminophen, a common painkiller, may cause liver damage.

- Some medicines, such as cough syrups and laxatives, have high alcohol content. If you drink at the same time, your alcohol level will go up.

- Alcohol used with some sleeping pills, pain pills, or anxiety/antidepression medicine can be deadly.

How much alcohol is too much?

The National Institute on Alcohol Abuse and Alcoholism, part of the National Institutes of Health, recommends that people who are healthy and over age 65 should have no more than seven drinks a week and no more than three drinks on any one day.

When does drinking become a problem?

Some people have been heavy drinkers for many years. But, just as with Uncle George, over time the same amount of alcohol packs a more powerful punch. Other people, like Grandma Betty, develop a drinking problem later in life. Sometimes this is a result of major life changes like death of dear friends or a loved one, moving to a new home, or failing health. These kinds of changes can cause loneliness, boredom, anxiety, or depression. In fact, depression in older adults often goes along with drinking too much.

Not everyone who drinks daily has a drinking problem. And, not all problem drinkers have to drink every day. You might want to get help if you, or a loved one, hides or lies about drinking, has more than seven drinks a week, or gets hurt or hurts others when drinking.

No one wants to get hurt or to hurt others as the result of too much alcohol. Yet, it can happen if you drink more than you should. Be aware of how your body changes as you age. Be alert to these changes, adjust how much alcohol you can safely drink, and continue to enjoy life to the fullest.

Section 5.5

Stress and the Abuse of Alcohol and Other Substances

Text in this section is excerpted from "Stress and Substance Abuse: A Special Report after the 9/11 Terrorist Attacks," National Institute on Drug Abuse (NIDA), September 9, 2009. The complete document with references is available online at http://www.drugabuse.gov/stressand drugabuse.html.

In the aftermath of the terrorist attacks on New York City and Washington DC, people across the country and abroad struggled with the emotional impact of large-scale damage and loss of life, as well as the uncertainty of what would happen next. These are stressful times and may be particularly difficult times for people who are more vulnerable to substance abuse or may be recovering from an addiction. For example, we know that stress is one of the most powerful triggers for relapse in addicted individuals, even after long periods of abstinence.

Stress and Drug Abuse; Stress and Relapse to Drug Abuse

Many clinicians and addiction medicine specialists suggest that stress is the number one cause of relapse to drug abuse, including smoking and alcoholism. Now, research is elucidating a scientific basis for these clinical observations. In both people and animals, stress leads to an increase in the brain levels of a peptide known as corticotrophin-releasing factor (CRF). The increased CRF levels in turn triggers a cascade of biological responses. Research also has shown that administering CRF or a chemical that mimics the action of CRF in animals produces increases in stress-related behaviors And, mice that lack a receptor for CRF (CRF1) have impaired stress responses and express less anxiety-related behavior. Furthermore, people subjected to chronic stress or those who show symptoms of PTSD often have hormonal responses that are not properly regulated and do not return to normal when the stress is over. This may make these individuals more prone to stress-related illnesses and may prompt patients to relapse to drug use.

Selected Research Findings on Stress and Drug Abuse; Stress and Relapse to Drug Abuse

- Studies have reported that individuals exposed to stress are more likely to abuse alcohol and other drugs or undergo relapse.

- In an analysis of studies regarding factors that can lead to continued drug use among opiate addicts, high stress was found to predict continued drug use.

- Research has shown that in animals not previously exposed to illicit substances, stressors increase vulnerability for drug self-administration.

- Acute stress can improve memory, whereas chronic stress can impair memory and may impair cognitive function.

- Research has shown that there is overlap between neurological circuits that respond to drugs and those that respond to stress.

- Researchers have shown that, among drug-free cocaine abusers in treatment, exposure to personal stress situations led to consistent and significant increases in cocaine craving, along with activation of emotional stress and a physiological stress response. In another study of cocaine abusers in treatment, significant increases in cocaine and alcohol craving were observed with stress and drug cues imagery but not with neutral-relaxing imagery.

- A follow-up study of smokers who had completed a national smoking cessation program showed that there is a strong relationship between stress coping resources and the ability to sustain abstinence.

- Animal studies have shown that stress induces relapse to heroin, cocaine, alcohol, and nicotine self-administration.

Posttraumatic Stress Disorder (PTSD) and Substance Abuse

Research shows that posttraumatic stress disorder (PTSD), a psychiatric disorder, may develop in people after they experience or witness life-threatening events such as terrorist incidents, military combat, natural disasters, serious accidents, or violent personal assaults like rape. Research also shows that PTSD is a risk factor for substance abuse and addiction. Symptoms of PTSD can include reexperiencing the trauma; avoidance of people, places, and thoughts connected to the event;

and arousal, which may include trouble sleeping, exaggerated startle response, and hypervigilance. People who develop such symptoms may be more prone to escape from the realities of the day by self-medicating with drugs. In fact, clinical observations suggest that PTSD patients may use psychoactive substances without a physician's directions to relieve traumatic memories and other symptoms associated with PTSD.

Selected Research Findings on PTSD and Substance Use Disorders

- High rates of comorbidity of PTSD and substance use disorders were first reported in war-related studies, in which as many as 75% of combat veterans with lifetime PTSD also met criteria for alcohol abuse or dependence.

- In a general population study, the overall lifetime rate of PTSD was 7.8%. Among men with a lifetime history of PTSD, 34.5% reported drug abuse or dependence at some point in their lives versus 15.1% of men without PTSD. For women, 26.9% with a lifetime history of PTSD reported drug abuse or dependence during their lives versus 7.6% of women without PTSD.

- Among adolescents lifetime rates of PTSD have been found ranging from 6.3%, in a community sample of older adolescents, to 29.6%, in substance-dependent adolescents aged 15 to 19 receiving treatment. And, among the substance-dependent adolescents, 19.2% currently had PTSD.

- Persons with a lifetime history of PTSD have elevated rates of co-occurring disorders. Among men with PTSD during their lives, rates of co-occurring alcohol abuse or dependence are the highest, followed by depression, conduct disorder, and drug abuse or dependence. Among women with PTSD during their lives, rates of comorbid depression are highest, followed by some anxiety disorders, alcohol abuse or dependence, and drug abuse or dependence.

- Patients with PTSD commonly have substance use disorders, particularly abuse of and dependence on central nervous system depressants. This frequent co-occurrence of PTSD and substance use, suggests that the two are related.

- The most recent thinking about the association between PTSD and substance use disorders suggests that for combat veterans and civilians, the onset of PTSD typically precedes the onset of substance use disorders.

- In a study of 1007 young adults designed to look for a causal relationship between PTSD and substance use disorders, researchers found that when they reevaluated the participants at three and five years after an initial assessment, PTSD was associated with a more than four-fold increased risk of drug abuse and dependence. The risk for abuse or dependence was highest for prescribed psychoactive drugs. The results suggest that drug abuse or dependence in persons with PTSD might be caused by efforts to self-medicate.

Chapter 6

Understanding the Development of an Addiction

Chapter Contents

Section 6.1

How Do Addictions Develop?

This section includes text from "Understanding Drug Abuse and Addiction," National Institute on Drug Abuse (NIDA), updated May 19, 2010.

Understanding Substance Abuse and Addiction

Many people do not understand why individuals become addicted to drugs or how drugs change the brain to foster compulsive drug abuse. They mistakenly view drug and substance abuse and addiction as strictly a social problem and may characterize those who take drugs as morally weak. One very common belief is that individuals should be able to just stop taking drugs or alcohol if they are only willing to change their behavior. What people often underestimate is the complexity of drug addiction—that it is a disease that impacts the brain and because of that, stopping drug abuse is not simply a matter of willpower. Through scientific advances we now know much more about how exactly drugs work in the brain, and we also know that drug addiction can be successfully treated to help people stop abusing drugs and resume their productive lives.

Drug abuse and addiction are a major burden to society. Estimates of the total overall costs of substance abuse in the United States—including health- and crime-related costs as well as losses in productivity—exceed half a trillion dollars annually. This includes approximately $181 billion for illicit drugs, $168 billion for tobacco, and $185 billion for alcohol. Staggering as these numbers are, however, they do not fully describe the breadth of deleterious public health—and safety—implications, which include family disintegration, loss of employment, failure in school, domestic violence, child abuse, and other crimes.

What is drug addiction?

Addiction is a chronic, often relapsing brain disease that causes compulsive drug seeking and use despite harmful consequences to the individual who is addicted and to those around them. Drug addiction is a brain disease because the abuse of drugs leads to changes in the structure and function of the brain. Although it is true that for most people the initial decision to take drugs is voluntary, over time the changes in the brain caused by repeated drug abuse can affect a person's self control and ability to make sound decisions, and at the same time send intense impulses to take drugs.

It is because of these changes in the brain that it is so challenging for a person who is addicted to stop abusing drugs. Fortunately, there are treatments that help people to counteract addiction's powerful disruptive effects and regain control. Research shows that combining addiction treatment medications, if available, with behavioral therapy is the best way to ensure success for most patients. Treatment approaches that are tailored to each patient's drug abuse patterns and any co-occurring medical, psychiatric, and social problems can lead to sustained recovery and a life without drug abuse.

Similar to other chronic, relapsing diseases (such as diabetes, asthma, or heart disease), drug addiction can be managed successfully. And, as with other chronic diseases, it is not uncommon for a person to relapse and begin abusing drugs again. Relapse, however, does not signal failure—rather, it indicates that treatment should be reinstated, adjusted, or that alternate treatment is needed to help the individual regain control and recover.

What happens to your brain when you take drugs?

Drugs are chemicals that tap into the brain's communication system and disrupt the way nerve cells normally send, receive, and process information. There are at least two ways that drugs are able to do this: (1) by imitating the brain's natural chemical messengers, and/or (2) by overstimulating the reward circuit of the brain.

Nearly all drugs, directly or indirectly, target the brain's reward system by flooding the circuit with dopamine. Dopamine is a neurotransmitter present in regions of the brain that control movement, emotion, motivation, and feelings of pleasure. The overstimulation of this system which normally responds to natural behaviors that are linked to survival (eating, spending time with loved ones, and so forth) produces euphoric effects in response to the drugs. This reaction sets in motion a pattern that teaches people to repeat the behavior of abusing drugs. As a person continues to abuse drugs, the brain adapts to the overwhelming surges in dopamine by producing less dopamine or by reducing the number of dopamine receptors in the reward circuit. As a result, dopamine's impact on the reward circuit is lessened, reducing the abuser's ability to enjoy the drugs and the things that previously brought pleasure. This decrease compels those addicted to drugs to keep abusing drugs in order to attempt to bring their dopamine function back to normal. And, they may now require larger amounts of the drug than they first did to achieve the dopamine high—an effect known as tolerance.

Long-term abuse causes changes in other brain chemical systems and circuits as well. Glutamate is a neurotransmitter that influences the reward circuit and the ability to learn. When the optimal concentration of glutamate is altered by drug abuse, the brain attempts to compensate, which can impair cognitive function. Drugs of abuse facilitate unconscious (conditioned) learning, which leads the user to experience uncontrollable cravings when they see a place or person they associate with the drug experience, even when the drug itself is not available. Brain imaging studies of drug-addicted individuals show changes in areas of the brain that are critical to judgment, decision making, learning and memory, and behavior control. Together, these changes can drive an abuser to seek out and take drugs compulsively despite adverse consequences—in other words, to become addicted to drugs.

Why do some people become addicted, while others do not?

No single factor can predict whether or not a person will become addicted to drugs. Risk for addiction is influenced by a person's biology, social environment, and age or stage of development. The more risk factors an individual has, the greater the chance that taking drugs can lead to addiction.

- **Biology:** The genes that people are born with—in combination with environmental influences—account for about half of their addiction vulnerability. Additionally, gender, ethnicity, and the presence of other mental disorders may influence risk for drug abuse and addiction.

- **Environment:** A person's environment includes many different influences—from family and friends to socioeconomic status and quality of life in general. Factors such as peer pressure, physical and sexual abuse, stress, and parental involvement can greatly influence the course of drug abuse and addiction in a person's life.

- **Development:** Genetic and environmental factors interact with critical developmental stages in a person's life to affect addiction vulnerability, and adolescents experience a double challenge. Although taking drugs at any age can lead to addiction, the earlier that drug use begins, the more likely it is to progress to more serious abuse. And because adolescents' brains are still developing in the areas that govern decision making, judgment, and self-control, they are especially prone to risk-taking behaviors, including trying drugs of abuse.

Prevention Is the Key

Drug addiction is a preventable disease. Results from National Institute on Drug Abuse (NIDA)-funded research have shown that prevention programs that involve families, schools, communities, and the media are effective in reducing drug abuse. Although many events and cultural factors affect drug abuse trends, when youths perceive drug abuse as harmful, they reduce their drug taking. It is necessary, therefore, to help youth and the general public to understand the risks of drug abuse, and for teachers, parents, and healthcare professionals to keep sending the message that drug addiction can be prevented if a person never abuses drugs.

Section 6.2

The Science Behind Addiction

This section includes text from "Drugs, Brains, and Behavior: The Science of Addiction (Part 1)," National Institute on Drug Abuse (NIDA), April 2007.

Drugs, Brains, and Behavior

In general, people begin taking drugs for a variety of reasons:

- **To feel good:** Most abused drugs produce intense feelings of pleasure. This initial sensation of euphoria is followed by other effects, which differ with the type of drug used. For example, with stimulants such as cocaine, the high is followed by feelings of power, self-confidence, and increased energy. In contrast, the euphoria caused by opiates such as heroin is followed by feelings of relaxation and satisfaction.

- **To feel better:** Some people who suffer from social anxiety, stress-related disorders, and depression begin abusing drugs in an attempt to lessen feelings of distress. Stress can play a major role in beginning drug use, continuing drug abuse, or relapse in patients recovering from addiction.

- **To do better:** The increasing pressure that some individuals feel to chemically enhance or improve their athletic or cognitive performance can similarly play a role in initial experimentation and continued drug abuse.

- **Curiosity and because others are doing it:** In this respect adolescents are particularly vulnerable because of the strong influence of peer pressure; they are more likely, for example, to engage in thrilling and daring behaviors.

The initial decision to take drugs is mostly voluntary. However, when drug abuse takes over, a person's ability to exert self control can become seriously impaired. Brain imaging studies from drug-addicted individuals show physical changes in areas of the brain that are critical to judgment, decision making, learning and memory, and behavior control. Scientists believe that these changes alter the way the brain works, and may help explain the compulsive and destructive behaviors of addiction.

Table 6.1. Examples of Risk and Protective Factors

Risk Factors	Domain	Protective Factors
Early aggressive behavior	Individual	Self-control
Poor social skills	Individual	Positive relationships
Lack of parental supervision	Family	Parental monitoring and support
Substance abuse	Peer	Academic competence
Drug availability	School	Anti-drug use policies
Poverty	Community	Strong neighborhood attachment

Why do some people become addicted to drugs, while others do not?

As with any other disease, vulnerability to addiction differs from person to person. In general, the more risk factors an individual has, the greater the chance that taking drugs will lead to abuse and addiction. Protective factors reduce a person's risk of developing addiction.

No single factor determines whether a person will become addicted to drugs. The overall risk for addiction is impacted by the biological makeup of the individual—it can even be influenced by gender or ethnicity, his or her developmental stage, and the surrounding social environment (for example, conditions at home, at school, and in the neighborhood).

Scientists estimate that genetic factors account for between 40% and 60% of a person's vulnerability to addiction, including the effects of environment on gene expression and function. Adolescents and individuals with mental disorders are at greater risk of drug abuse and addiction than the general population.

Environment factors that increase the risk of addiction include the following:

- **Home and family:** The influence of the home environment is usually most important in childhood. Parents or older family members who abuse alcohol or drugs, or who engage in criminal behavior, can increase children's risks of developing their own drug problems.

- **Peers and school:** Friends and acquaintances have the greatest influence during adolescence. Drug-abusing peers can sway even those without risk factors to try drugs for the first time. Academic failure or poor social skills can put a child further at risk for drug abuse.

What other factors increase the risk of addiction?

Early use: Although taking drugs at any age can lead to addiction, research shows that the earlier a person begins to use drugs the more likely they are to progress to more serious abuse. This may reflect the harmful effect that drugs can have on the developing brain; it also may result from a constellation of early biological and social vulnerability factors, including genetic susceptibility, mental illness, unstable family relationships, and exposure to physical or sexual abuse. Still, the fact remains that early use is a strong indicator of problems ahead, among them, substance abuse and addiction.

Method of administration: Smoking a drug or injecting it into a vein increases its addictive potential. Both smoked and injected drugs enter the brain within seconds, producing a powerful rush of pleasure. However, this intense high can fade within a few minutes, taking the abuser down to lower, more normal levels. It is a starkly felt contrast, and scientists believe that this low feeling drives individuals to repeated drug abuse in an attempt to recapture the high pleasurable state.

Brain development: The brain continues to develop into adulthood and undergoes dramatic changes during adolescence. One of the brain areas still maturing during adolescence is the prefrontal cortex—the part of the brain that enables us to assess situations, make sound decisions, and keep our emotions and desires under control. The fact that this critical part of an adolescent's brain is still a work-in-progress puts them at increased risk for poor decisions (such as trying drugs or continued abuse). Thus, introducing drugs while the brain is still developing may have profound and long-lasting consequences.

Section 6.3

Frequently Asked Questions about Addiction

Excerpted from "Frequently Asked Questions," National Institute on Drug Abuse (NIDA), updated May 11, 2010.

What are the physical signs of abuse or addiction?

The physical signs of abuse or addiction can vary depending on the person and the drug being abused. For example, someone who abuses marijuana may have a chronic cough or worsening of asthmatic symptoms. Each drug has short-term and long-term physical effects. Stimulants like cocaine increase heart rate and blood pressure, whereas opioids like heroin may slow the heart rate and reduce respiration.

How quickly can I become addicted to a drug?

There is no easy answer to this. If and how quickly you might become addicted to a drug depends on many factors including the biology of your body. All drugs are potentially harmful and may have life-threatening consequences associated with their abuse. There are also vast differences among individuals in sensitivity to various drugs. While one person may use a drug one or many times and suffer no ill effects, another person may be particularly vulnerable and overdose with first use. There is no way of knowing in advance how quickly someone may become addicted—but there are some clues, one important one being whether there is a family history of addition.

How do I know if someone is addicted to drugs?

If a person is compulsively seeking and using a drug despite negative consequences, such as loss of job, debt, physical problems brought on by drug abuse, or family problems, then he or she probably is addicted. And while people who are addicted may believe they can stop any time, most often they cannot, and will need professional help—first to determine if they in fact are addicted, and then to obtain drug abuse treatment. Support from friends and family can be critical in getting people into treatment and helping them to maintain abstinence following treatment.

Are there effective treatments for drug addiction?

Drug addiction can be effectively treated with behavioral-based therapies. Treatment will vary for each person depending on the type of drug(s) being used, and multiple courses of treatment may be needed to achieve success. For referrals to treatment programs:

Substance Abuse and Mental Health Services Administration (SAMHSA)

Toll-Free: 800-662-HELP (4357)
Website: http://findtreatment.samhsa.gov

Chapter 7

The Genetics of Alcoholism

Chapter Contents

69

Section 7.1

Genes and Addiction

Excerpted from "Genetics of Addiction," National Institute on Drug Abuse (NIDA), May 8, 2009.

Genetics: The Blueprint of Health and Disease

Why do some people become addicted, while others do not? Studies of identical twins indicate that as much as half of an individual's risk of becoming addicted to nicotine, alcohol, or other drugs depends on his or her genes. Pinning down the biological basis for this risk is an important avenue of research for scientists trying to solve the problem of drug abuse.

Genes—functional units that make up our deoxyribonucleic acid (DNA)—provide the information that directs our bodies' basic cellular activities. Research on the human genome has shown that the DNA sequences of any two individuals are 99.9% identical. However, that 0.1% variation is profoundly important, contributing to visible differences, like height and hair color, and to invisible differences, such as increased risks for, or protection from, heart attack, stroke, diabetes, and addiction.

Some diseases, like sickle cell anemia or cystic fibrosis, are caused by an error in a single gene. Medical research has been strikingly successful at unraveling the mechanisms of these single-gene disorders. However, most diseases, including addiction, are more complicated with variations in many different genes contributing to an individual's overall level of risk or resistance.

Recent advances in DNA analysis are enabling researchers to untangle complex genetic interactions by examining a person's entire genome at once. These genome-wide association studies (GWAS) identify subtle variations in DNA sequence called single-nucleotide polymorphisms (SNPs)—places where individuals differ in just a single letter of the genetic code. If a SNP appears more often in individuals with a disease than those without, it is presumed to be located in or near a gene that influences susceptibility to that disease.

GWAS are extremely powerful because they are unbiased and comprehensive—they can implicate a known gene in a disorder, and they can identify genes which may have been overlooked or previously unknown. Building on GWAS results, scientists gather additional evidence from affected families, animal models, and biochemical experiments to verify and understand the link between a gene and risk for a disease.

What role does the environment play in a disease like addiction?

That old saying nature or nurture might be better phrased nature and nurture because research shows that individual health is the result of dynamic interactions between genes and environmental conditions. For example, susceptibility to high blood pressure is influenced by both genetics and lifestyle including diet, stress, and exercise. Environmental influences, such as exposure to drugs or stress, can alter both gene expression and gene function. In some cases, these effects may persist throughout a person's life. Research suggests that genes can also influence how a person responds to his or her environment, placing some individuals at higher risk than others.

The promise of personalized medicine: The emerging science of pharmacogenomics promises to harness the power of genomic information to improve treatments for addiction. Clinicians often find substantial variability in how individual patients respond to treatment. Part of that variability is due to genetics. Genes influence the numbers and types of receptors in our brains, how quickly our bodies metabolize drugs, and how well we respond to different medications. Armed with an understanding of genetics, health providers will be better equipped to match patients with the most suitable treatments, adjust medication dosages, and avoid or minimize adverse reactions.

Research advance: A National Institute on Drug Abuse (NIDA)-sponsored study of alcohol dependent patients treated with naltrexone found that patients with a specific variant in an opioid receptor gene, Asp40, had a significantly lower rate of relapse (26.1%) than patients with the Asn40 variant (47.9%). In the future, identifying which mu-opioid receptor gene variant a patient possesses may help predict the most effective choice of medication for alcohol addiction.

Section 7.2

Is There a Genetic Link between Alcoholism and Other Drug Use Disorders?

This section includes excerpts from "The Genetics of Alcohol and Other Drug Dependence," National Institute on Alcohol Abuse and Alcoholism (NIAAA), 2008. The complete document with references is available at http://pubs.niaaa.nih.gov/publications/arh312/111-118.htm.

Identifying Specific Genes Related to Alcohol and Other Drug (AOD) Dependence

With robust evidence indicating that genes influence both alcohol dependence and dependence on illicit drugs, efforts now are underway to identify specific genes involved in the development of these disorders. This identification, however, is complicated by many factors. For example, numerous genes are thought to contribute to a person's susceptibility to alcohol and/or drug dependence, and affected people may carry different combinations of those genes. Additionally, environmental influences have an impact on substance use, as does gene–environment interaction. Finally, the manifestation of AOD dependence varies greatly among affected people, for example, with respect to age of onset of problems, types of symptoms exhibited (symptomatic profile), substance use history, and presence of comorbid disorders.

Despite the complications mentioned, the rapid growth in research technologies for gene identification in recent years has led to a concomitant increase in exciting results. After suffering many disappointments in early attempts to identify genes involved in complex behavioral outcomes (phenotypes), researchers now are frequently succeeding in identifying genes that help determine a variety of clinical phenotypes. These advances have been made possible by several factors:

- First, advances in technologies to identify a person's genetic makeup (genotyping technology) have dramatically lowered the cost of genotyping, allowing for high-throughput analyses of the entire genome.

- Second, the completion of several large-scale research endeavors, such as the Human Genome Project, the International HapMap Project, and other government and privately funded efforts, have made a wealth of information on variations in the human genome publicly available. The International HapMap Project is a multicountry effort to identify and catalog genetic similarities and differences in human beings by comparing the genetic sequences of different individuals in order to identify chromosomal regions where genetic variants are shared. Using the information obtained in the HapMap Project, researchers will be able to find genes that affect health, disease, and individual responses to medications and environmental factors.

- Third, these developments have been complemented by advances in the statistical analysis of genetic data.

Several large collaborative projects that strive to identify genes involved in AOD dependence currently are underway. The first large-scale project aimed at identifying genes contributing to alcohol dependence was the National Institute on Alcohol Abuse and Alcoholism (NIAAA)-sponsored Collaborative Study on the Genetics of Alcoholism (COGA), which was initiated in 1989. This study, which involves collaboration of investigators at several sites in the United States, examines families with several alcohol-dependent members who were recruited from treatment centers across the United States. This study has been joined by several other gene identification studies focusing on families affected with alcohol dependence, including the following:

- A sample of Southwestern American Indians (Long et al. 1998)

- The Irish Affected Sib Pair Study of Alcohol Dependence (Prescott et al. 2005a)

- A population of Mission Indians (Ehlers et al. 2004)

- A sample of densely affected families collected in the Pittsburgh area (Hill et al. 2004)

- An ongoing data collection from alcohol-dependent individuals in Australia

Importantly, most of these projects include comprehensive psychiatric interviews that focus not only on alcohol use and alcohol use disorders but which also allow researchers to collect information about other drug use and dependence. This comprehensive approach permits researchers to address questions about the nature of genetic influences on AOD dependence.

More recently, additional studies have been initiated that specifically seek to identify genes contributing to various forms of illicit drug dependence as well as general drug use problems Through these combined approaches, researchers should be able to identify both genes with drug-specific effects and genes with more general effects on drug use.

Genes Encoding Proteins Involved in Alcohol Metabolism

The genes that have been associated with alcohol dependence most consistently are those encoding the enzymes that metabolize alcohol (chemically known as ethanol). The main pathway of alcohol metabolism involves two steps. In the first step, ethanol is converted into the toxic intermediate acetaldehyde; this step is mediated by the alcohol dehydrogenase (ADH) enzymes. In a second step, the acetaldehyde is further broken down into acetate and water by the actions of aldehyde dehydrogenase (ALDH) enzymes. The genes that encode the ADH and ALDH enzymes exist in several variants (alleles) that are characterized by variations (polymorphisms) in the sequence of the deoxyribonucleic acid (DNA) building blocks. In people carrying these alleles, ethanol is more rapidly converted to acetaldehyde. Rapid acetaldehyde production can lead to acetaldehyde accumulation in the body which results in highly unpleasant effects, such as nausea, flushing, and rapid heartbeat, that may deter people from drinking more alcohol.

Interestingly, the effects of these genes do not appear to be limited to alcohol dependence. One study compared the frequency of alleles that differed in only one DNA building block (single nucleotide polymorphisms [SNPs]) throughout the genome between people with histories of illicit drug use and/or dependence and unrelated control participants. This study detected a significant difference for a SNP located near the ADH gene cluster. More recent evidence suggests that genetic variants in the ADH1A, ADH1B, ADH1C, ADH5, ADH6, and ADH7 genes are associated with illicit drug dependence and that this association is not purely attributable to comorbid alcohol dependence. The mechanism by which these genes may affect risk for illicit drug dependence is not entirely clear. However, other observations also indicate that enzymes involved in alcohol metabolism may contribute to illicit drug dependence via pathways that currently are unknown but independent of alcohol metabolism.

Genes encoding proteins involved in neurotransmission: AODs exert their behavioral effects in part by altering the transmission of signals among nerve cells (neurons) in the brain. This transmission is mediated by chemical messengers (neurotransmitters) that are released by the signal-emitting neuron and bind to specific proteins (receptors) on the signal-receiving neuron. AODs influence the activities of several neurotransmitter systems, including those involving the neurotransmitters gamma-aminobutyric acid (GABA), dopamine, and acetylcholine, as well as naturally produced compounds that structurally resemble opioids and cannabinoids. Accordingly, certain genes encoding components of these neurotransmitter systems may contribute to the risk of both alcohol dependence and illicit drug dependence.

GABA is the major inhibitory neurotransmitter in the human central nervous system—it affects neurons in a way that reduces their activity. Several lines of evidence suggest that GABA is involved in many of the behavioral effects of alcohol, including motor coordination dysfunction, anxiety reduction, sedation, withdrawal signs, and preference for alcohol.

Genes involved in the endogenous opioid system: Endogenous opioids are small molecules naturally produced in the body that have similar effects as the opiates (such as morphine and heroin) and which, among other functions, modulate the actions of other neurotransmitters. The endogenous opioid system has been implicated in contributing to the reinforcing effects of several drugs of abuse, including alcohol, opiates, and cocaine. This is supported by the finding that the medication naltrexone (which prevents the normal actions of endogenous opioids) for example, is an opioid antagonist, is useful in the treatment of alcohol dependence and can reduce the number of drinking days, amount of alcohol consumed, and risk of relapse.

Conclusions

For both alcohol dependence and drug dependence, considerable evidence suggests that genetic factors influence the risk of these disorders, with heritability estimates of 50% and higher. Moreover, twin studies and studies of electrophysiological characteristics indicate that the risk of developing AOD dependence, as well as other disinhibitory disorders (such as antisocial behavior), is determined at least in part by shared genetic factors. These observations suggest that some of a person's liability for AOD dependence will result from a general externalizing factor and some will result from genetic factors that are more disorder specific.

Several genes have been identified that confer risk to AOD dependence. Some of these genes—such as GABRA2 and CHRM2—apparently act through a general externalizing phenotype. For other genes that appear to confer risk of AOD dependence—such as genes involved in alcohol metabolism and in the endogenous opioid and cannabinoid systems—however, the pathways through which they affect risk remain to be elucidated. Most of the genes reviewed in this section originally were found to be associated with alcohol dependence and only subsequently was their association with risk for dependence on other illicit drugs discovered as well. Furthermore, studies that primarily aim to identify genes involved in dependence on certain types of drugs may identify different variants affecting risk, underscoring the challenge of understanding genetic susceptibility to different classes of drugs.

This review does not exhaustively cover all genes that to date have been implicated in alcohol and illicit drug dependence. For example, several genes encoding receptors for the neurotransmitter dopamine have been suggested to determine at least in part a person's susceptibility to various forms of drug dependence.

The increasingly rapid pace of genetic discovery also has resulted in the identification of several genes encoding other types of proteins that appear to be associated with alcohol use and/or dependence. These include, for example, two genes encoding taste receptors (i.e., the TAS2R16 gene and the TAS2R38 gene) and a human gene labeled ZNF699 that is related to a gene previously identified in the fruit fly Drosophila as contributing to the development of tolerance to alcohol in the flies. Future research will be necessary to elucidate the pathways by which these genes influence alcohol dependence and/or whether they are more broadly involved in other forms of drug dependence.

Section 7.3

Alcohol Metabolism Is Controlled by Genetic Factors

This section is excerpted from "Alcohol Metabolism: An Update," *Alcohol Alert, Number 72*, National Institute on Alcohol Abuse and Alcoholism (NIAAA), July 2007. The complete document with references is available at http://pubs.niaaa.nih.gov/publications/AA72/AA72.htm.

Drinking heavily puts people at risk for many adverse health consequences, including alcoholism, liver damage, and various cancers. But some people appear to be at greater risk than others for developing these problems. Why do some people drink more than others? And why do some people who drink develop problems, whereas others do not?

Research shows that alcohol use and alcohol-related problems are influenced by individual variations in alcohol metabolism, or the way in which alcohol is broken down and eliminated by the body. Alcohol metabolism is controlled by genetic factors, such as variations in the enzymes that break down alcohol; and environmental factors, such as the amount of alcohol an individual consumes and his or her overall nutrition. Differences in alcohol metabolism may put some people at greater risk for alcohol problems, whereas others may be at least somewhat protected from alcohol's harmful effects.

This section describes the basic process involved in the breakdown of alcohol, including how toxic byproducts of alcohol metabolism may lead to problems such as alcoholic liver disease, cancer, and pancreatitis. It also describes populations who may be at particular risk for problems resulting from alcohol metabolism as well as people who may be genetically protected from these adverse effects.

The Chemical Breakdown of Alcohol

Alcohol is metabolized by several processes or pathways. The most common of these pathways involves two enzymes—alcohol dehydrogenase (ADH) and aldehyde dehydrogenase (ALDH). These enzymes help break apart the alcohol molecule, making it possible to eliminate it from the body. First, ADH metabolizes alcohol to acetaldehyde, a highly toxic substance and known carcinogen. Then, in a second step, acetaldehyde is further metabolized down to another, less active by-product called acetate, which then is broken down into water and carbon dioxide for easy elimination.

Other enzymes: The enzymes cytochrome P450 2E1 (CYP2E1) and catalase also break down alcohol to acetaldehyde. However, CYP2E1 only is active after a person has consumed large amounts of alcohol, and catalase metabolizes only a small fraction of alcohol in the body. Small amounts of alcohol also are removed by interacting with fatty acids to form compounds called fatty acid ethyl esters (FAEE). These compounds have been shown to contribute to damage to the liver and pancreas.

Acetaldehyde, a toxic byproduct: Much of the research on alcohol metabolism has focused on an intermediate byproduct that occurs early in the breakdown process—acetaldehyde. Although acetaldehyde is short lived, usually existing in the body only for a brief time before it is further broken down into acetate, it has the potential to cause significant damage. This is particularly evident in the liver, where the bulk of alcohol metabolism takes place. Some alcohol metabolism also occurs in other tissues, including the pancreas and the brain, causing damage to cells and tissues. Additionally, small amounts of alcohol are metabolized to acetaldehyde in the gastrointestinal tract, exposing these tissues to acetaldehyde's damaging effects.

In addition to its toxic effects, some researchers believe that acetaldehyde may be responsible for some of the behavioral and physiological effects previously attributed to alcohol. For example, when acetaldehyde is administered to lab animals, it leads to coordination dysfunction, memory impairment, and sleepiness, effects often associated with alcohol.

On the other hand, other researchers report that acetaldehyde concentrations in the brain are not high enough to produce these effects. This is because the brain has a unique barrier of cells (the blood-brain barrier) that help to protect it from toxic products circulating in the bloodstream. It is possible, however, that acetaldehyde may be produced in the brain itself when alcohol is metabolized by the enzymes catalase and CYP2E1.

The Genetics behind Metabolism

Regardless of how much a person consumes, the body can only metabolize a certain amount of alcohol every hour. That amount varies widely among individuals and depends on a range of factors, including liver size and body mass.

In addition, research shows that different people carry different variations of the ADH and ALDH enzymes. These different versions can be traced to variations in the same gene. Some of these enzyme variants work more or less efficiently than others; this means that some people can break down alcohol to acetaldehyde, or acetaldehyde to acetate, more quickly than others. A fast ADH enzyme or a slow ALDH enzyme can cause toxic acetaldehyde to build up in the body, creating dangerous and unpleasant effects that also may affect an individual's risk for various alcohol-related problems—such as developing alcoholism.

The type of ADH and ALDH an individual carries has been shown to influence how much he or she drinks, which in turn influences his or her risk for developing alcoholism. For example, high levels of acetaldehyde make drinking unpleasant, resulting in facial flushing, nausea, and a rapid heartbeat. This flushing response can occur even when only moderate amounts of alcohol are consumed. Consequently, people who carry gene varieties for fast ADH or slow ALDH, which delay the processing of acetaldehyde in the body, may tend to drink less and are thus somewhat protected from alcoholism (although, they may be at greater risk for other health consequences when they do drink).

Genetic differences in these enzymes may help to explain why some ethnic groups have higher or lower rates of alcohol-related problems. For example, one version of the ADH enzyme, called ADH1B*2, is common in people of Chinese, Japanese, and Korean descent but rare in people of European and African descent. Another version of the ADH enzyme, called ADH1B*3, occurs in 15–25% of African Americans. These enzymes protect against alcoholism by metabolizing alcohol to acetaldehyde very efficiently, leading to elevated acetaldehyde levels that make drinking unpleasant. On the other hand, a recent study by Spence and colleagues found that two variations of the ALDH enzyme, ALDH1A1*2 and ALDH1A1*3, may be associated with alcoholism in African-American people.

Although these genetic factors influence drinking patterns, environmental factors also are important in the development of alcoholism and other alcohol-related health consequences. For example, Higuchi and colleagues found that as alcohol consumption in Japan increased between 1979 and 1992, the percentage of Japanese alcoholics who carried the protective ADH1B*2 gene version increased from 2.5–13%. Additionally, despite the fact that more Native American people die of alcohol-related causes than do any other ethnic group in the United States, research shows that there is no difference in the rates of alcohol metabolism and enzyme patterns between Native Americans and Whites. This suggests that rates of alcoholism and alcohol-related problems are influenced by other environmental and/or genetic factors.

Health Consequences of Alcohol Use

Alcohol metabolism and cancer: Alcohol consumption can contribute to the risk for developing different cancers, including cancers of the upper respiratory tract, liver, colon or rectum, and breast. This occurs in several ways, including through the toxic effects of acetaldehyde.

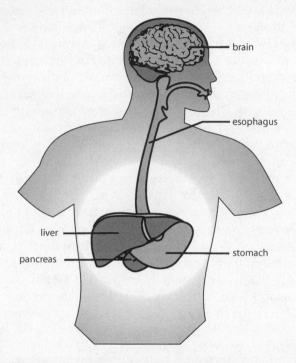

Figure 7.1. *Where Alcohol Metabolism Takes Place: Alcohol is metabolized in the body mainly by the liver. The brain, pancreas, and stomach also metabolize alcohol.*

Many heavy drinkers do not develop cancer, and some people who drink only moderately do develop alcohol-related cancers. Research suggests that just as some genes may protect individuals against alcoholism, genetics also may determine how vulnerable an individual is to alcohol's carcinogenic effects.

Ironically, the very genes that protect some people from alcoholism may magnify their vulnerability to alcohol-related cancers. The International Agency for Research on Cancer asserts that acetaldehyde should be classified as a carcinogen. Acetaldehyde promotes cancer in several ways—for example, by interfering with the copying (replication) of deoxyribonucleic acid (DNA) and by inhibiting a process by which the body repairs damaged DNA. Studies have shown that people who are exposed to large amounts of acetaldehyde are at greater risk for developing certain cancers, such as cancers of the mouth and throat. Although these individuals often are less likely to consume large amounts of alcohol, Seitz and colleagues suggest that when they do drink their risk for developing certain cancers is higher than drinkers who are exposed to less acetaldehyde during alcohol metabolism.

Acetaldehyde is not the only carcinogenic byproduct of alcohol metabolism. When alcohol is metabolized by CYP2E1, highly reactive, oxygen-containing molecules—or reactive oxygen species (ROS)—are produced. ROS can damage proteins and DNA or interact with other substances to create carcinogenic compounds.

Fetal alcohol spectrum disorder (FASD): Pregnant women who drink heavily are at even greater risk for problems. Poor nutrition may cause the mother to metabolize alcohol more slowly, exposing the fetus to high levels of alcohol for longer periods of time. Increased exposure to alcohol also can prevent the fetus from receiving necessary nutrition through the placenta. In rats, maternal malnutrition has been shown to contribute to slow fetal growth, one of the features of FASD, a spectrum of birth defects associated with drinking during pregnancy. These findings suggest that managing nutrition in pregnant women who drink may help to reduce the severity of FASD.

Alcoholic liver disease: As the chief organ responsible for the breakdown of alcohol, the liver is particularly vulnerable to alcohol metabolism's effects. More than 90% of people who drink heavily develop fatty liver, a type of liver disease. Yet only 20% will go on to develop the more severe alcoholic liver disease and liver cirrhosis.

Alcoholic pancreatitis: Alcohol metabolism also occurs in the pancreas, exposing this organ to high levels of toxic byproducts such as acetaldehyde and fatty acid ethyl esters (FAEE). Still, less than 10% of heavy alcohol users develop alcoholic pancreatitis—a disease that irreversibly destroys the pancreas—suggesting that alcohol consumption alone is not enough to cause the disease. Researchers speculate that environmental factors such as smoking and the amount and pattern of drinking and dietary habits, as well as genetic differences in the way alcohol is metabolized, also contribute to the development of alcoholic pancreatitis, although none of these factors has been definitively linked to the disease.

Conclusion

Researchers continue to investigate the reasons why some people drink more than others and why some develop serious health problems because of their drinking. Variations in the way the body breaks down and eliminates alcohol may hold the key to explaining theses differences. New information will aid researchers in developing metabolism-based treatments and give treatment professionals better tools for determining who is at risk for developing alcohol-related problems.

Part Two

The Problem of
Underage Drinking

Chapter 8

Underage Drinking in America: Scope of the Problem

Underage alcohol consumption (referring to persons under the minimum legal drinking age of 21) in the United States (U.S.) is a widespread and persistent public health and safety problem that creates serious personal, social, and economic consequences for adolescents, their families, communities, and the nation as a whole. Alcohol is the drug of choice among America's adolescents, used by more young people than tobacco or illicit drugs. The prevention and reduction of underage drinking and treatment of underage youth—those under the age of 21—with alcohol use disorders (AUDs) are therefore important public health and safety goals.

Research has demonstrated the potential negative consequences of underage alcohol use on human maturation, particularly on the brain which recent studies show continues to develop into a person's twenties. Although considerable attention has been focused on the serious consequences of underage drinking and driving, accumulating evidence indicates that the range of adverse consequences is much more extensive than that and should also be comprehensively addressed. For example, the highest prevalence of alcohol dependence in the U.S. population is among 18- to 20-year-olds who typically began drinking years earlier. This finding underscores the need to consider problem

This chapter is excerpted from "The Surgeon General's Call to Action to Prevent and Reduce Underage Drinking: Section 1," U.S. Department of Health and Human Services (HHS), 2007. The complete document with references is available at http://www.surgeongeneral.gov/topics/underagedrinking/calltoaction.pdf.

drinking within a developmental framework. Furthermore, early and especially early heavy drinking are associated with increased risk for adverse lifetime alcohol-related consequences. Research also has provided a more complete understanding of how underage drinking is related to factors in the adolescent's environment, cultural issues, and an adolescent's individual characteristics. Taken together, these data demonstrate the compelling need to address alcohol problems early, continuously, and in the context of human development using a systematic approach that spans childhood through adolescence into adulthood.

Underage drinking remains a serious problem despite laws against it in all 50 states; decades of federal, state, tribal, and local programs aimed at preventing and reducing underage drinking; and efforts by many private entities. Underage drinking is deeply embedded in the American culture, is often viewed as a rite of passage, is frequently facilitated by adults, and has proven to be stubbornly resistant to change. A new, more comprehensive and developmentally sensitive approach is warranted. The growing body of research in the developmental area, including identification of risk and protective factors for underage alcohol use, supports the more complex prevention and reduction strategies that are proposed.

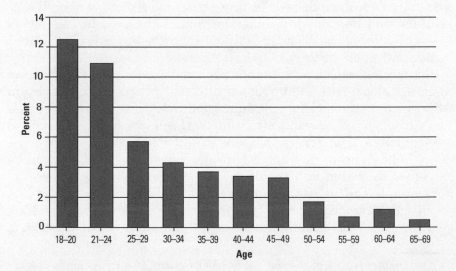

Figure 8.1. *Prevalence of Past-Year DSM-IV Alcohol Dependence–United States (Source: Grant et al. 2004; data from the National Epidemiologic Survey on Alcohol and Related Conditions)*

The Nature of Underage Drinking

Underage alcohol use is a pervasive problem with serious health and safety consequences for the nation. The nature and gravity of the problem is best described in terms of the number of children and adolescents who drink, when and how they drink, and the negative consequences that result from drinking.

Alcohol is the most widely used substance of abuse among America's youth: As indicated in Figure 8.2, a higher percentage of youth in 8th, 10th, and 12th grades used alcohol in the month prior to being surveyed than used tobacco or marijuana—the illicit drug most commonly used by adolescents.

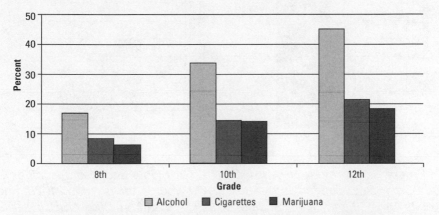

Figure 8.2. Past-Month Adolescent Alcohol, Cigarette, and Marijuana Use by Grade (Source: Data from 2006 Monitoring the Future Survey)

A substantial number of young people begin drinking at very young ages: A number of surveys ask youth about the age at which they first used alcohol. Because the methodology in the various surveys differs, the data are not consistent across them. Nonetheless, they do show that a substantial number of youth begin drinking before the age of 13. For example, data from recent surveys indicate that:

• Approximately 10% of 9- to 10-year-olds have started drinking.

• Nearly one-third of youth begin drinking before age 13.

• More than one-tenth of 12- or 13-year-olds and over one-third of 14- or 15-year-olds reported alcohol use (a whole drink) in the past year.

• The peak years of alcohol initiation are 7th and 8th grades.

Adolescents drink less frequently than adults, but when they do drink, they drink more heavily than adults: When youth between the ages of 12 and 20 consume alcohol, they drink on average about five drinks per occasion about six times a month, as indicated in Figure 8.3. This amount of alcohol puts an adolescent drinker in the binge range which, depending on the study, is defined as five or more drinks on one occasion or five or more drinks in a row for men and four or more drinks in a row for women. By comparison, adult drinkers age 26 and older consume on average two to three drinks per occasion about nine times a month.

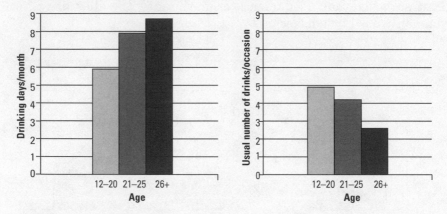

Figure 8.3. *Number of Drinking Days per Month and Usual Number of Drinks per Occasion for Youth Ages 12–20, Young Adults Ages 21–25, and Adults Ages 26 and Older (Source: SAMHSA data from 2005 NSDUH)*

Differences in underage alcohol use exist between the sexes and among racial and ethnic groups. Despite differences between the sexes and among racial and ethnic groups, overall rates of drinking among most populations of adolescents are high. In multiple surveys, underage males generally report more alcohol use during the past month than underage females. Boys also tend to start drinking at an earlier age than girls, drink more frequently, and are more likely to binge drink. When youth ages 12–20 were asked about how old they were when they started drinking, the average age was 13.90 for boys and 14.36 for girls for those adolescents who reported drinking. Interestingly, the magnitude of the sex-related difference in the frequency of binge drinking varies substantially by age (see Figure 8.4). Further, data from the Monitoring the Future survey show that while the percentages of boys and girls in the 8th and 10th grades who binge drink are similar (10.5 and 10.8, and 22.9 and 20.9, respectively), among 12th graders, boys have a higher prevalence of binge drinking compared to girls (29.8 compared to 22.8).

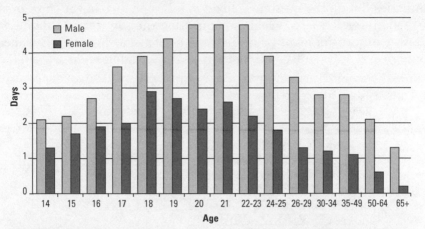

Figure 8.4. *Number of Days in the Past 30 in which Drinkers Consumed Five or More Drinks, by Age and Gender (Source: SAMHSA data from 2005 NSDUH)*

While the percentage of adolescents of all racial/ethnic subgroups who drink is high, Black or African American and Asian youth tend to drink the least, as shown in Figure 8.5.

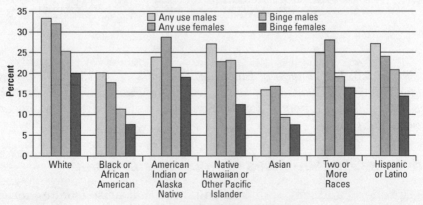

Figure 8.5. *Alcohol Use and Binge Drinking in the Past Month among Persons Ages 12–20 by Race/Ethnicity and Gender, Annual Averages Based on 2002–2005 Data (Source: SAMHSA, Office of Applied Studies, NSDUH— special data analysis)*

Binge drinking by teens is not limited to the United States: As shown in Figure 8.6, in many European countries a significant proportion of young people ages 15–16 report binge drinking. In all of the countries listed, the minimum legal drinking age is lower than in the United States. These data call into question the suggestion that having a lower minimum legal drinking age, as they do in many European countries, results in less problem drinking by adolescents.

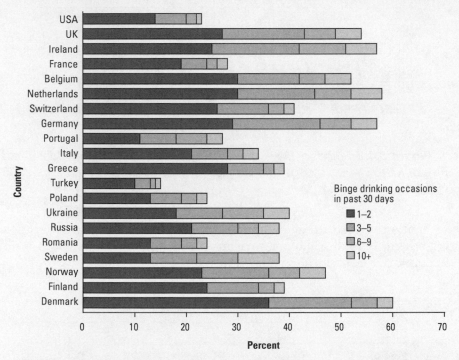

Figure 8.6. Percentage of European Students Ages 15–16 Who Have Engaged in Binge Drinking (5+ Drinks) within the Past 30 Days (Source: Hibell et al, 2004–data from European School Survey Project on Alcohol and Drugs, 2003)

Adverse Consequences of Underage Drinking

The short- and long-term consequences that arise from underage alcohol consumption are astonishing in their range and magnitude, affecting adolescents, the people around them, and society as a whole. Adolescence is a time of life characterized by robust physical health and low incidence of disease, yet overall morbidity and mortality rates increase 200% between middle childhood and late adolescence/early adulthood. This dramatic rise is attributable in large part to the increase in risk taking, sensation seeking, and erratic behavior that follows the onset of puberty and which contributes to violence, unintentional injuries, risky sexual behavior, homicide, and suicide. Alcohol frequently plays a role in these adverse outcomes and the human tragedies they produce. Among the most prominent adverse consequences of underage alcohol use are the following:

- Death from injuries which are the main cause of death for people under age 21. Annually, about 5,000 people under age 21 die from alcohol-related injuries involving underage drinking. About 1,900 (38%) of the 5,000 deaths involve motor vehicle crashes, about 1,600 (32%) result from homicides, and about 300 (6%) result from suicides.

- Risky sexual behavior, including unwanted, unintended, and unprotected sexual activity, and sex with multiple partners. Such behavior increases the risk for unplanned pregnancy and for contracting sexually transmitted diseases (STDs), including infection with human immunodeficiency virus (HIV), the virus that causes acquired immunodeficiency syndrome (AIDS).

- Increased risk of physical and sexual assault.

Underage alcohol use is also associated with academic failure, illicit drug use, tobacco use, and alterations in the structure and function of the developing brain which continues to mature into the mid to late twenties. Underage drinking is also a risk factor for heavy drinking later in life and continued heavy use of alcohol leads to increased risk across the lifespan for acute consequences and for medical problems such as cancers of the oral cavity, larynx, pharynx, and esophagus; liver cirrhosis; pancreatitis; and hemorrhagic stroke.

Early onset of drinking: Approximately 40% of individuals who report drinking before age 15 also describe their behavior and drinking at some point in their lives in ways consistent with a diagnosis for alcohol dependence. This is four times as many as among those who do not drink before age 21.

Alcohol consumption by underage college students is commonplace: Indeed, many college students, as well as some parents and administrators, accept alcohol use as a normal part of student life. Studies consistently indicate that about 80% of college students drink alcohol, about 40% engage in binge drinking, and about 20% engage in frequent episodic heavy consumption, which is bingeing three or more times over the past two weeks.

Children of alcoholics (COAs): COAs are between four and ten times more likely to become alcoholics than children from families with no alcoholic adults and therefore require special consideration when addressing underage drinking. COAs are at elevated risk for earlier onset of drinking and earlier progression into drinking problems. Some of the elevated risk is attributable to the socialization effects of living in an alcoholic household, some to genetically transmitted differences in response to alcohol that make drinking more pleasurable and/or less aversive, and some to elevated transmission of risky temperamental and behavioral traits that lead COAs, more than other youth, into increased contact with earlier drinking and heavier drinking peers.

Chapter 9

Current Drinking Patterns among Underage Drinkers

Chapter Contents

Section 9.1

Quantity and Frequency of Alcohol Use among Underage Drinkers

Excerpted from "Quantity and Frequency of Alcohol Use among Underage Drinkers," Substance Abuse and Mental Health Services Administration (SAMHSA), March 31, 2008.

In 2006, a majority (53.9%) of American adolescents and young
adults aged 12 to 20 had used an alcoholic beverage at least once in
their lifetime. Young people aged 12 to 20 consumed approximately
11.2% of the alcoholic drinks consumed in the United States in the
past month by persons aged 12 or older. Research shows that underage
drinkers tend to consume more alcohol per occasion than those over
the legal minimum drinking age of 21. Studies also have linked early
drinking to heavy alcohol consumption and alcohol-related problems in
adulthood. For example, in 2006, 16.3% of adults aged 21 or older who
had first used alcohol before the age of 15 met the criteria for alcohol
dependence or abuse in the past year compared with 2.4% of adults
who first used alcohol at age 21 or older. Research also shows that
early initiation of alcohol use is associated with higher likelihood of
involvement in violent behaviors, suicide attempts, unprotected sexual
intercourse, and multiple sex partners.

The National Survey on Drug Use and Health (NSDUH) asks persons aged 12 or older to report the frequency and quantity of their
alcohol use during the 30 days prior to the interview. Respondents
who drank alcohol in the past 30 days also are asked for the number
of days they consumed alcohol in the past month and the average
number of drinks consumed per day on the days they drank. All findings presented in this report are based on combined 2005 and 2006
NSDUH data.

Past month alcohol use: Combined 2005 and 2006 data indicate
that an annual average of 28.3% of persons aged 12 to 20 in the United
States (an estimated 10.8 million persons annually) drank alcohol in
the past month. Rates of past month alcohol use among persons aged
12 to 20 varied by demographic characteristics. Young adults aged 18

94

to 20 were three times as likely as youths aged 12 to 17 to have used alcohol in the past month (51.4% versus 16.6%). Underage males were more likely than their female counterparts to have drunk alcohol in the past month (29.1% versus 27.5%). Across racial/ethnic groups, the rate of past month alcohol use among persons aged 12 to 20 ranged from 17.6% among Asians to 32.3% among Whites.

Number of days of alcohol use in the past month: Past month alcohol users aged 12 to 20 drank on an average of 5.9 days in the past month. Underage drinkers aged 18 to 20 consumed alcohol on more days in the past month than those aged 12 to 17 (6.7 versus 4.6 days). Male underage drinkers used alcohol on more days in the past month than their female counterparts (6.6 versus 5.1 days). The number of days of alcohol use in the past month varied by race/ethnicity, ranging from an average of 4.2 days among Asians to an average of 8.3 days in the past month among native Hawaiians or Other Pacific Islanders.

Section 9.2

Where Do Youth Obtain and Consume Alcohol?

Text in this section is excerpted from the following Substance Abuse and Mental Health Services Administration (SAMHSA) documents: "Results from the 2008 NSDUH National Findings: Chapter 3," September 2009; "Underage Alcohol Use: Where Do Young People Drink?" August 28, 2008; and "Underage Alcohol Use: Where Do Young People Get Alcohol?" November 20, 2008.

Alcohol Use: Results from the National Survey on Drug Use and Health

- Across geographic regions in 2008, underage current alcohol use rates were higher in the Northeast (30.0%) than in the Midwest (27.1%), and both rates were higher than in the South (24.7%). The rate in the West (25.8%) was similar to rates in the South and Midwest regions, but was significantly lower than the rate in the Northeast.

- In 2008, underage current alcohol use rates were higher in small metropolitan areas (27.9%) compared with large metropolitan areas (25.9%) and similar in large metropolitan areas and non-metropolitan areas (25.3%). The rate in nonmetropolitan areas decreased from 2007, when it was 28.8%.

- In 2008, 81.7% of current drinkers aged 12 to 20 were with two or more other people the last time they drank alcohol, 13.6% were with one other person the last time they drank, and 4.7% were alone.

- A majority of underage current drinkers in 2008 reported that their last use of alcohol in the past month occurred either in someone else's home (56.2%) or their own home (29.6%). Under-age males were more likely than females to have been at a con-cert or sports game on their last drinking occasion (2.5% versus 1.1%), whereas females were more likely than males to have been in a restaurant, bar, or club on their last drinking occasion (10.3% versus 7.0%).

- Among underage current drinkers in 2008, 30.8% paid for the alcohol the last time they drank, including 8.3% who purchased the alcohol themselves and 22.3% who gave money to someone else to purchase it.

- Among underage drinkers who did not pay for the alcohol the last time they drank, the most common source was an unrelated person aged 21 or older (37.4%). Other underage persons pro-vided the alcohol on the last occasion 21.1% of the time. Parents, guardians, or other adult family members provided the alcohol 21.0% of the time. Other sources of alcohol for underage drinkers included: 5.8% who took the alcohol from home; 3.2% who took it from someone else's home; and, 6.9% who got it some other way.

Where do young people drink?

In 2006, a majority (53.4%) of current alcohol users aged 12 to 20 drank at someone else's home the last time they used alcohol, and an-other 30.3% drank in their own home. This overall pattern of last using alcohol in their own home or at someone else's home held for drinkers at each age from 13 to 20. More than 60% of drinkers aged 16 or 17 used alcohol in someone else's home the last time they drank. About

36% or more of drinkers aged 13, 14, and 20 last used alcohol in their own homes; and, 10.0% of 13-year-old drinkers last consumed alcohol in public places (such as a park, a beach, or a parking lot).

The percentage of underage alcohol users who had their most recent drink in a car or other vehicle peaked at 10.1% at age 16. An estimated 15.0% of those aged 20 last drank in a restaurant, bar, or club. Approximately 7% to 10% of alcohol users aged 13 to 17 last drank in public places, with the percentages decreasing to fewer than 4% of drinkers aged 18 to older. In contrast, most recent use of alcohol in a restaurant, bar, or club started to increase at age 18 and was at its highest point at age 20.

Do age-related changes in drinking locations differ for males and females?

Among male alcohol users, the percentage reporting that they drank most recently in a car or other vehicle did not differ significantly by age between ages 15 and 20, but it did differ for females. An estimated 12.8% of female alcohol users who were aged 16 last drank alcohol in a car or other motor vehicle, a rate that was eight times greater than the rate for female drinkers who were aged 20 (1.6%). At age 16, 7.3% of male current drinkers had their last drink in a car or other vehicle.

Among 15-year-old drinkers, females were twice as likely as males to have last used alcohol in a public place, such as a park, beach, or parking lot (10.6% versus 5.0%). Among males, alcohol consumption in public places peaked at age 16 and then declined. Among females, alcohol consumption in public places declined after age 15.

Where Young People Get Alcohol

Nearly one-third (30.6%) of current alcohol users aged 12 to 20 in 2006 and 2007 (an estimated 3.2 million persons) paid for the last alcohol they used, and 69.4% (an estimated 7.3 million persons) got the last alcohol they used for free. More than one in four (26.4%) got the last alcohol they used for free from a non-relative aged 21 or older, 14.6% got it for free from another underage person, 5.9% got it from a parent or guardian, 8.5% got it from another relative aged 21 or older, and 3.9% took it from their own home without asking.

How do underage males and females obtain alcohol?

Underage male alcohol users were more likely than their female counterparts to have paid for the last alcohol they used (36.8% versus 23.6%). Conversely, more than three-fourths of female underage drinkers (76.4%)

obtained their last alcohol for free compared with 63.2% of males. Female underage drinkers were more likely than their male counterparts to have gotten the last alcohol they used for free from a non-relative of legal drinking age (31.0% versus 22.1%).

Table 9.1. Source of Alcohol Obtained for Free for the Last Use in the Past Month among Alcohol Users Aged 12 to 20, by Age Group: Annual Averages, 2006 and 2007*

	Age group		
Source of alcohol	12–14	15–17	18–20
From parent or guardian	16.6%	7.3%	4.2%
From another family member aged 21 or older	12.8%	9.3%	7.7%
From someone not related aged 21 or older	13.4%	20.3%	30.5%
From someone under age 21	18.6%	20.9%	11.1%
Took it from own home	14.0%	5.3%	2.2%

Source: SAMHSA, 2006 and 2007 NHDUHs.

How many drinks do underage drinkers have, depending on how they obtain alcohol?

Current alcohol users aged 12 to 20 consumed more drinks on average the last time if they paid for the last alcohol they used (6.0 drinks) compared with those who did not pay for their last alcohol (3.9 drinks). Underage current drinkers who got alcohol for free from a non-relative of legal drinking age consumed more drinks on average (4.3 drinks) than those who got the last alcohol they used from a parent or guardian (2.5 drinks).

Chapter 10

Does Advertising Play a Role in Underage Drinking?

Chapter Contents

Section 10.1

Advertising Regulations for Alcoholic Beverages

This section is excerpted from "Self-Regulation in the Alcohol Industry," Federal Trade Commission (FTC), June 2008.

Self-Regulation in the Alcohol Industry
Executive Summary

Underage alcohol use is a widespread problem with significant health and safety consequences. This report of the efforts by the alcohol industry to reduce the likelihood that alcohol advertising will target youth, by its placement or content, was prepared by the Federal Trade Commission and provides data about how industry members allocate promotional dollars and data on compliance with the industry's advertising placement standard (requiring that at least 70% of the audience for advertising consist of adults 21 and older).

Allocation of promotional expenditures and related self-regulatory efforts: The data provided by the suppliers show that about 42% of promotional funds are used for television, radio, print, and outdoor advertising; about 40% are used to help wholesalers and retailers promote alcohol to consumers; about 16% are used for sponsorships; and the final 2% are directed to other efforts, such as Internet advertising, other digital promotions, and product placement. It appears that the suppliers keep self-regulatory responsibilities in mind as they engage in promotional efforts, even in cases where the self-regulatory codes do not expressly apply.

Compliance with the 70% placement standard: Prior to 2003, the industry codes permitted placing advertisements in media where as little as 50% of the audience was composed of adults and did not specify any placement protocol to support this standard. Between 2000 and 2003, at the Commission's recommendation, the alcohol industry modified its self-regulatory codes to require suppliers to check reliable audience composition data before placing an ad and to make a placement only if that data showed that, historically, at least 70% of the audience consisted of adults 21 and older. The Special Orders required the companies to describe their placement practices, and to provide data showing the composition of the audience (that is, number and percent of persons below and above the legal drinking age [LDA]) for each individual television, radio, magazine, and newspaper advertising placement disseminated in the first six months of 2006.

The responses showed that the suppliers directed their media buyers to follow the steps set forth in the self-regulatory codes, and to conduct periodic after-the-fact audits to determine whether the placements had, in fact, met the 70% standard. Advertising placement can be an uncertain process, as it relies on data about past audiences to predict the future. Nevertheless, more than 92% of all television, radio, and print advertising placements for which data were available had an LDA audience composition of 70% or better when they ran. Further, about 97% of total alcohol advertising impressions (that is, individual exposures to an advertisement) were due to placements that met the 70% target, as placements that missed the target were concentrated in media with smaller audiences. In the first half of 2006, more than 85% of the aggregate audience for the twelve suppliers' advertising consisted of adults above the LDA, although some individual companies' aggregates were a few points lower.

External review of advertising: Self-regulation is most effective when an advertiser's internal mechanisms for fostering code compliance are supplemented by a system in which another entity provides consistent, impartial, objective, and public resolution of disputes about whether a particular practice violates code standards. Per earlier Federal Trade Commission (FTC) recommendations, the three major industry trade associations now have systems for external review of complaints about code compliance. In 2006, the review boards considered twenty-six complaints. Trade association members complied with review board conclusions in all cases where the review board determined that a member had violated the code.

Underage access to alcohol: Restrictions on teen access to alcohol are a proven way to reduce teen drinking. The FTC developed the "We Don't Serve Teens" (WDST) program to provide parents and other responsible adults with information about the importance of restricting teen alcohol access. A wide range of public and private entities, including federal and state government representatives, consumer groups, the advertising industry, and the alcohol industry, joined the Commission in 2007 to spread the word, "Don't serve alcohol to teens. It's unsafe. It's illegal. It's irresponsible."

Section 10.2

Youth Exposure to Alcohol Advertising

This section is excerpted from "Youth Exposure to Alcohol Advertising in Magazines–United States, 2001–2005," *Morbidity and Mortality Weekly Report* (*MMWR*), August 3, 2007, Centers for Disease Control and Prevention (CDC).

Studies have documented the contribution of alcohol marketing to underage drinking. In 2000, the trade association for the wine industry changed its voluntary marketing code to stop advertising in magazines in which youths aged 12–20 years were greater than 30% of the audience. In 2003, this threshold was adopted by the trade associations for beer and liquor producers. To determine the proportion of alcohol advertisements placed in magazines with disproportionately large youth readerships (for example, greater than 15% of readers aged 12–20 years) and to assess the proportion of youths exposed to these advertisements, the Center on Alcohol Marketing and Youth (Health Policy Institute, Georgetown University, District of Columbia) evaluated the placement of alcohol advertisements in 143 national magazines for which readership composition data were available for 2001–2005; these 143 publications accounted for approximately 90% of expenditures for all alcohol advertising in national print magazines. This section summarizes the results of that study, which indicated that alcohol advertising remained common in magazines with greater than 15% youth readership but decreased substantially in magazines with greater than 30% youth readership. These results suggest that although voluntary industry standards have reduced youth exposure to alcohol advertising in magazines, strengthening these standards by establishing a greater than 15% youth readership threshold would further reduce exposure. In addition, independent monitoring of youth exposure to alcohol advertising should continue, as recommended by the U.S. Congress and Surgeon General.

During 2001–2005, total youth exposure to alcohol advertising in magazines decreased 46.9% (from approximately 5.74 billion impressions in 2001 to 3.05 billion in 2005). During this period, exposure among those aged less than 21 years decreased 25.0%. The proportion of youth exposure to alcohol advertising in magazines with greater than 15% youth readership decreased 7.6% (from 89.3% in 2001 to 82.5% in 2005). The proportion of youth exposure to alcohol advertising in magazines with greater than 30% youth readership decreased 95.5% (from 20.8% in 2001 to 0.9% in 2005), whereas the proportion of youth exposure in magazines with greater than 15% to 30% youth readership increased 19.1% (from 68.5% in 2001 to 81.6% in 2005).

Liquor accounted for most alcohol advertising in magazines in all study years and for 1,909 (65.9%) of 2,897 advertisements in 2005. In 2005, nine (0.3%) alcohol advertisements appeared in magazines with greater than 30% youth readership. In magazines with greater than 15% to 30% youth readership, liquor accounted for 879 (69.1%) of 1,272 advertisements, and beer accounted for 291 (22.9%) of advertisements. However, premixed alcoholic beverages (also known as alcopops, which are flavored, premixed drinks such as hard lemonade) had the largest proportion of advertisements in magazines with greater than 15% to 30% youth readership (90.9%), followed by beer (56.0%), liquor (46.0%), and wine (18.4%). Liquor (67.9%) and beer (23.8%) advertisements accounted for most youth exposure to alcohol advertising overall. The beverage-specific proportions of youth exposure accounted for by advertising in magazines with greater than 15% to 30% youth readership ranged from 64.6% for wine to 98.7% for premixed alcoholic beverages.

The proportion of alcohol advertisements placed in magazines with disproportionately large youth audiences varied considerably by brand, even within beverage categories. Of the 201 alcohol brands advertised in magazines in 2005, a total of 36 brands placed all of their advertising in magazines with greater than 15% youth readership, 38 brands placed more than half of their advertising in these magazines, 39 had half or less of their advertising in these magazines, and 88 brands had no advertising in these magazines.

Section 10.3

How to Identify, Analyze, and Evaluate Media Messages

Text in this section is excerpted from "Media Literacy Ladder," Substance Abuse and Mental Health Services Administration (SAMHSA), February 24, 2009.

The media literacy ladder is a visual organizer to help teens identify, analyze, and evaluate media messages. The information presented in the ladder can empower your teen by helping them become a critical consumer of information. Each step on the ladder introduces teens to one of five basic principles of media education. Ask your teen to pick any media message—a movie, a magazine article, a television (TV) or magazine advertisement, a T-shirt, or song lyrics. Next, starting at the bottom of the ladder and working to the top, ask your teen to answer the questions at each step on the ladder. The first two steps (identifying form and purpose) require your teen to identify details in the media message. For example, a TV news broadcast presents information differently than a billboard or a bumper sticker does. Those differences in form help shape not only what is said but also how it is said.

The top three steps encourage your teen to analyze information in the media message. In other words, they can make comparisons, link cause and effect, distinguish fact from opinion, and investigate bias and slant. In doing so, your teen may begin to understand how messages are constructed to shape meaning and how the construction process itself is shaped by assumptions about culture, gender, race, social class, and age.

Finally, when your teen has reached the top of the ladder, encourage them to evaluate the media message. That is, ask them to draw conclusions and form opinions about the media message. Is the message accurate and complete, or is important information missing from the message? You and your teen can climb the ladder together to discuss the latest movie, breaking headline, a favorite music video, hit song, or advertising campaign.

Identify, Analyze, Evaluate

5. Reality: Media messages represent (someone's) social reality. What is the message maker's point of view?

4. Interpretation: People interpret media messages differently. How does the message make you feel?

3. Construction: Each media message is a construction. What words, images, or sounds are used to create the message?

2. Purpose: Each media message has a purpose. Who created the message and why?

1. Form: Media messages come in different forms. Through what medium is the message delivered?

Chapter 11

How Alcohol Affects Development

Chapter Contents

Section 11.1

Developmental Perspective on Underage Alcohol Use

Text in this section is excerpted from "Developmental Perspective on Underage Alcohol Use," *Alcohol Alert Number 78*, National Institute on Alcohol Abuse and Alcoholism (NIAAA), July 2009.

Dramatic developmental changes unfold as individuals mature from birth to childhood, from childhood to adolescence, and from adolescence to early adulthood. These include physiological changes such as physical growth, brain development, and puberty; as well as psychological and social changes such as an evolving sense of self, forming more mature relationships with friends, and transitioning from middle school to high school.

Developmental changes factor into underage drinking. For example, as a high school student transitions to college, he or she may experience greater freedom and autonomy, creating more opportunities to use alcohol. Underage drinking also can influence development, potentially affecting the course of a person's life. For example, alcohol use can interfere with school performance and/or negatively affect peer relationships.

Key Stages in Human Development

As children mature, they achieve key developmental milestones such as changing the way they relate to parents and peers, beginning school and moving through different grades and school settings, undergoing puberty, gaining greater independence, and taking on more responsibilities. These milestones may come earlier for some individuals than others, depending on how quickly they mature, but tend to correspond, in general, to certain ages and developmental stages:

- Prenatal: Prior to birth

- Ages 0–10: Childhood

- Ages 10–15: Early to mid-adolescence

108

- Ages 16–20: Late adolescence

- Ages 21–25: Transition to early adulthood

Each stage in development carries risks for alcohol use and its consequences. Studies show that alcohol use typically begins in early adolescence (ages 12–14) and that between ages 12 and 21, rates of alcohol use and binge drinking increase sharply before leveling off in the twenties.

How Developmental Factors Influence Drinking and Risk for Drinking

Researchers are investigating the complex relationship between developmental factors and alcohol use to better understand how the risks for drinking and alcohol-related problems emerge across development.

Personality and behavior: Aspects of personality/temperament and certain behaviors that are evident early in life—often before children enter elementary school—such as antisocial behavior, poor self-regulation, poor self-control, anxiety, a tendency toward depression, and shyness may predict initiation of alcohol use in early adolescence, as well as future heavy use and alcohol use disorders (AUDs). Individuals with the most persistent personality and behavior problems are those most likely to experience more chronic and severe forms of AUDs in adulthood.

Family dynamics: Family dynamics also factor into a child's risk for underage drinking. When parents respond well to their child's needs, that child is better able to regulate his or her emotions and behavior. The most effective family environments are characterized by greater warmth, moderate discipline, and limited stress. Conversely, parents who are depressed, antisocial, or aggressive toward their children or who create a family atmosphere marked by conflict may hinder their child's ability to regulate and control his or her own behavior. Problems with behavioral control, in turn, increase the risk for involvement with alcohol and other drugs (AODs). Early exposure to AOD use by parents and siblings also increases the risk for underage alcohol use.

Peer relationships and culture: As they mature, adolescents place increased importance on peer relationships. Peers who drink may encourage experimentation with alcohol use. This experimentation can have potentially dangerous consequences. Yet, as researchers note, the increased risk-taking and experimentation that is characteristic of adolescence marks an important developmental progression, as individuals begin to form their own identities and to develop strong bonds with peers.

Gene and environment interaction: Research suggests that the interaction of inherited and environmental factors strongly influences drinking behavior and that their relative influence varies across adolescence. For example, the initiation of alcohol use is tied more to environmental than to genetic influences. In contrast, across middle to late adolescence, the relative influence of genetic factors on underage drinking increases, although there are important individual differences. Some of the genetic factors that influence problem drinking are specific to alcohol, whereas others influence a range of behaviors that reflect a general lack of impulse control in late adolescence and early adulthood.

Adolescent brain development and gaps in maturity: All regions of the brain do not mature at the same time or at the same pace. For example, a region deep within the brain that governs emotions and mediates fear and anxiety (the limbic system) matures in early adolescence. Its development is believed to be triggered by the hormones that set puberty in motion. In contrast, the frontal cortex—the region responsible for self-regulation, decision-making, and behavioral control—develops more gradually, as a result of age and experience. This creates a period of time during adolescence in which emotions are heightened, but the ability to regulate these emotions and regulate one's behavior still is developing. Some researchers believe this differential maturation of brain regions may contribute to the increased risk-taking behavior common during adolescence.

Differences in sensitivity to alcohol: Research with animals suggests that compared with adults, adolescents are less sensitive to the negative effects of alcohol intoxication—such as sedation, hangover, and loss of coordination—but are more sensitive to the way alcohol eases social situations. Because human adolescents may be less sensitive than adults to certain aversive effects of alcohol, they may be at higher risk for consuming more drinks per drinking occasion. This developmental phenomenon may help explain why adolescents are able to drink larger amounts of alcohol (as in binge drinking) without experiencing the same levels of physiological effects (such as sleepiness and poor coordination) as adults.

Section 11.2

Alcohol Use and Adolescent Development

Text in this section is excerpted from "The Surgeon General's Call to Action to Prevent and Reduce Underage Drinking: Section 2," U.S. Department of Health and Human Services (HHS), 2007. The complete report with references is available at http://www.surgeongeneral.gov/topics/underage drinking/calltoaction.pdf.

Adolescence, the period between the onset of puberty and the assumption of adult roles, is a time of particular vulnerability to alcohol use and its consequences for a variety of developmental reasons, some specific to the individual and others related to the biological and behavioral changes produced by adolescence itself. It also is a time when the developing brain may be particularly susceptible to long-term negative effects from alcohol use. New research indicates that the brain continues to develop into the twenties, creating a significant and extended period during its development of potential exposure to alcohol's harmful effects, particularly because so many youth drink alcohol, so many start drinking relatively early, and so many binge drink. For the purpose of this document, puberty is defined as a sequence of events by which a child becomes a young adult characterized by secretions of hormones, development of secondary sexual characteristics, reproductive functions, and growth spurts.

Because adolescents are involved in multiple systems, all of which may affect their decision to use alcohol, each system plays a part in that decision. For example, a stable family environment contributes to positive outcomes, as does a supportive community. To properly protect adolescents from alcohol use, parents and other adults must engage in multiple social systems as individuals, citizens, and voters. By understanding the role these systems play in the teen's life and by acting strategically on the basis of established and emerging research, the Nation can reduce the risk and consequences of underage alcohol use.

A Developmental Framework

Underage alcohol use is best addressed and understood within a developmental framework, because this behavior is directly related

111

to the processes that occur during adolescence. Advances in the fields of epidemiology, developmental psychopathology, human brain development, and behavioral genetics have provided new insights into adolescent development and its relationship to underage alcohol use. Research indicates that adolescent alcohol consumption is a complex behavior influenced by the following:

- Normal maturational changes that all adolescents experience (biological and cognitive changes, such as sexual development and differential maturation of specific regions of the brain, and psychological and social changes, such as increased independence and risk taking)

- Multiple social and cultural contexts (the social systems) in which adolescents live (family, peers, and school)

- Genetic, psychological, and social factors specific to each adolescent

- Environmental factors that influence the availability and appeal of alcohol

The Developing Adolescent Brain

Age, experience, and overall physical maturation, including puberty, are among the multiple factors influencing brain development. In adolescence, brain development is characterized by dramatic changes to the brain's structure, neuron connectivity (wiring), and physiology. For example, during late childhood and early adolescence the number of neural connections increases. By contrast, in later adolescence the number of connections is reduced through selective pruning at the same time that myelination of neurons is increasing, thereby enhancing the efficiency of the brain. These changes in the brain affect everything from emerging sexuality to emotionality and judgment. Because not all parts of the adolescent brain mature at the same time, the adolescent may be at a disadvantage in certain situations. For example, the limbic areas of the brain, which are thought to regulate emotions and are associated with an adolescent's lowered sensitivity to risk and propensity for novelty and sensation seeking, mature earlier than the frontal lobes, which are thought to be responsible for self-regulation, judgment, reasoning, problem-solving, and impulse control. This difference in maturational timing across the brain can result in impulsive decisions or actions, a disregard for consequences, and emotional reactions that can put teenagers at serious risk in ways that may surprise even the

112

adolescents themselves. There is, however, tremendous individual variability among adolescents, the pathways they follow, and the outcomes they experience.

Adolescent Decision-Making around Alcohol

Despite a body of literature suggesting that adolescents have not yet reached full cognitive maturity, they generally do as well as adults when called upon to make reasoned decisions using abstract processes in emotionally neutral situations. Differences in decision-making between adults and adolescents are most evident in situations with heightened social or emotional overtones. Such contexts may intensify the innate drive adolescents experience for novelty and sensation seeking. As a result, they may be more likely to make decisions that place themselves at greater risk when peers are present and/or in emotionally charged settings. Given that certain situations can override an adolescent's good intentions and sound decision-making capacity, it is important to structure the social system surrounding youth to minimize negative outcomes. Relevant to underage drinking, studies show that adolescents who spend more time with peers who consume alcohol are more likely to drink.

Stress, Puberty, and Significant Adolescent Transitions

The physical effects of puberty create dramatic changes in the sexual and social experience of maturing adolescents that require significant psychological and social adaptation. Together with hormonally induced mood and behavior changes, these sexual and social maturation stressors may contribute to increased consumption of alcohol during the adolescent period. Transitions lead to increased responsibilities and academic expectations, which are also potential sources of stress. This is important because research shows a link between stress and alcohol consumption. Significant contextual transitions and achievement of milestones for adolescents often occur at specific ages, not at specific developmental periods. As a result, some adolescents may be developmentally out of step with the majority of their peers or with the demands of their social environment, particularly in the case of early- and late-maturing adolescents. A mismatch between social pressures and the cognitive and emotional abilities of an adolescent may increase vulnerability to involvement with alcohol. During significant transitions, adolescents can benefit from extra support to avoid alcohol use.

The Effects of Alcohol on Physiological Processes and Biological Development

A question of primary concern is whether adolescent alcohol consumption can disrupt physiological processes and biological development to produce long-term negative consequences. Recent research shows that adolescent alcohol use has the potential to trigger long-term biological changes that may alter an adolescent's development as well as affect the adolescent's immediate behavior. The resulting adverse outcomes may include mental disorders such as anxiety and depressive disorders. Furthermore, early alcohol use may have detrimental effects on the developing brain, including neuro-cognitive impairment.

Moreover, human studies indicate that long-term, heavy alcohol use continued throughout one's lifetime can result in more severe effects on the brain's structure and functioning. Although there have been only a few studies, there is some indication that adolescents who drink heavily may experience adverse effects that disrupt normal growth and affect liver, bone, and endocrine development.

Chapter 12

Factors That Place Teens at Risk for Alcohol-Related Problems

Chapter Contents

Section 12.1

Adolescents at Risk for Substance Use Disorders

Excerpted from "Adolescents at Risk for Substance Use Disorders," National Institute on Alcohol Abuse and Alcoholism (NIAAA), 2008. The complete document with references is available at http://pubs.niaaa.nih.gov/publications/arh312/168-176.htm.

Adolescence is the developmental period of highest risk for the onset of problematic alcohol and other drug (AOD) use. Some experimentation with alcohol may be considered normal during adolescence; however, people who engage in binge drinking or who have developed alcohol use disorders typically also engage in other drug use, most frequently cigarettes and marijuana. AOD use behaviors are multifaceted and complex and are influenced by a multiplicity of genetic and environmental liabilities.

Risk factors for adolescent AOD use and substance use disorders (SUDs) can be divided into heritable, environmental, and phenotypic factors. Heritable risk factors are reflected in familial patterns of SUDs and other psychiatric disorders. Environmental risk factors include family-related characteristics, such as family functioning, parenting practices, and child maltreatment, as well as other contextual factors, such as peer influences, substance availability, and consumption opportunities. These heritable and environmental factors then interact to determine a person's observable characteristics and behaviors (phenotypes), such as AOD use.

Heritable risks: Historically, a person's genetic risk for developing a certain disorder has been estimated by establishing a family history of the disorder, and this approach remains important for research on SUDs. Presence of an SUD in a parent has consistently been shown to be a strong risk factor for adolescent AOD use and SUDs. However, the transmission of SUDs from parent to offspring occurs through both genetic and environmental influences.

In general, children of alcoholic parents (COAs) have been studied more extensively than children of parents with other addictive disorders.

The existing studies identified both common and distinct features between COAs and children of parents with other SUDs. For example, compared with children whose parents have no SUDs, COAs exhibit increased rates of alcohol use disorders. Similarly, children of parents with SUDs involving cocaine, heroin, or other illicit drugs tend to start using tobacco earlier than reference children and to have increased rates of illicit drug use and SUD symptoms.

Psychological dysregulation: Psychological dysregulation is defined as deficiency in three domains—cognitive, behavioral, and emotional—when adapting to environmental challenges. These three domains of dysregulation are statistically related to one overall dimension, conceptualized as psychological dysregulation. Variations in psychological dysregulation at specific developmental stages may be important for understanding adolescent SUDs. For example, an increasing number of studies indicate that childhood psychological dysregulation predicts adolescent SUDs. Furthermore, childhood psychological dysregulation significantly discriminates boys with and without parental SUDs.

As described by Tarter and colleagues, psychological dysregulation can be thought of as a single construct that comprises distinct but related components—executive cognitive dysfunction, behavioral impulsivity, and emotional lability. However, it also is important to note that alternative conceptualizations of these dimensions and their relationship to childhood and adolescent disorders exist.

The view that psychological dysregulation is one construct comprising several components also is consistent in several important ways with another concept—the externalizing spectrum—which was proposed by Krueger and colleagues. Using data from studies of twins as well as mother reports, these investigators found evidence for a hierarchical model linking SUDs, conduct disorder (CD), and antisocial personality disorder. In a factor analysis, these disorders all were related to one general factor, which the investigators labeled an externalizing factor. In addition to this general factor, the model also posits that distinct etiological characteristics pertaining to each disorder are involved.

However, psychological dysregulation in different manifestations can be observed at all developmental stages, including CD and attention deficit hyperactivity disorder (ADHD) during childhood, SUDs during adolescence, and borderline personality disorder or antisocial personality disorder during adulthood.

CD during childhood is one of the most important predictors of adolescent SUDs. Among a sample of about 500 boys, 250 of whom demonstrated antisocial behavior, White and colleagues investigated associations among early psychopathology and trajectories of AOD use during adolescence. The investigators found that higher levels of several disorders—including CD, oppositional defiant disorder (ODD), ADHD, and depression—predicted higher levels of alcohol use, although only CD predicted increased alcohol use over time.

The cognitive dimension of psychological dysregulation, also known as executive cognitive dysfunction, is particularly relevant for understanding SUDs. For example, in a study of 66 high-risk adolescents, Tapert and colleagues (2002) demonstrated that a high level of executive cognitive dysfunction predicted AOD use and SUDs eight years later, even when controlling for other factors, such as level of baseline AOD use, family history of SUDs, and CD in the child. Executive cognitive function might be one of the primary components underlying the relationship between psychological dysregulation and AOD involvement.

In summary, the construct of psychological dysregulation strongly predicts AOD use initiation, acceleration, and related problems during adolescence. Various brain structures, such as the prefrontal cortex in the outer layer of the brain and subcortical regions located deeper within the brain, may be involved in the development of psychological dysregulation.

Brain structures related to psychological dysregulation as endophenotypes: Chambers and colleagues (2003) have described adolescence as the critical period of addiction vulnerability, because during this period the brain pathways (neural circuits) that enable people to experience motivation and rewarding experiences still are developing. Moreover, the adolescent and adult brains appear to differ with respect to the brain regions that primarily respond to novel stimuli. It appears that the adolescent brain responds to novel stimuli largely through a brain structure known as amygdala. This is part of the brain's limbic system, which, among other functions, is involved in controlling emotions. In contrast, the adult brain increasingly uses higher cognitive functions (executive functions) mediated by the frontal cortex to interpret novel stimuli. Variations in how these neural pathways develop may contribute to the risk for AOD drug use during adolescence. Specifically, researchers have suggested that psychological dysregulation may be related to the function of the prefrontal cortex.

Environmental influences on risk of adolescent SUD: Several environmental influences have been identified that affect the risk of accelerated AOD involvement and the development of adolescent SUDs. Major environmental influences include child maltreatment and other traumatic events; parental influences, such as parenting practices; and peer influences. Some of these also lead to manifestations of psychological dysregulation, such as CD, ADHD, and major depressive disorder.

Parenting practices: Low levels of parental monitoring are a significant predictor of adolescent SUDs across all age, gender, and ethnic groups. The association of parental monitoring and both alcohol and marijuana use also has been demonstrated in a sample of low-income teens in a health clinic setting. Moreover, this relationship is found regardless of whether parental monitoring is assessed based on adolescents' perceptions or on adult reports of monitoring. Clark and colleagues found that among community adolescents who had never had an SUD, those who reported low levels of parental supervision were more likely to subsequently develop an alcohol use disorder.

Peer influences: Peers are an important environmental factor in the development of adolescent SUDs, although peers seem to have a more modest role relative to parents. Longitudinal studies have demonstrated that peer AOD use predicts adolescent alcohol use and marijuana use. Moreover, affiliation with peers who generally engage in deviant behaviors predicted adolescent SUDs in a longitudinal study. A longitudinal study of more than 6,000 adolescents found that peer alcohol use at the beginning of the study was significantly related to increases in adolescent alcohol use over time; moreover, the reverse also was true in that adolescent alcohol use at the beginning of the study also was related to increases in peer alcohol use. This study suggests that both directions of influence likely contribute to the association of adolescent and peer AOD use.

Aggregation of risk factors: Risk studies typically have assessed the impact of one or more variables on risk in a large group of people, often at only one point in time. Conversely, longitudinal studies that follow individual people over time have typically focused on single risk factors, such as parental AUDs. Relatively few studies, however, have examined multiple risk factors over time in a way that is directly applicable to specific individuals.

A few informative studies have demonstrated how multiple factors from different domains combine to determine an individual's risk for accelerated AOD use and SUDs. For example, Clark and colleagues used an approach called cluster analysis to divide 560 children into five risk groups. For this analysis, the investigators used the variables of parental SUDs early use of alcohol or tobacco; and psychological dysregulation integrated across affective, behavioral, and cognitive domains. The children in the highest risk group (having two parents with an SUD, early use of one or two substances, and the highest levels of psychological dysregulation) demonstrated significantly earlier use of and associated problems with tobacco, alcohol, marijuana, and cocaine. These results demonstrate that it may be necessary to combine multiple risk characteristics to comprehensively identify the children and adolescents at greatest risk of accelerated AOD use.

Section 12.2

Paternal Alcohol Use Increases Substance Use among Adolescents

This section is excerpted from "Fathers' Alcohol Use and Substance Use among Adolescents," Substance Abuse and Mental Health Services Administration (SAMHSA), June 18, 2009.

Alcohol dependence or abuse—and even moderate alcohol use—among fathers living with adolescents (youths aged 12 to 17) may increase the risk of substance use among those children. Increasing public awareness of the association between paternal alcohol use and adolescent substance use may help to focus attention on providing treatment for affected fathers and support for their children to prevent or reduce adolescent substance use.

This section examines rates of adolescent substance use and substance use disorders (dependence on or abuse of alcohol or illicit drugs) by level of alcohol use in the past year among fathers (for example: no alcohol use, alcohol use but no alcohol use disorder, and alcohol use disorder). It focuses on biological, step-, adoptive, and foster children aged 12 to 17 who were living with their fathers at the time of the survey interview. All findings are based on annual averages from combined 2002 to 2007 National Survey on Drug Use and Health (NSDUH) data.

Fathers' Alcohol Use

Almost one in twelve (7.9%) fathers living with adolescents aged 12 to 17 had an alcohol use disorder, while 68.1% used alcohol in the past year but did not have an alcohol use disorder; 24.1% did not use alcohol in the past year. Nearly one-third (31.2%) of fathers living with adolescents indicated binge alcohol use in the past month.

Adolescent Alcohol Use and Alcohol Use Disorder

The rate of past year alcohol use among adolescents was lower for those who lived with a father who did not use alcohol in the past year than for those who lived with a father who used alcohol but did not have an alcohol use disorder and for those who lived with a father with an alcohol use disorder (21.1% versus 33.2% and 38.8%, respectively). Adolescents' past year alcohol use rates did not differ significantly between those who lived with fathers who had an alcohol use disorder and those who lived with fathers who used alcohol but who did not have an alcohol use disorder.

The rates of past month binge alcohol use and past year alcohol use disorder among adolescents increased with the level of paternal alcohol use. For example, the rate of alcohol use disorder among adolescents who lived with a father who did not use alcohol in the past year was lower than the rate among those who lived with a father who used alcohol in the past year but did not have an alcohol use disorder (3.0% versus 4.7%), which in turn was lower than the rate among those who lived with a father with an alcohol use disorder (10.3%).

Adolescent Illicit Drug Use and Drug Use Disorder

Paternal alcohol use also was related to adolescent illicit drug use. The percentage of adolescents using illicit drugs in the past year increased with the level of paternal alcohol use, with illicit drug use reported by 14.0% of adolescents who lived with a father who did not use alcohol in the past year, 18.4% of those who lived with a father who used alcohol but did not have an alcohol use disorder, and 24.2% of those who lived with a father with an alcohol use disorder. The rate of past year illicit drug use disorder among adolescents was 2.6% among those who lived with a father who did not use alcohol in the past year, 3.9% among those who lived with a father who used alcohol but did not have an alcohol use disorder, and 4.2% among those who lived with a father with an alcohol use disorder.

Section 12.3

Alcohol, Energy Drinks, and Youth: A Dangerous Mix

Excerpted from "Alcohol, Energy Drinks, and Youth: A Dangerous Mix," © 2007 The Marin Institute (www.marininstitute.org). Reprinted with permission.

Energy Drinks: Rapidly Expanding Market

The story of alcoholic energy drinks begins with the introduction and rapidly developing popularity of nonalcoholic energy drinks in the marketplace. High-caffeine soft drinks have existed in the United States since at least the 1980s beginning with Jolt Cola. Energy drinks, which have caffeine as their primary energy component, began being marketed as a separate beverage category in the United States in 1997 with the introduction of the Austrian import Red Bull. Energy drink consumption and sales have exploded since then, with more than $3.2 billion in sales in 2006, a 516% inflation-adjusted increase since 2001.

This explosion has encouraged a proliferation of new brands: as many as 500 new energy drink products were introduced worldwide in 2006. Yet the market in the United States is dominated by five producers, which account for 93.8% of sales. Although Red Bull's share has been slipping, it still is by far the largest manufacturer, with 42.7% of the market, followed by Hansen Natural Corporation (Monster brands–16%), PepsiCo (SoBe and Amp brands–13.2%), Rockstar International (12.1%), and Coca-Cola (Full Throttle and Tab brands–9.8%). Mintel International Group, a leading marketing research firm, anticipates continued, although less dramatic, growth of 84% in sales by 2011. It also predicts rapid consolidation of the industry. This market growth has largely come at the expense of soft drinks, and soft drink manufacturers such as Coca-Cola and Pepsi have responded by aggressively entering the market, developing new hybrid soda/energy drinks, shifting marketing strategies, and distributing and then buying up new brands.

Negative Health Impacts of Caffeine and Energy Drinks

Although there is debate regarding the benefits of energy drink and caffeine consumption, there is consensus among health researchers that caffeine consumption can have adverse health consequences, particularly at high doses. Among the most common negative effects are increased anxiety, panic attacks, increased blood pressure, increased gastric acid, bowel irritability, and insomnia. According to an article published by the American Society of Addiction Medicine, caffeine is considered an addictive drug under standard drug diagnosis criteria, and doses of 500 milligrams (mg) or more (four to eight servings of most energy drink brands) can result in caffeine intoxication. Dependent users report an inability to quit or to cut down their consumption, despite having medical or psychological problems made worse by caffeine, and they report continued use of caffeine to avoid experiencing caffeine withdrawal symptoms. Contrary to popular belief and industry marketing claims, caffeine does not enhance sports performance and can have a negative impact at high doses because of its diuretic effects.

With the rising popularity of energy drinks and with more young people ingesting high levels of caffeine, more serious health problems are now being reported in the nation's poison centers. One three-year study by a Chicago poison center found more than 250 cases of caffeine overdose, with 12% of those requiring hospitalization. Nearly two-thirds of the hospitalizations involved the intensive care unit. Symptoms included insomnia, palpitations, tremors, sweating, nausea, vomiting, diarrhea, chest pains, and neurological symptoms. The average age of patients was 21.

Another poison center study focused on Redline, a high potency nonalcoholic energy drink containing 250 mg of caffeine per serving. Nine cases requiring hospitalization related to this specific drink were reported in the California Poison Control System Database in a two-year period, with severe symptoms involved.

A nonalcoholic energy drink called Spike Shooter, containing 300 mg of caffeine per serving, caused an uproar in Colorado Springs. In just one week, 18 high school students there reported becoming sick after drinking this product. The principal of the high school became so alarmed that she banned the drink on campus and convinced the nearby convenience store to stop selling it.

The product's label warns that those under 18 and anyone with health concerns should not use it. According to the news account:

Despite the warning, 14-year-old Rachel Woodrow, a diabetic, drank one can and started shaking. Two days later, she was hospitalized for a seizure. Rachel's parents say doctors told them the drink increased her metabolism and may have triggered the seizure. Rachel admits she didn't read the label. Rachel says, "I thought it would make me feel hyper and everything, but I didn't think I would have a seizure." Another student wanted to "get a little hype" by drinking "spike shooter." Instead, Chris Weir says, "My stomach started to cramp up. I had a headache and I started vomiting."

Systematic studies assessing the impact of caffeine overdose do not yet exist, although anecdotal reports from other countries suggest potentially serious consequences. In 2000, an 18-year-old Irish student died after sharing four cans of Red Bull with friends and then playing basketball. In 2001, Swedish officials investigated the deaths of three young people who had been drinking Red Bull; two of them had mixed the product with alcohol. Ultimately, no clear connections in the deaths were made and the Swedish government simply recommended that energy drinks not be used to quench thirst or be combined with alcohol. Other countries have followed Sweden's lead and put restrictions on the availability of energy drinks. Norway has limited sales to drug stores, and France and Denmark have banned the drinks altogether.

In summary, although research is limited, we can conclude that people who consume caffeine experience similar (although less severe) effects on the body—addiction, withdrawal, and tolerance—as do consumers of other psychoactive drugs. Potentially serious health consequences occur when the drugs are consumed in high doses, and these occurrences are being reported more frequently by health providers as high-potency energy drinks become more available in the market. Yet, despite these health concerns, the primary focus of most research literature on caffeine and energy drinks is on whether the beverages enhance performance, with recent research questioning the industry's marketing claims. Largely ignored are the health implications of sustained consumption of high levels of caffeine, particularly among youth, and the impact of combining energy drinks with alcohol.

Research on the Health Effects of Other Energy Drink Additives

Energy drink manufacturers also make marketing claims (or rely on the claims of others) that ingredients besides caffeine (for example: taurine, gingko, ginseng, and guarana) enhance energy drinks' positive effects, including improved mental alertness and physical performance. According to Mintel, one in three surveyed said they drink nonalcoholic energy drinks for ingredients other than caffeine, noting that "most of these ingredients consist of herbs such as guarana and taurine, which create a mysterious aura that intrigues some energy drink users."

These marketing claims are not supported in the research literature. For example, taurine supplements may have modest beneficial health impacts in some carefully defined situations, depending on individual health conditions and dosage. Energy drinks are a poor vehicle for gaining these possible benefits because dosage levels (which are often not disclosed) vary widely across beverages, their possible impacts depend on individual characteristics of users, and safe upper dosage limits have not been established.

Similarly, gingko and ginseng are popular among many alternative health providers and advocates for their potential to improve long-term health. Research has not confirmed any long- or short-term health benefits of these supplements, and providing unspecified dosages of them in energy drinks is unlikely to have any immediate effect on mental or physical performance. Guarana is a powerful herbal stimulant that enhances the stimulating effects of caffeine. Research does not suggest any mental or physical effects beyond those attributable to caffeine.

In summary, despite manufacturers' claims, there is no scientific basis for concluding that the noncaffeine additives in energy drinks contribute to either long-term health benefits or short-term mental alertness and physical performance. They may create health risks, particularly since dosage levels are often not disclosed. As suggested by Mintel, these ingredients appear to be included mainly for marketing purposes.

Health Implications of Adding Alcohol to Energy Drinks

Energy drinks clearly have potential negative health consequences, and marketing claims regarding their benefits have limited support in the research literature. What health and safety implications exist for adding alcohol to the mix? Alcohol is a leading cause of death and injury, from driving under the influence of alcohol to violence, sexual assault, and suicide, and contributes to family and community disruption, poor school performance, and other psychological and sociological dysfunctions. These problems are particularly acute for young people. Does mixing alcohol with energy drinks create more risks than alcohol alone?

While the health research literature here is limited, the studies that do exist suggest cause for concern. At least four studies on humans have examined the interaction of some energy drink additives with alcohol. In one study, researchers gave 15 subjects either doses of caffeine and alcohol or alcohol alone and then tested them on a variety of performance measures. Subjects who ingested caffeine reported reduced depressant effects of alcohol, but showed only limited improvement in motor skills over the other subjects.

The remaining three studies, using similar designs, found no such improvements. The second found that energy drinks did not reduce alcohol's deleterious impact on heart rate, oxygen uptake, and other physiological variables during strenuous exercise. The third found that while energy drinks did reduce some subjects' perception of alcohol intoxication, motor coordination, and visual reaction tests, they had no impact on alcohol's negative effects. The subjects' performance was significantly worse after ingesting the alcohol–energy drink mix despite the volunteers' perception of increased alertness and reduced intoxication.

The fourth study also concluded that caffeine does not counteract alcohol's effect, but went a step further, assessing the importance of consumers' expectancies. Those who were not aware of the caffeine in the beverage compensated to some degree for alcohol's intoxicating effects, while those who were aware of the presence of caffeine did not. In other words, the belief that caffeine will counteract the alcohol may undermine the capacity to compensate for one's intoxication.

These findings support a truism among alcoholism recovery and prevention specialists that drinking coffee does not in itself counteract intoxication but rather results in a "wide awake drunk." Public health and alcohol treatment experts generally advise against mixing energy drinks and alcohol, because, as suggested by research that is available, the combination may lead intoxicated persons to conclude mistakenly that they are capable of potentially dangerous activities, such as driving. These risks may be particularly acute for young people, who are inexperienced and more likely to engage in risk-taking behavior.

The available research focuses on short-term intoxicating effects. Alcohol is also associated with a wide array of negative long-term consequences, including alcoholism and alcohol abuse, liver damage, cancer, and birth defects. It can also adversely affect brain development among teenagers and young adults. Does routine consumption of high doses of caffeine exacerbate these problems? The research literature has thus far failed to investigate the potential physiological risks of combining caffeine and alcohol, a stimulant and a depressant, over time. Likewise, there is no literature on the triple combination of alcohol, caffeine, and sweeteners, all of which have the potential for leading to addiction.

Conclusion: Combining Alcohol and Caffeine Is Potentially Harmful

As the available research suggests, alcoholic energy drinks create a dangerous mix. Yet the alcohol industry markets the beverages with messages that fail to alert users to the potential for misjudging one's intoxication and, instead, suggest that the beverages will enhance alertness and energy. The industry promotes their use precisely in circumstances that may lead to alcohol-related harm: in social situations that may involve driving, as an enhancement to sexual encounters, and in late-night partying environments that may result in violence. At least one industry executive is aware of the misleading marketing messages. According to Mark Hall, sales executive for Hansen, discussing its alcoholic energy drink Hard E: "The effect is a heightened level of awareness. You will get intoxicated at the same rate as with any other alcoholic beverage. The difference is that you will seem more alert and more awake."

Chapter 13

Alcohol Use on College Campuses

Chapter Contents

Section 13.1

Drinking on Campus: Scope of the Problem

Excerpted from *Alcohol and Other Drugs on Campus: The Scope of the Problem*, by Daniel Ari Kapner (Washington, DC: U.S. Department of Education, Office of Safe and Drug-Free Schools, Higher Education Center for Alcohol and Other Drug Abuse and Violence Prevention, August 2008). For more information, please contact the Center at 800-676-1730 or visit the Center's website at www.higheredcenter.org.

The most widespread health problem on college and university campuses in the United States is high-risk alcohol and other drug (AOD) use. Recent reports confirm that the nation's campuses continue to encounter significant consequences as a result of this problem.

College student drinking is widespread. Studies suggest that between 1993 and 2001, approximately 44% of college students were heavy drinkers, defined for men as five or more drinks in a row on at least one occasion in the past two weeks, and for women as four or more drinks.

In addition, drinking behavior has become increasingly polarized since 1993, with more students abstaining but also more students frequently drinking heavily. The percentage of students who abstained from alcohol increased from 16% in 1993 to 22.8% in 2007, while the percentage of those engaged in frequent heavy drinking decreased from 19.7% in 1993 to 19% in 2006. At the same time, the percentage of non-heavy drinking students decreased from 39.7% in 1993 to 36.3% in 2001, while that of occasional heavy drinkers increased from 24.3% in 1993 to 45.5% in 2006. Campuses should take a look at how such a polarization in drinking behavior may affect their student population.

Additionally, students report getting drunk more frequently in 2001 than in 1993. In 1993, nearly a quarter of students said they became drunk more than three times during the past 30 days; this rate increased to 29.4% in 2001. The percentage of students who said they drank alcohol to get drunk climbed from 39.9% in 1993 to 48.2% in 2001.

Drinking rates vary considerably on different campuses. For instance, the 2000 College Alcohol Study (CAS) report suggests that campuses in the Northeast and the Midwest have higher rates of drinking than campuses elsewhere. In addition, drinking varies among different populations on campus. Men are more likely to drink heavily than are women. According to studies, fraternity members and athletes are more likely to drink heavily and to suffer negative consequences than are other groups on campus. According to a special analysis of 2005 data from the Core Institute, high-risk drinking is highest among American Indian students (52.6%), followed by White (50.2%), and Hispanic students (49.3%), with Black (23.3%) and Asian and Pacific Islander students (33.7%) reporting the lowest levels.

Consequences of Alcohol Use

The consequences that both drinking and nondrinking students suffer due to alcohol use are even more alarming. Compiling results from a number of studies, as a result of alcohol use, every year:

- 1,700 college students die from alcohol-related causes, and 1,300 of these deaths involve drinking and driving.

- 600,000 students suffer nonfatal injuries.

- Nearly 500,000 students have unprotected sex.

- More than 100,000 students are too intoxicated to know whether they consented to sexual intercourse.

- 1.2%–1.5% of students attempt suicide because of alcohol or other drug use.

- More than 150,000 students develop a health problem related to alcohol.

- 11% of students damage property.

- 2.8 million students drive while under the influence of alcohol.

Drinking on campus undermines the mission of higher education, with heavy drinking leading to a decline in academic performance. The National Institute on Alcohol Abuse and Alcoholism (NIAAA) reports that about 25% of college students report academic problems caused by alcohol use, such as earning lower grades, doing poorly on exams or papers, missing class, and falling behind. Several AOD prevention experts suggest that heavy drinking can have a negative effect on the institution as a whole, reducing retention rates, increasing expenses from incidents of vandalism, and branding the institution a party school. This party school image may encourage more alcohol-related problems, as it attracts students who choose to be in high-risk settings. For example, researchers have found fraternities to be a social setting that draws students who desire to be in heavy drinking environments.

Secondary effects of alcohol use: Students who abstain or are moderate drinkers frequently suffer from the behavior of other students who drink heavily. Even though the majority of college and university students are not heavy drinkers, with 65.5% abstaining from all alcohol use, more than three-quarters of the students living in residence halls, fraternities, or sororities report that they have experienced at least one secondary effect due to another student's drinking.

Following are prominent secondary effects reported by students who live on campus or in sorority or fraternity houses and who abstain or drink moderately:

- 60.0% had study or sleep interrupted.
- 47.6% had to take care of a drunken student.
- 29.2% had been insulted or humiliated.
- 19.5% of female respondents experienced an unwanted sexual advance.
- 19.0% had a serious argument or quarrel.
- 15.2% had property damaged.
- 8.7% had been pushed, hit, or assaulted.
- 1.0% of female respondents had been a victim of sexual assault or acquaintance rape.

Alcohol is also associated with riots, hazing, and various forms of nonsexual violence on campus. Student riots have become a serious problem for campuses, usually taking place following sporting events or after new campus alcohol policies are created. Riots pose challenges for campus administrators and law enforcement officers and can lead to unexpected economic burdens. Numerous campus riots point to alcohol as a key contributing factor.

Community consequences of alcohol use: Communities neighboring campuses also experience the secondary effects of college student drinking. Studies show that those living within one mile of a campus are much more likely to report alcohol-related noise and disturbances, vandalism, public drunkenness, and vomit and public urination by students on their property than are people living more than one mile from a campus.

Neighborhoods closer to campus have a much higher density of alcohol outlets than neighborhoods farther from campus. Fully 92.1% of neighborhood residents within one mile of campus and 74.9% of those more than one mile from campus report the presence of a nearby alcohol outlet. These outlets are especially abundant near campuses that have higher levels of heavy drinking. A reduction in the number of alcohol outlets near campuses may significantly lower the secondary effects experienced by individuals residing in those areas.

Section 13.2

Campus Safety Issue: Violence and Alcohol Use

Excerpted from *Interpersonal Violence and Alcohol and Other Drug Use,* (Washington, DC: U.S. Department of Education, Office of Safe and Drug-Free Schools, Higher Education Center for Alcohol and Other Drug Abuse and Violence Prevention, August 2008). For more information, please contact the Center at 800-676-1730 or visit the Center's website at www.higheredcenter.org.

Interpersonal Violence and Alcohol and Other Drug Use

Under increasing pressure from parents, students, and lawmakers to ensure the safety of campus communities, colleges and universities have improved security measures in residence halls and other buildings and have made an effort to raise awareness of the ways in which people can protect themselves against crime.

To spur these crime prevention efforts, the federal *Student Right-to-Know and Campus Security Act* mandates that colleges and universities publish reports of crime statistics so that campus community members, prospective students, and their parents can become better informed of crime rates at different institutions.

Campus crime statistics from more than 6,000 institutions of higher education indicate that in 2003 there were more than 155,000 liquor law violations, more than 26,000 drug arrests, approximately 3,000 aggravated assaults, more than 2,500 forcible sex offenses, and ten murders on these campuses. Experts agree, however, that these figures, which are based on reported crimes, underestimate actual crimes on America's campuses. In fact, the *National College Women Sexual Victimization* (NCWSV) study, a 1996 survey of 4,446 women sponsored by the U.S. Department of Justice, found that fewer than 5% of completed and attempted rapes were reported to law enforcement officials.

Contrary to common belief, most violence on campus cannot be attributed to outsiders intruding on an otherwise peaceful environment. In fact, some experts estimate that at least 70% of violent acts are perpetrated by students. The majority of college students fall within the age group (18–24) most likely to be the victims of nonfatal assault. This age group is also overrepresented among perpetrators of violence.

Experts suggest that efforts to prevent violence must be comprehensive, beginning with an assessment of those most affected by various types of interpersonal violence and the identification of risk factors in the campus environment that foster or perpetuate violence, such as alcohol use, fraternity hazing practices, and intolerance of individual differences. This much-needed assessment can be a difficult process, however, because the vast majority of violent acts go unreported. Often victims fear reprisal from their assailants or believe that university or law enforcement officials will not respond adequately.

Types of violence most affecting colleges and universities: Interpersonal violence can take many forms on campuses. Three of the most prevalent types are rape and sexual assault; nonsexual physical assault, including fights, muggings, hazing, and dating violence; and hate crimes.

Alcohol and Violence

The National Institute on Alcohol Abuse and Alcoholism (NIAAA) 2002 report on college drinking estimates that more than 70,000 students between the ages of 18 and 24 survive alcohol-related sexual assault or date rape each year. This same report estimates that more than 600,000 students are assaulted by drinking students on a yearly basis.

In their 1993 study of 530 undergraduate men, Koss and Gaines found alcohol to be one of the most significant contributors to sexual aggression among male college students. Students are more likely to become aggressive when their blood alcohol level rises rapidly (for example, following heavy drinking), lessening capacity for conflict resolution and decreasing inhibitions. In addition, many students use intoxication as an excuse for inappropriate and violent behavior. Several studies estimate that between 50% and 80% of violence on campus is alcohol-related. One study of residence halls found that 71% of violent acts directed toward resident advisers were alcohol-related. In a study of students who were victims of sexual aggression while in college, from intimidation and illegal restraint to rape, the women surveyed reported that 68% of their male assailants had been drinking at the time of the attack.

A national survey of more than 14,000 students found that 11% of students who do not drink heavily but live on campuses with high levels of drinking have been victims of assault. This rate is nearly double the number of victims of assault on campuses with lower levels of drinking. A study of college men in New England found that those who drink heavily are four times as likely as moderate drinkers to be involved in physical fights.

Section 13.3

Sexual Violence and Alcohol Use on Campus

Excerpted from *Sexual Violence and Alcohol and Other Drug Use on Campus*, (Washington, DC: U.S. Department of Education, Office of Safe and Drug-Free Schools, Higher Education Center for Alcohol and Other Drug Abuse and Violence Prevention, August 2008). For more information, please contact the Center at 800-676-1730 or visit the Center's website at www.higheredcenter.org.

The term sexual assault encompasses a continuum of behaviors from unwanted touching to rape. Definitions of rape and sexual assault vary, with each state having its own legal definitions. The *National College Women Sexual Victimization* (NCWSV) study, a 1997 telephone survey of 4,446 women sponsored by the U.S. Department of Justice, defined rape as follows:

Forced sexual intercourse including both psychological coercion as well as physical force. Forced sexual intercourse means vaginal, anal, or oral penetration by the offender(s). This category also includes incidents where the penetration is from a foreign object such as a bottle. Includes attempted rapes, female and male victims, and rape by individuals of the opposite sex and same sex. Attempted rape includes verbal threats of rape.

The NCWSV study found that 1.7% of college women had experienced a completed rape and 1.1% an attempted rape in the seven months prior to the study. Projecting these figures over an entire calendar year, the survey's authors concluded that nearly 5% of college women might be victimized annually and that up to 25% might be assaulted during their college years.

Sexual assault is defined more broadly than rape, as "the full range of forced sexual acts, including forced touching or kissing; verbally coerced intercourse; and vaginal, oral, or anal penetration." Because sexual assault encompasses many behaviors and is widely underreported, the actual number of sexual assaults on campus in a year is unknown, but the number is believed to be large.

Sexual assault does not affect victims only physically but also may leave lasting psychological and emotional scars. Moreover, assaults affect the entire campus, not just individual students. Sexual violence compromises the integrity of the safe, welcoming environment campuses are supposed to provide, impinging on the academic and social success of all students

Causes and Contributors

Sexual aggression is a complex behavior resulting from multiple causes. Many of those who are victims of sexual assault are made to feel that they were somehow responsible for the assault, either through their behavior or appearance or by somehow inviting an assault to occur. In fact, the only victim characteristic that predicts sexual assault is a previous assault. The victim-blaming mentality is unjustified and stands in the way of understanding the true antecedents and determinants of sexual assault.

Alcohol use: Alcohol is a frequently cited situational contributor to sexual violence. More than 97,000 students between the ages of 18 and 24 experience alcohol-related sexual assault or date rape each year in the United States. Researcher Antonia Abbey reports that, on average, at least 50% of sexual assaults among college students involve alcohol use, with exact estimates varying based on the study sample and methods. While alcohol and other drug use maybe present in violent incidents, it does not justify or excuse assault.

Alcohol use may increase the risk of sexual assault through several pathways. For example, drinkers may use alcohol as an excuse to engage in sexually aggressive behavior or as a coercive tactic to obtain sex. In addition, alcohol may result in increased misperceptions of the woman's sexual interest, decreased concern about her experience, or decreased ability to evaluate accurately whether consent has been obtained. Many men falsely believe that alcohol increases sexual arousal and legitimates nonconsensual sexual aggression. Perpetrators perceive drinking women as more sexually available, for example, believing that women who have two or more drinks are more interested than other women in having sex. Intoxication by the victim can decrease her ability to resist assault effectively. This is especially true if a victim becomes unconscious after drinking. Additionally, alcohol use sometimes fosters a double standard in which women are held more responsible, and men held less responsible, if an assault occurs.

Rape-facilitating drugs: In addition to alcohol, various other drugs are used to facilitate rape. These include marijuana, cocaine, gamma hydroxybutyrate (GHB), benzodiazepines (including Rohypnol), ketamine, barbiturates, chloral hydrate, methaqualone, heroin, morphine, lysergic acid diethylamide (LSD), and other hallucinogens. Sometimes referred to as date rape drugs, these substances may be taken knowingly or may be slipped surreptitiously into someone's drink or otherwise given to an unsuspecting person who is then assaulted. When combined with alcohol, as is frequently the case, these drugs can lead to blackout.

While alcohol is by far the most commonly used rape-facilitating drug, Rohypnol and GHB also are well known for their incapacitating effects. The effects of Rohypnol are felt within 30 minutes after use and may persist for many hours. Rohypnol is very dangerous when mixed with alcohol or other depressants. Possible adverse outcomes include difficulty breathing, coma, and even death.

Sexual harassment: As with rape and sexual assault, legal definitions of sexual harassment vary from state to state, as do campus policies addressing the problem. Sexual harassment, like sexual assault, can involve many types of behavior, including unwanted displays of sexually explicit material, suggestive looks or gestures, sexual teasing or comments, exposure, and deliberate touching or physical closeness.

One study of campus housing asked whether students had experienced unwanted looks and gestures, sexual teasing, or deliberate touching while in coed residence halls. About 50% of women residents answered yes for at least one of these three categories. In addition, nearly 40% had experienced unwanted social contact and 30% unwanted kissing or fondling. Men living in residence halls also suffered harassment. Almost half reported unwanted sexual teasing and more than 20% experienced unwanted deliberate touching.

Section 13.4

Academic Performance and Alcohol Use

Excerpted from *College Academic Performance and Alcohol and Other Drug Use*, (Washington, DC: U.S. Department of Education, Office of Safe and Drug-Free Schools, Higher Education Center for Alcohol and Other Drug Abuse and Violence Prevention, August 2008). For more information, please contact the Center at 800-676-1730 or visit the Center's website at www.higheredcenter.org.

Difficulty meeting academic responsibilities is one of the most common consequences of alcohol use. The National Institute on Alcohol Abuse and Alcoholism (NIAAA) Task Force on College Drinking reports that about 25% of college students report academic problems caused by alcohol use, such as earning lower grades, doing poorly on exams or papers, missing class, and falling behind.

According to a national study of more than 14,000 students, 21.6% of students who drank during the year prior to the study had fallen behind in their schoolwork and 29.5% had missed class because of their alcohol use.

In a national survey of 33,379 college students from 53 two- and four-year colleges located in the United States, 21.8% of students reported performing poorly on a test or assignment, and 30.7% said they had missed a class due to alcohol use in the previous 12 months.

A national survey of nearly 94,000 students from 197 colleges and universities conducted over three years found in the third year that students with an A average consume a little more than four drinks per week, B students have six drinks per week, C students average almost eight drinks per week, and students with Ds or Fs consume almost ten drinks per week. Other studies also found a direct relationship between drinking on campus and poor academic performance.

In addition to well-documented consequences such as poor performance on assignments and missed classes, studies suggest that college drinking is a major factor in student dropout rates.

Heavy drinking also has a negative effect on the image of an institution, branding it a party school. This image may encourage more alcohol-related problems, as it attracts students who choose to be in high-risk environments.

Given alcohol's detrimental effect on student performance, a decrease in drinking on campus should enhance the quality of higher education. Research suggests that the most effective way to change the culture of drinking is through environmental management, that is, by changing the physical, social, legal, and economic environment on and around campus that fosters alcohol use.

Section 13.5

What Policy-Makers Need to Know about College Drinking

Excerpted from "What Colleges Need to Know Now: An Update on College Drinking Research," National Institute on Alcohol Abuse and Alcoholism (NIAAA), November 2007. The complete report with references is available at http://www .collegedrinkingprevention.gov/1College_Bulletin-508_361C4E.pdf.

Alcohol-related problems on campus still exist, but there is encouraging news. Research shows that several initiatives aimed at reducing alcohol problems among college-age youth have been effective, leading to reductions in underage drinking, alcohol-related assaults, emergency department visits, and alcohol-related crashes.

A close collaboration between colleges and their surrounding communities is key. This includes environmental approaches (such as more vigorous enforcement of zero tolerance laws, other drinking and driving laws, and strategies to reduce the availability of alcohol) as well as approaches that target the individual drinker (such as wider implementation of alcohol screening, counseling, and treatment programs).

Individual approaches: According to several new studies, strategies that focus on preventing drinking and alcohol problems in individual students continue to have significant research support. However, these findings also offer some new insights. A number of new studies have examined measures to reduce drinking among mandated students—or students who have been identified as having a problem with alcohol and who have been mandated to receive intervention and/or treatment for their problems. One strategy for increasing

139

participation in these interventions is to make screening a routine event in university health centers and to use new technology, particularly the Internet, to reach larger percentages of students. The use of computer- or Web-delivered brief interventions is showing promise in a college setting.

Multi-component approach: Short of completely banning alcohol use on campus, research shows that the best prevention programs use multiple approaches. One such multi-component approach, the *A Matter of Degree* program (AMOD), was launched in 1997 at ten colleges in the United States. AMOD focused on reducing alcohol availability, raising prices, and limiting alcohol promotions and advertising on and around campus.

Sites where this program was implemented saw improvements in two measures—the percentage of students missing class as a result of alcohol use and the percentage of students driving after heavy alcohol use—compared with colleges that acted as control sites. When researchers assessed the interventions more closely, they found that those sites which instituted more interventions had greater success, reducing both alcohol-related problems, such as binge drinking, and the secondhand effects of drinking, such as alcohol-related assaults.

Social norms: The social norms approach is based on the view that many college students think campus attitudes are much more permissive toward drinking than they really are and believe other students drink much more than they actually do. The phenomenon of perceived social norms—or the belief that everyone is drinking and drinking is acceptable—is one of the strongest correlates of drinking among young adults and the subject of considerable research. By and large, the approach most often used on campuses to change students' perception of drinking focuses on the use of social norms campaigns. These campaigns attempt to communicate the true rate of student alcohol use on campus, with the assumption that as students' misperceptions about other students' alcohol use are corrected, their own levels of alcohol use will decrease. Just as environmental approaches work best when multiple interventions are used, social norms campaigns have demonstrated the most success when they are teamed with other prevention efforts.

Chapter 14

Family Guide to Underage Drinking Prevention

Chapter Contents

Section 14.1

Parental Involvement in Alcohol Use Prevention

Excerpted from "Parental Involvement in Preventing Youth Substance Use,"
Substance Abuse and Mental Health Services Administration (SAMHSA),
May 28, 2009. The complete document is available at http://www.oas.samhsa
.gov/2k9/159/ParentInvolvementHTML.pdf.

Preventing youth substance use requires a comprehensive approach
involving communities, schools, peers, and families. Research indicates
that parents are an influential factor in whether youths use alcohol, tobacco, and illicit drugs. Expression of disapproval of substance use and
engagement in their children's day-to-day activities are key tools parents
can use to help to protect their children against substance use. The National Survey on Drug Use and Health (NSDUH) can help to shed light
on youths' perceptions of parental disapproval of substance use as well
as parental involvement in the day-to-day activities of their children. All
findings presented in this report are based on 2007 NSDUH data.

Perceived parental disapproval of substance use: Most youths
aged 12 to 17 believed that their parents would strongly disapprove
of their using substances. In 2007, 89.6% thought their parents would
strongly disapprove of their having one or two drinks of an alcoholic
beverage nearly every day, and 92.1% thought their parents would
strongly disapprove of their smoking one or more packs of cigarettes
per day. Also, 93.3% thought their parents would strongly disapprove
of their using marijuana or hashish once a month or more.

Youths' perceptions that their parents would strongly disapprove of
their substance use varied by age and gender. Perceptions of parental
disapproval generally decreased with age. For example, 95.8% of youths
aged 12 or 13 thought their parents would strongly disapprove of their
smoking one or more packs of cigarettes per day compared with 93.4%
of those aged 14 or 15 and 87.4% of those aged 16 or 17. Females were
more likely than males to think that their parents would strongly
disapprove of their smoking one or more packs of cigarettes per day
(92.6% versus 91.6%) and of their drinking an alcoholic beverage nearly

every day (90.4% versus 88.8%). There was no difference by gender in perceptions of parental disapproval of using marijuana or hashish once a month or more.

Parental involvement: The majority of youths indicated that their parents were involved in their day-to-day activities. Over four-fifths (85.7%) said that their parents always or sometimes let them know they were proud of something they had done, and 86.2% said that their parents always or sometimes let them know when they had done a good job; 87.8% said that their parents always or sometimes made them do chores around the house. Fewer youths said their parents always or sometimes limited the amount of time they watched television (39.7%). Among youths enrolled in school in the past year, 80.9% said their parents always or sometimes provided help with homework, and 70.4% indicated that their parents always or sometimes limited their time out with friends on school nights.

Perceptions of parental involvement also varied by age and gender: Younger youths were generally more likely than their older counterparts to indicate parental involvement. For example, 90.7% of those aged 12 or 13 felt that their parents always or sometimes let them know they were proud of something they had done compared with 84.5% of those aged 14 or 15 and 82.2% of those aged 16 or 17. Males were more likely than females to think that their parents always or sometimes let them know they had done a good job (87.7% versus 84.6%) and to let them know they were proud of something they had done (87.2% versus 84.2%). Among those enrolled in school in the past year, males were more likely than females to report that their parents always or sometimes provided help with homework (82.6% versus 79.1%), but males were less likely than females to report that their parents always or sometimes limited their time out with friends on a school night (68.7% versus 72.1%).

Discussion: Families, peers, schools, and communities are all key components in substance use prevention among youths. Previous research shows that youths who perceive that their parents disapprove of substance use and who report that their parents are involved in their day-to-day activities are less likely than those who do not to use alcohol, tobacco, or illicit drugs. Parents need to understand that they are an integral and effective part of substance use prevention. Findings in this report suggest that most parents do clearly express their disapproval of youth substance use and are actively engaged in the day-to-day life of their children. However, these data also indicate that perceived disapproval of youth substance use and parental involvement are more prevalent for younger than for older youths.

Section 14.2

Talk to Your Child about Alcohol

Text in this section is excerpted from "Make a Difference: Talk to Your Child about Alcohol," National Institute on Alcohol Abuse and Alcoholism (NIAAA), March 2007.

For many parents, bringing up the subject of alcohol is no easy matter. Your young teen may try to dodge the discussion, and you yourself may feel unsure about how to proceed. To make the most of your conversation, take some time to think about the issues you want to discuss before you talk with your child. Consider too how your child might react and ways you might respond to your youngster's questions and feelings. Then choose a time to talk when both you and your child have some down time and are feeling relaxed.

You don't need to cover everything at once. In fact, you're likely to have a greater impact on your child's decisions about drinking by having a number of talks about alcohol use throughout his or her adolescence. Think of this talk with your child as the first part of an ongoing conversation. And remember to make it a conversation, not a lecture. You might begin by finding out what your child thinks about alcohol and drinking.

Your child's views about alcohol: Ask your young teen what he or she knows about alcohol and what he or she thinks about teen drinking. Ask your child why he or she thinks kids drink. Listen carefully without interrupting. Not only will this approach help your child to feel heard and respected, but it can serve as a natural lead-in to discussing alcohol topics.

Important facts about alcohol: Although many kids believe that they already know everything about alcohol, myths and misinformation abound. Here are some important facts to share:

- Alcohol is a powerful drug that slows down the body and mind. It impairs coordination; slows reaction time; and impairs vision, clear thinking, and judgment.

- Beer and wine are not safer than hard liquor. A 12-ounce can of beer, a 5-ounce glass of wine, and 1.5 ounces of hard liquor all

144

contain the same amount of alcohol and have the same effects on the body and mind.

- On average, it takes 2–3 hours for a single drink to leave a person's system. Nothing can speed up this process, including drinking coffee, taking a cold shower, or walking it off.

- People tend to be very bad at judging how seriously alcohol has affected them. That means many individuals who drive after drinking think they can control a car—but actually cannot.

- Anyone can develop a serious alcohol problem, including a teenager.

Good reasons not to drink: In talking with your child about reasons to avoid alcohol, stay away from scare tactics. Most young teens are aware that many people drink without problems, so it is important to discuss the consequences of alcohol use without overstating the case. Some good reasons why teens should not drink:

- **You want your child to avoid alcohol:** Clearly state your own expectations about your child's drinking. Your values and attitudes count with your child, even though he or she may not always show it.

- **To maintain self-respect:** Teens say the best way to persuade them to avoid alcohol is to appeal to their self-respect—let them know that they are too smart and have too much going for them to need the crutch of alcohol. Teens also are likely to pay attention to examples of how alcohol might lead to embarrassing situations or events—things that might damage their self-respect or alter important relationships.

- **Drinking is illegal:** Because alcohol use under the age of 21 is illegal, getting caught may mean trouble with the authorities. Even if getting caught doesn't lead to police action, the parents of your child's friends may no longer permit them to associate with your child.

- **Drinking can be dangerous:** One of the leading causes of teen deaths is motor vehicle crashes involving alcohol. Drinking also makes a young person more vulnerable to sexual assault and unprotected sex. And while your teen may believe he or she wouldn't engage in hazardous activities after drinking, point out that because alcohol impairs judgment, a drinker is very likely to think such activities won't be dangerous.

- **You have a family history of alcoholism:** If one or more members of your family has suffered from alcoholism, your child may be somewhat more vulnerable to developing a drinking problem.

- **Alcohol affects young people differently than adults:** Drinking while the brain is still maturing may lead to long-lasting intellectual effects and may even increase the likelihood of developing alcohol dependence later in life.

The "magic potion" myth: The media's glamorous portrayal of alcohol encourages many teens to believe that drinking will make them cool, popular, attractive, and happy. Research shows that teens who expect such positive effects are more likely to drink at early ages. However, you can help to combat these dangerous myths by watching television shows and movies with your child and discussing how alcohol is portrayed in them. For example, television advertisements for beer often show young people having an uproariously good time, as though drinking always puts people in a terrific mood. Watching such a commercial with your child can be an opportunity to discuss the many ways that alcohol can affect people—in some cases bringing on feelings of sadness or anger rather than carefree high spirits.

How to handle peer pressure: It's not enough to tell your young teen that he or she should avoid alcohol—you also need to help your child figure out how. What can your daughter say when she goes to a party and a friend offers her a beer? Or what should your son do if he finds himself in a home where kids are passing around a bottle of wine and parents are nowhere in sight? What should their response be if they are offered a ride home with an older friend who has been drinking?

Brainstorm with your teen for ways that he or she might handle these and other difficult situations, and make clear how you are willing to support your child. An example: "If you find yourself at a home where kids are drinking, call me and I'll pick you up—and there will be no scolding or punishment." The more prepared your child is, the better able he or she will be to handle high-pressure situations that involve drinking.

Mom, Dad, did you drink when you were a kid?

This is the question many parents dread—yet it is highly likely to come up in any family discussion of alcohol. The reality is that many parents did drink before they were old enough to legally do so. So how can one be honest with a child without sounding like a hypocrite who advises, "Do as I say, not as I did"?

This is a judgment call. If you believe that your drinking or drug use history should not be part of the discussion, you can simply tell your child that you choose not to share it. Another approach is to admit that you did do some drinking as a teenager, but that it was a mistake—and give your teen an example of an embarrassing or painful moment that occurred because of your drinking. This approach may help your child better understand that youthful alcohol use does have negative consequences.

How to host a teen party:

- Agree on a guest list—and don't admit party crashers.

- Discuss ground rules with your child before the party.

- Encourage your teen to plan the party with a responsible friend so that he or she will have support if problems arise.

- Brainstorm fun activities for the party.

- If a guest brings alcohol into your house, ask him or her to leave.

- Serve plenty of snacks and non-alcoholic drinks.

- Be visible and available—but don't join the party.

Section 14.3

Family-Based Prevention among Teens with Genetic Risk Factors for Substance Abuse

Excerpted from "Prevention Program Helps Teens Override a Gene Linked to Risky Behavior," National Institute on Alcohol Abuse and Alcoholism (NIAAA), May 15, 2009.

A family-based prevention program designed to help adolescents avoid substance use and other risky behavior proved especially effective for a group of young teens with a genetic risk factor contributing toward such behavior, according to a study by researchers at the University of Georgia.

For two-and-a-half years, investigators monitored the progress of 11-year-olds enrolled in a family-centered prevention program called Strong African American Families (SAAF), and a comparison group. A deoxyribonucleic acid (DNA) analysis showed some youths carried the short allele form of 5-HTTLPR. This fairly common genetic variation, found in over 40% of people, is known from previous studies to be associated with impulsivity, low self-control, binge drinking, and substance use.

The researchers found that adolescents with this gene who participated in the SAAF program were no more likely than their counterparts without the gene to have engaged in drinking, marijuana smoking, and sexual activity. Moreover, youths with the gene in the comparison group were twice as likely to have engaged in these risky behaviors as those in the prevention group.

"The findings underscore that nurture can influence nature during adolescence, a pivotal time when delaying the start of alcohol consumption and other risky behaviors can have a significant impact on healthy child development," says NIAAA Acting Director Kenneth R. Warren, PhD. "This study is one of the first to combine prevention research with a gene-environment study design."

"This study is an excellent example of how we can target prevention interventions based on a person's genetic make-up to reduce their substance abuse risk," says National Institute on Drug Abuse (NIDA) Director Nora Volkow, MD.

The research team recruited 641 families in rural Georgia with similar demographic characteristics. They were divided randomly into two groups: 291 were assigned to a control group that received three mailings of health-related information, and 350 were assigned to the SAAF program, in which parents and children participated in seven consecutive weeks of two-hour prevention sessions. The parents learned about effective caregiving strategies that included monitoring, emotional support, family communication, and handling racial discrimination, which can contribute to substance abuse. The children were taught how to set and attain positive goals, deal with peer pressure and stress, and avoid risky activities.

Researchers conducted home visits with the families when the children were ages 11, 12, and 14 and collected data on parent-child relationships, peer relationships, youth goals for the future, and youth risk behavior. Two years later, the scientists collected DNA from saliva samples provided by the adolescents to determine whether they carried the short allele of 5HTTLPR. The results confirmed that the adolescents carrying this risk gene who were in the control group engaged in risky behaviors at a rate double that of their peers in the SAAF program.

"We found that the prevention program proved especially beneficial for children with a genetic risk factor tied to risky behaviors," says the lead author, Gene H. Brody, PhD, Regents Professor and Director of the Center for Family Research at the University of Georgia. "The results emphasize the important role of parents, caregivers, and family-centered prevention programs in promoting healthy development during adolescence, especially when children have a biological makeup that may pose a challenge."

Dr. Brody also notes that much of the protective influence of SAAF results from enhancing parenting practices. "The ability of effective parenting to override genetic predispositions to risky behaviors demonstrates the capacity of family-centered prevention programs to benefit developing adolescents," he says. The study team, which included researchers from the University of Iowa and Vanderbilt University, concluded that the results validate the use of randomized, controlled prevention trials to test hypotheses about the ways in which genes and environments interact.

Chapter 15

Efforts to Prevent and Reduce Alcohol Problems in Adolescents

Chapter Contents

Section 15.1

School Interventions to Prevent Alcohol Abuse

Text in this section is excerpted from "Keep Kids Alcohol Free: Strategies for Action," National Institutes of Health (NIH), 2007.

As school-based prevention programs have become more guided by research, they have broadened their focus from the individual to include environmental influences and social norms, in particular the effects of peers. For example, studies show that sixth graders who think that more of their peers are drinking than actually are drinking are more likely to drink when compared with those students who learn that their peers do not approve of drinking.

Project Northland, developed by researchers at the University of Minnesota with a grant from the National Institute on Alcohol Abuse and Alcoholism (NIAAA), is a comprehensive alcohol use prevention program for students in grades six through eight. This program has successfully reduced alcohol use in this age group. The participants learn that fewer of their peers drink alcohol than they thought, how to resist pressure to drink, and to talk with their parents about what happens if they do drink.

School district action results in a community coalition: The Troy, Michigan, school district put in place a three-pronged prevention effort when the town started seeing more youths using alcohol. It included a peer pressure resistance program in the schools, a parent group, and a community program. The federally funded Troy Community Coalition that resulted from this initial effort worked with groups from preschoolers to senior citizens. The coalition offered a class to help parents talk to their children about alcohol and encouraged police to make sure bars and stores were not selling alcohol to minors. Because youth were stealing alcohol from grocery store shelves, the coalition also successfully worked for legislation requiring retailers to safeguard the alcohol in their stores. In addition, the coalition trained pediatricians to help parents understand the problems associated with underage drinking.

Reinforce acceptable social norms: Schools can establish alcohol policies that clearly state expectations and penalties regarding alcohol use by students. Such policies reinforce the norm that underage drinking will not be tolerated. School staff, students, parents, and the community must support and enforce such policies consistently in order to shape appropriate attitudes about alcohol among students.

A good school alcohol policy:

- States that alcohol and alcohol use are not allowed on school grounds, at school-sponsored activities, and while students are representing the school.

- Describes the consequences for violating the policy.

- Explains how to assess and refer students who abuse alcohol and guarantees that self-referral will be treated confidentially and will not be punished.

- Pays attention to due process issues in dealing with violators.

- Is cautious about imposing suspension and expulsion for violators because students who are away from school and unsupervised may spend the time drinking alcohol.

Offer students feedback about use rates: Schools can teach students actual alcohol use rates through education programs. Participants discuss how many students actually drink and whether drinking is a good idea. Students taught with this approach use alcohol less and have fewer related problems because they want to be in the majority.

For More Information

Normative Education
Website: http://www.tanglewood.net/products/allstars/article1995.htm

School-Based Curricula (such as Project Northland)
Website: http://modelprograms.samhsa.gov

School Alcohol Policy Information
Website: http://www.epi.umn.edu/alcohol/policy/schools.shtm

Section 15.2

Comprehensive Principles for Interventions Aimed at Underage Alcohol Use

This section is excerpted from "The Surgeon General's Call to Action to Prevent and Reduce Underage Drinking: Sections 3 and 4," U.S. Department of Health and Human Services (HHS), 2007.

Prevention and Reduction of Alcohol Use and Alcohol Use Disorders in Adolescents

To succeed, prevention and reduction efforts must take into account the dynamic developmental processes of adolescence, the influence of an adolescent's environment, and the role of individual characteristics in the adolescent's decision to drink. The goals of interventions aimed at underage alcohol use are to:

- change societal acceptance, norms, and expectations surrounding underage drinking;

- prevent adolescents from starting to drink;

- delay initiation of drinking;

- intervene early, especially with high risk youth;

- reduce drinking and its negative consequences, including progression to alcohol use disorders (AUD), when initiation already has occurred;

- identify adolescents who have developed AUD and who would benefit from additional interventions, including treatment and recovery support services.

In essence, these efforts form a continuum designed to help children and adolescents make sound choices about alcohol use. Scientific research provides the foundation for the design of interventions that accomplish these goals and the means for determining which interventions are effective.

154

Prevention efforts have typically approached the issue of underage drinking through two avenues: by seeking to change the adolescent and by seeking to change the adolescent's environment. Interventions aimed at adolescents themselves seek to change expectations, attitudes, and intentions; impart knowledge and skills; and provide the necessary motivation to better enable adolescents to resist influences that would lead them to drink. Environmental interventions seek to reduce opportunities for underage drinking (for example, the availability of and access to alcohol for adolescent consumption). Examples include:

- increasing enforcement of and penalties for violating the minimum legal drinking age for youth who drink or attempt to purchase alcohol, for merchants who sell to youth, and for people who provide alcohol to underage youth; and

- reducing community tolerance for underage alcohol use.

Underage alcohol use is a complex problem that has proved resistant to solution for decades. Established and emerging research, however, suggests a new evidence-based approach with considerable promise. The principles derived from this research include the following:

1. Underage alcohol use is a phenomenon that is directly related to human development. Because of the nature of adolescence itself, alcohol poses a powerful attraction to adolescents, with unpredictable outcomes that can put any child at risk.

2. Factors that protect adolescents from alcohol use as well as those that put them at risk change during the course of adolescence. Internal characteristics, developmental issues, and shifting factors in the adolescent's environment all play a role.

3. Protecting adolescents from alcohol use requires a comprehensive, developmentally based approach that is initiated before puberty and continues throughout adolescence with support from families, schools, colleges, communities, the health care system, and government.

4. The prevention and reduction of underage drinking is the collective responsibility of the nation. Scaffolding the nation's youth is the responsibility of all people in all of the social systems in which adolescents operate: family, schools, communities, health care systems, religious institutions, criminal and juvenile justice systems, all levels of government, and society as a whole. Each social system has a potential impact on the adolescent, and the active involvement of all systems is necessary to

155

fully maximize existing resources to prevent underage drinking and its related problems. When all the social systems work together toward the common goal of preventing and reducing underage drinking, they create a powerful synergy that is critical to realize the vision.

5. Underage alcohol use is not inevitable, and parents and society are not helpless to prevent it.

Section 15.3

Alcohol Use Prevention and Intervention in Underage Populations

Excepted from "Young Adult Drinking," National Institute on Alcohol Abuse and Alcoholism (NIAAA), April 2006.

What researchers have learned about the different trajectories that drinkers follow as they progress through young adulthood has important implications for prevention. Studies have shown that people follow a variety of pathways across the adolescent and young adult years; alcohol use behaviors change differently for different people; and factors that predict alcohol use patterns emerge and disappear at different ages. One approach to prevention simply will not fit every need. Recognizing the varied and ever-changing trajectories that alcohol use can take offers scientists a solid developmental foundation on which to build effective interventions. One way to prevent alcohol-related problems—among young people or the population as a whole—is to establish policies that reduce overall alcohol consumption rates or reduce the rates of high-risk drinking. Alcohol control policies influence the availability of alcohol, the social messages about drinking that are conveyed by advertising and other marketing approaches, and the enforcement of existing alcohol laws.

Most alcohol control policies target either young people under the legal drinking age of 21 or the drinking behavior of the population as a whole, rather than specific subpopulations such as young adults. Nevertheless, some of these policies have a larger effect on young adult drinkers compared with the rest of the population such as measures that address drinking in bars and clubs, because young adults are more likely than other age groups to patronize these establishments.

Prevention on college campuses: In recent years, an increasing number of colleges have implemented policies to reduce alcohol consumption and alcohol-related problems. Examples include establishing alcohol-free college residences and campuses, prohibiting self-service of alcohol at campus events, prohibiting beer kegs on campus, and banning sales or marketing of alcohol on campus. Though research on the success of these programs is limited, studies have shown that students living in substance-free residences are less likely to engage in heavy episodic or binge drinking, and underage students at colleges that ban alcohol are less likely to engage in heavy episodic drinking and more likely to abstain from alcohol.

Prevention in the military: Current strategies to prevent alcohol problems among military personnel are similar to strategies being used with other populations of drinkers, including instituting and enforcing policies that regulate alcohol availability and pricing, deglamorizing alcohol use, and promoting personal responsibility and overall good health.

Prevention among the general population: Some of the principal strategies for influencing the drinking behavior of the general population are raising taxes on alcoholic beverages, limiting the number of alcohol establishments in a particular geographic area, training the staff of bars and stores to sell alcohol responsibly, and restricting alcohol marketing and advertising. Of these strategies, the effects of raising alcohol prices have been the most extensively studied. Studies show that underage youth are particularly sensitive to increased prices, decreasing their alcohol consumption by a greater amount than older drinkers.

Prevention of drinking and driving: Traffic crashes are the leading cause of death among teens, and more than half of drivers ages 21–24 who died in traffic crashes in 2003 tested positive for alcohol. Raising the minimum legal drinking age (MLDA) to 21 has produced significant reductions in traffic crashes among 18- to 20-year-olds, and it appears to have had a spillover effect on the drinking behavior of 21- to 25-year-olds. Another effective strategy to reduce drinking and driving is to lower the legal limit for allowable blood alcohol content (BAC) for drivers. In the past two decades, all states in the United States have adopted a BAC limit of 0.08% for adult drivers and a BAC limit of zero, or slightly higher, for youth under age 21. These often are referred to as zero tolerance laws. Studies have found that laws setting the legal allowable BAC at 0.08% have resulted in 5% to 8% reductions in alcohol-related fatal traffic crashes among all drivers. Laws setting the limit at 0.02% have led to a 19% reduction in drinking and driving and a 20% reduction in fatal traffic crashes among young drivers.

Comprehensive community prevention approaches: Perhaps the best way to reduce harmful drinking and alcohol-related problems in young adults is through comprehensive approaches that rely heavily on community action. Whether they are working, attending college, or in the military, young adults typically are part of a community. And young people's usual sources of alcohol—retail outlets, restaurants, bars, and social settings such as parties—also operate within the environment of the community. To be effective, community prevention interventions require a mix of research-tested programs and policy strategies, along with strong enforcement of those laws.

Section 15.4

Adolescent Exposure to Substance Use Prevention Messages

Excerpted from "Exposure to Substance Use Prevention Messages and Substance Use among Adolescents," Substance Abuse and Mental Health Services Administration (SAMHSA), April 2, 2009.

Adolescents are subjected to influences that may increase their risk for substance use or protect them from it. Substance use prevention programs generally are designed to lessen the influence of risk factors and increase the influence of protective factors. Substance use prevention messages and programs are provided through parents, the media, schools, and other sources. Gaining a better understanding of how many and which types of adolescents receive prevention messages and programs through each of the many potential sources is essential for the development of effective prevention programming.

The National Survey on Drug Use and Health (NSDUH) asks adolescents (youths aged 12 to 17) whether they have been exposed to prevention messages in the past 12 months through parental sources (for example: talked with at least one of their parents during the past year about the dangers of tobacco, alcohol, or drug use) and media sources (they saw or heard any alcohol or drug prevention messages from sources such as posters, pamphlets, radio, or television). In addition, adolescents are asked whether they have been exposed to prevention messages in the past 12 months through school sources (such as a special class about drugs or alcohol in school; films, lectures, discussions, or printed information about drugs or alcohol in one of their regular school classes such as health or physical education; and films, lectures, discussions, or printed information about drugs or alcohol outside of regular classes such as in a special assembly), as well as whether they have participated in the past 12 months in an alcohol, tobacco, or drug prevention program outside of school.

Trends in Adolescent Exposure to Prevention Messages

From 2002 to 2007, there were decreases in the percentages of adolescents reporting exposure to drug or alcohol use prevention messages through media sources (from 83.2% to 77.9%) and prevention programs outside of school (from 12.7% to 11.3%). Conversely, the percentage who had talked with their parents about the dangers of alcohol, drug, or tobacco use in the past year increased from 58.1% in 2002 to 59.6% in 2007. The percentage of adolescents exposed to school-based prevention messages in 2007 (70.2%) did not differ significantly from the percentage exposed in 2002 (71.4%).

Exposure to Prevention Messages, by Demographic Characteristics

Combined data from 2002 to 2007 indicate that females were more likely than males to have talked with a parent about the dangers of substance use, to have received prevention messages through media sources, and to have received prevention messages through school sources in the past year. For example, 61.5% of females talked with a parent about the dangers of substance use compared with 57.4% of males. Males and females were equally likely to have participated in a substance use prevention program outside of school (12.2%).

The percentage of adolescents who talked with a parent about the dangers of substance use decreased with age, with 61.6% of those aged 12 or 13, 59.5% of those aged 14 or 15, and 57.1% of those aged 16 or 17 indicating that they had talked with a parent about substance use in the past year. The percentage who participated in a prevention program outside of school also decreased with age (15.0%, 11.8%, and 9.9% for those aged 12 or 13, 14 or 15, and 16 or 17, respectively). Conversely, the percentage receiving prevention messages through media sources in the past year increased with age (77.0%, 82.7%, and 84.2% for those aged 12 or 13, 14 or 15, and 16 or 17, respectively). The percentage receiving prevention messages through school was highest among those aged 14 or 15 (74.2%).

Relationship between Exposure to Prevention Messages and Substance Use

Adolescents who reported having conversations with parents about the dangers of substance use were less likely than those who did not have such conversations to have been past month users of cigarettes (10.6% versus 12.5%), alcohol (16.2% versus 18.3%), and illicit drugs (9.5% versus 11.7%). Similarly, those who received prevention messages at school were less likely than those who did not to have used cigarettes (10.4% versus 13.7%), alcohol (16.6% versus 17.9%), and illicit drugs (9.7% versus 12.2%).

Findings were mixed on the relationship between substance use and exposure to prevention messages through sources outside of school and through media sources. Past month alcohol use was lower among adolescents who received prevention messages through prevention programs outside of school than among those who did not (14.7% versus 17.3%), but there was no difference in cigarette or illicit drug use. The prevalence of past month use of cigarettes or illicit drugs was lower among adolescents who reported having received prevention messages from media sources than among those who reported having no such exposure, but past month alcohol use was slightly higher among those who received messages from media sources than among those who did not receive them (17.2% versus 16.4%).

Discussion

In each year of data presented in this report, the majority of adolescents received substance use prevention messages through the media, school, and parents. Although this is encouraging, it is important for practitioners, policymakers, educators, and parents to note the percentage of adolescents who did not receive prevention messages through these sources—in 2007, about 30% of adolescents did not receive prevention messages through school sources, and 40% did not talk with one of their parents about the dangers of substance use. Taken together with the mixed results on trends (increases in exposure for some sources, decreases for some, and no change for others), these findings suggest the need for continued vigilance in ensuring that our nation's adolescents are receiving prevention messages.

This report also reinforces findings from previous studies that emphasize the impact of parental and school involvement on the prevention of substance use. The prevalence of substance use was lower among adolescents exposed to prevention messages through parental and school sources than among those who were not exposed.

Chapter 16

Community-Based Alcohol Abuse Prevention

Chapter Contents

Section 16.1

Strategies for Local Alcohol-Related Policies and Practices

This section is excerpted from "Keep Kids Alcohol Free: Strategies for Action," National Institutes of Health (NIH), 2007.

Alcohol is a regular feature of leisure activities in most communities. Alcohol ads and billboards commonly display attractive, youthful models. Neighborhoods allow alcohol companies to sponsor local fairs, races, sports activities, and other family-focused events. And communities often turn a blind eye to underage drinking and sales to minors. In all these ways, society tells children that alcohol use is accepted, expected, and even essential to having a good time. Many communities are using a variety of strategies to control the visibility and availability of alcohol in their children's environment.

For example, in an experimental program funded by the National Institute on Alcohol Abuse and Alcoholism, seven participating communities made changes in local alcohol-related policies and practices when compared to eight nonparticipating communities. The changes involved local institutional policies as well as practices of law enforcement agencies, licensing departments, community and civic groups, houses of worship, schools, and the local media. The direct impact of this program, called Communities Mobilizing for Change on Alcohol (CMCA), required more checking of age identifications (IDs) by alcohol retailers, resulting in fewer purchases of alcohol by 18- to 20-year-olds. CMCA shows that changing the alcohol-related social and policy environment in communities is essential to long-term prevention.

Raise the price of alcoholic beverages: Higher prices can reduce alcohol purchases, particularly those by minors. Most studies have found that when the price of alcohol goes up, consumption by young people goes down. In addition, research shows that an increase in the price of alcohol is linked to reductions in alcohol-related problems among adolescents. The most efficient means of increasing the price of alcohol is by increasing taxes.

Control the number of alcohol outlets: Studies show that the more alcohol outlets there are in a community, the more citizens drink and the greater the probability of alcohol-related problems. Large numbers of alcohol outlets make it easier to buy alcohol and make it a more visible part of the community. Large numbers of outlets can also stretch the resources of enforcement agencies, making it harder to enforce minimum age laws. Communities can control the number of alcohol outlets through planning and zoning ordinances and conditional use permits.

Train and license servers and sellers: In many states and jurisdictions, alcohol licensees and their employees must be trained before they can do business. Training may cover the importance of checking IDs, how to identify false IDs, how to refuse politely to sell to underage persons, and who is liable (sellers or employees) when sales are made to minors. This training is more effective when alcohol managers and owners are also trained in how to establish alcohol policies and practices for their businesses. Some states and jurisdictions are also setting a minimum age for servers and sellers of alcohol and requiring them to be licensed or certified.

Register kegs: Large, unsupervised parties where alcohol is served, both in private homes and in other settings, have become a common part of the youth scene in many communities. Too often these parties take the form of keggers—parties where beer is available to everyone who attends. With keg registration, each keg is engraved with a unique identifier that is linked to the purchaser's ID. If the keg turns up at a party where underage people are drinking, the authorities can use the keg ID to trace the person responsible and impose appropriate penalties.

Enforce establishment policies: One way to reduce sales to minors is to check the age identification of all individuals who appear to be younger than 30. Establishments that regularly check IDs and closely supervise sales by employees have lower rates of underage sales. Communities can request owners and managers of alcohol establishments to require ID checks as a standard policy and to make sure their employees understand this policy. Communities that publicize and praise retailers who do not sell to anyone under 21 encourage retailers to become partners in the effort to prevent underage drinking.

Conduct compliance checks: Compliance checks can show whether sellers and servers of alcohol are obeying minimum age laws. The buyer should preferably be age 18 to 19. Using multiple buyers provides a more accurate check of the business and allows the business a greater opportunity to have at least partial success. If a sale is made, the police can take appropriate action. Police incident reports can also point to the merchants who made the underage sales. These enforcement strategies work better if they are widely publicized to outlet owners and their staff.

Deter third-party sales: Surveys suggest that many minors get alcohol from adults of legal age who buy it for them. Such third-party sales are illegal in most states. In those states, adults who buy alcohol for underage persons can be warned, cited, or arrested by the police. Merchants can also inform their customers about criminal and civil liabilities for providing alcohol to individuals under the age of 21.

Section 16.2

Town Hall Meetings Mobilize Communities to Prevent and Reduce Underage Alcohol Use

Excerpted from "2008 Town Hall Meetings: Mobilizing Communities to Prevent and Reduce Underage Alcohol Use," Substance Abuse and Mental Health Services Administration (SAMHSA), 2009.

The U.S. Surgeon General has called on communities across the country to come together to encourage a new attitude about underage drinking. According to *The Surgeon General's Call to Action to Prevent and Reduce Underage Drinking*, communities that take a firm stance against underage drinking can help change how people think and act. Together, communities can support teen decisions not to drink.

To help mobilize communities, the Substance Abuse and Mental Health Services Administration (SAMHSA) has supported community-based organizations (CBOs) in hosting more than 3,000 Town Hall Meetings (THMs) since 2006. SAMHSA has reported an increase of more than 30% in participating CBOs. In 2008, 1,604 CBOs hosted 1,811 meetings, compared with 1,230 CBOs and 1,510 meetings in 2006, the first year of the initiative.

CBOs have given high ratings to the events and, more importantly, have already demonstrated intentions of continuing to work on underage drinking as a community health and safety problem that everyone can solve together.

THMs were held in every state, five U.S. territories, and the District of Columbia. CBOs made a concerted effort to engage people with different backgrounds, experience, and perspectives to ensure a well-rounded discussion. Participation from the community was diverse and included parents, prevention specialists, community leaders, law enforcement personnel, education professionals, teachers, local elected officials, business leaders, state elected officials, athletes, celebrities, human service staff, medical professionals, health officials, and youth. Some meetings attracted as many as 1,350 adults although the average was about 45. The average number of youth attending a meeting was 41.

The settings, formats, and contents of the THMs were as diverse and creative as the participants. THMs were conducted in community centers, public libraries, hotels, public and private schools, colleges, and religious institutions in rural, metropolitan, and urban areas. Many included presentations from community leaders and public officials on the incidence and prevalence of local underage drinking and related problems. All meetings reflected the concern that underage alcohol use is a critical problem affecting our communities and that every effort should be made to employ comprehensive approaches to addressing it. Sixty-three THMs were convened in Spanish. Individuals from many racial and ethnic groups attended meetings, including African American, Alaska Native, American Indian, Chinese, Ethiopian, Hispanic, and Somalian.

According to the data gathered on THMs:

- Sixty percent of the CBO respondents plan to host future events.

- Nearly half (46%) will conduct more THMs.

- Twenty-eight percent of the CBO respondents have already held follow-up meetings.

- Twenty-one percent have held discussion groups.

- Six percent have started a coalition.

THM planners and participants are adding coalition members, forming safe home parent network groups, collaborating with other programs, expanding youth advisory boards, and creating underage drinking task forces.

CBOs reported that virtually all attendees expressed interest in becoming more involved in working on decreasing alcohol use in their communities. Attendees also expected to develop more alcohol-free activities for themselves and their children.

Involving youth in planning and participating in the THMs ensured that their perspectives and input were included. This active engagement had a direct effect on the youth who participated. Adolescents who attended or led meetings reported that they have plans to:

- become more involved in reducing underage drinking by participating in positive and worthy activities;

- stay off drugs;

- avoid gangs and other negative influences; and

- join coalitions and youth groups such as Students Against Destructive Decisions (SADD).

Section 16.3

Communities That Care (CTC): An Evidence-Based Substance-Use Prevention System

Excerpted from "Innovative Community-Based Prevention System Reduces Risky Behavior in 10–14 Year Olds," National Institute on Drug Abuse (NIDA), September 7, 2009.

A randomized trial of Communities That Care (CTC), an evidence-based substance-use community-focused prevention system, showed significant reductions in the initiation of alcohol use, tobacco use, binge drinking, and delinquent behavior among middle schoolers as they progressed from the fifth through the eighth grades. The four-year trial, called the *Community Youth Development Study*, began in 2003.

Prevention research has produced programs with efficacy in reducing the risk of substance abuse among youth, but the process of getting these programs into communities has been difficult. CTC helps individual communities identify prevalent risk factors for future substance use among their youth and choose evidence-based programs to address those risk factors across the community. Recent research shows that for each dollar invested in research-based prevention programs, a savings of up to $10 in treatment for alcohol or other substance abuse can be seen.

To evaluate the CTC program, researchers studied a group of 4,407 fifth graders from 24 communities in Colorado, Illinois, Kansas, Maine,

Oregon, Utah and Washington. Twelve communities were randomly assigned to undergo CTC training and implementation, and 12 served as the control communities that did not implement CTC. In the CTC communities, stakeholders including educators, business and public leaders, health workers, religious leaders, social workers and other community volunteers received six training sessions over a year to help them identify the dominant risk and protective factors for substance use in their areas. The coalitions then chose and implemented from two to five evidence-based prevention programs tailored to their risk factors, from a menu of tested and effective prevention strategies. The strategies focus on a variety of topics depending on community need, including alcohol and drugs, violence prevention, reducing family conflict, life skills training, human immunodeficiency virus/acquired immunodeficiency syndrome (HIV/AIDS) prevention, dating safety, tobacco, and anger management. The youth were surveyed annually for four years concerning their risky behaviors to determine the impact of delivering programs through the CTC system.

By the eighth grade, students in the CTC communities were 32% less likely to begin using alcohol, 33% less likely to begin smoking, and 33% less likely to begin using smokeless tobacco than their peers in the control communities. Students from CTC communities were also 25% less likely to initiate delinquent behavior, itself a risk factor for future substance use and an important target for prevention.

The researchers plan to track the children from all 24 communities through the year following high school, to monitor the sustainability of the effects of CTC and whether the communities continue to employ their chosen prevention programs.

Chapter 17

The Minimum Legal Drinking Age (MLDA) Law

Overview of Underage Drinking Policy in the United States

State laws restricting access to alcoholic beverages by young people were first enacted early in the 20th century. These laws prohibited sales of alcohol to young people but did not directly prohibit consumption of alcoholic beverages by young people or provision of alcohol to youth by adults. Underage drinking policies in the United States have become more restrictive over time.

The 18th Amendment to the U.S. Constitution, ratified in 1919, prohibited the sale of all intoxicating liquors in the United States, superseding state laws on the sale of alcoholic beverages to young people. Following the repeal of the 18th Amendment in 1933, restrictions on possession and consumption of alcoholic beverages by youth and non-commercial provision of alcohol to youth by adults became the norm. Most states applied these restrictions to those under the age of 21, making the minimum legal drinking age the same as the minimum age then required for voting in federal elections.

Between 1970 and 1975, 29 states lowered their minimum drinking ages from 21 to 18, 19, or 20, following the enactment of the 26th Amendment to the U.S. Constitution, which granted 18- to 20-year-olds

This chapter includes text excerpted from "Highlight on Underage Drinking," Alcohol Policy Information System (APIS), September 28, 2008; and an excerpt from "Quick Stats: Age 21 Minimum Legal Drinking Age," Centers for Disease Control and Prevention (CDC), September 3, 2008.

the right to vote. In the 1980s, states began to return the minimum drinking age to 21. This reversal reflected both increased public concern about underage drinking and research findings linking lower minimum drinking ages with increases in alcohol-related motor vehicle crashes.

In 1984, Congress enacted the *National Minimum Drinking Age Act*, which remains in effect. This law requires that a portion of federal highway funds be withheld from any states that do not prohibit persons under 21 years of age from purchasing or publicly possessing alcoholic beverages. The U.S. Supreme Court held in 1987 that Congress was within constitutional bounds in attaching such conditions to the receipt of federal funds to encourage uniformity in states' drinking ages. By 1988, every state had passed legislation to meet the federal funding requirements. The result is that all states currently prohibit minors (a term widely used in this context to refer to persons under the age of 21) from possessing alcoholic beverages; most states also prohibit minors from purchasing and consuming alcoholic beverages. In addition, most states prohibit adults from furnishing alcoholic beverages to minors and some states prohibit "internal possession" of alcoholic beverages by minors. These prohibitions are subject to a number of exceptions that vary from state to state.

In addition to minimum drinking age laws, states have adopted a variety of policies to address underage drinking. Some of these policies apply to youth directly, for example, using false identification to purchase alcohol, loss of driving privileges for alcohol violations by minors(use/lose laws), and lower blood alcohol concentration levels for drivers under 21 (zero-tolerance laws). Other policies include minimum age for both alcohol sellers and for servers and bartenders, keg registration requirements, and criminal penalties for hosting underage parties.

In 2006, Congress enacted *The Sober Truth on Preventing Underage Drinking (STOP) Act* which authorized $18 million in federal funds to combat underage drinking. Provisions of the Act include: enhancement of an interagency committee to coordinate efforts by federal agencies to address the issue; annual reporting to Congress about state level efforts to combat underage drinking, including annual state report cards; a national media campaign aimed at adults; assessments of youth exposure to media messages; increased resources for community coalitions to enhance prevention efforts; and funding for new research on underage drinking, including short- and long-term effects on adolescent brain development.

Quick Stats about the Age 21 Minimum Legal Drinking Age

- The Task Force on Community Preventive Services recommends implementing and maintaining an age 21 minimum legal drinking age (MLDA) based on strong evidence of effectiveness, including a median 16% decline in motor vehicle crashes among underage youth in states that increased the legal drinking age to 21 years.

- The Task Force on Community Preventive Services also recommends enhanced enforcement of laws prohibiting the sale of alcohol to minors to reduce such sales.

- Age 21 MLDA laws result in lower levels of alcohol consumption among young adults age 21 years and older as well as those less than age 21 years.

- States with more stringent alcohol control policies tend to have lower adult and college binge drinking rates.

- In addition to the age 21 MLDA, other effective strategies for preventing underage drinking include increasing alcohol excise taxes and limiting alcohol outlet density. Youth exposure to alcohol marketing should also be reduced.

Part Three

The Physical Effects and Consequences of Alcohol Abuse

Chapter 18

Blood Alcohol Concentration (BAC)

Chapter Contents

Section 18.1

BAC and Alcohol Impairment

This section includes "The ABCs of BAC," National Highway Traffic Safety Administration, February 2005; "Estimating Blood Alcohol Levels in Children," National Institute of Alcohol Abuse and Alcoholism (NIAAA), 2009; and "Alcohol Impairment Charts," Substance Abuse and Mental Health Services Administration (SAMHSA), 2002.

BAC and Alcohol Impairment

What is BAC?

The amount of alcohol in a person's body is measured by the weight of the alcohol in a certain volume of blood. This is called the blood alcohol concentration, or BAC. Alcohol is absorbed directly through the walls of the stomach and the small intestine, goes into the bloodstream, and travels throughout the body and to the brain. Alcohol is quickly absorbed and can be measured within 30 to 70 minutes after a person has had a drink.

Does the type of alcohol I drink affect my BAC?

No. A drink is a drink, is a drink. A typical drink equals about half an ounce of alcohol (.54 ounces, to be exact). This is the approximate amount of alcohol found in: one shot of distilled spirits, or one 5-ounce glass of wine, or one 12-ounce beer.

What affects my BAC?

How fast a person's BAC rises varies with a number of factors:

- **The number of drinks:** The more you drink, the higher the BAC.

- **How fast you drink:** When alcohol is consumed quickly, you will reach a higher BAC than when it is consumed over a longer period of time.

- **Your gender:** Women generally have less water and more body fat per pound of body weight than men. Alcohol does not go into fat cells as easily as other cells, so more alcohol remains in the blood of women.

- **Your weight:** The more you weigh, the more water is present in your body. This water dilutes the alcohol and lowers the BAC.

- **Food in your stomach:** Absorption will be slowed if you've had something to eat.

What about other medications or drugs?

Medications or drugs will not change your BAC. However, if you drink alcohol while taking certain medications, you may feel, and be, more impaired which can affect your ability to perform driving-related tasks.

When am I impaired?

Because of the multitude of factors that affect BAC, it is very difficult to assess your own BAC or impairment. Though small amounts of alcohol affect one's brain and the ability to drive, people often swear they are fine after several drinks—but in fact, the failure to recognize alcohol impairment is often a symptom of impairment. While the lower stages of alcohol impairment are undetectable to others, the drinker knows vaguely when the buzz begins. A person will likely be too impaired to drive before looking—or maybe even feeling—drunk.

How will I know I'm impaired, and why should I care?

Alcohol steadily decreases a person's ability to drive a motor vehicle safely. The more you drink, the greater the effect. As with BAC, the signs of impairment differ with the individual. In single-vehicle crashes, the relative risk of a driver with BAC between .08 and .10 is at least 11 times greater than for drivers with a BAC of zero, and 52 times greater for young males. Further, many studies have shown that even small amounts of alcohol can impair a person's ability to drive. Every state has passed a law making it illegal to drive with a BAC of .08 or higher. A driver also can be arrested with a BAC below .08 when a law enforcement officer has probable cause, based on the driver's behavior.

What can I do to stay safe when I plan on drinking?

If you plan on drinking, plan not to drive. You should always:

- choose a non-drinking friend as a designated driver, or

- ask ahead of time if you can stay over at your host's house, or

- take a taxi (your community may have a Safe Rides program for a free ride home), and

- always wear your safety belt—it's your best defense against impaired drivers.

Table 18.1. Common Symptoms and Probable Effects of BAC on Driving Ability

Blood Alcohol Concentration (BAC)[1]	Typical Effects	Predictable Effects on Driving
.02%	Some loss of judgment, relaxation, slight body warmth, altered mood	Decline in visual functions (rapid tracking of a moving target), decline in ability to perform two tasks at the same time (divided attention)
.05%	Exaggerated behavior, may have loss of small-muscle control (focusing your eyes), impaired judgment, usually good feeling, lowered alertness, release of inhibition	Reduced coordination, reduced ability to track moving objects, difficulty steering, reduced response to emergency driving situations
.08%	Muscle coordination becomes poor (balance, speech, vision, reaction time, and hearing), harder to detect danger, judgment, self-control, reasoning, and memory are impaired	Concentration, short-term memory loss, speed control, reduced information processing capability (signal detection, visual search), impaired perception
.10%	Clear deterioration of reaction time and control; slurred speech, poor coordination, and slowed thinking	Reduced ability to maintain lane positions and brake appropriately
.15%	Far less muscle control than normal, vomiting may occur (unless this level is reached slowly or a person has developed a tolerance for alcohol), major loss of balance	Substantial impairment in vehicle control, attention to driving task, and in necessary visual and auditory information processing

[1]Information in this table shows the BAC level at which the effect usually is first observed, and has been gathered from a variety of sources including the National Highway Traffic Safety Administration, the National Institute on Alcohol Abuse and Alcoholism, the American Medical Association, the National Commission Against Drunk Driving, and www.webMD.com.

Estimating Blood Alcohol Levels in Children

Drink for drink, the average blood alcohol concentrations (BACs) attained by children and adolescents are much higher than those seen among college students or adults, according to a study supported by National Institute on Alcohol Abuse and Alcoholism (NIAAA) that appeared in the June 2009 issue of *Pediatrics*.

Using previously published health surveys and scientific reports, researchers derived total body water data and alcohol elimination rates—key variables in the BAC equation—for individuals ranging in age from 9–17. With that information, researchers were able to modify the equation used for estimating BACs in adults to estimate the BACs that theoretically would result after children and adolescents consume various numbers of drinks. No alcohol was provided to children or adolescents as part of this research.

Table 18.2. Alcohol Impairment Chart for Females

Approximate Blood Alcohol Percentage									
Drinks*	Body Weight in Pounds								Effect on Person
	90	100	120	140	160	180	200	220	240	
0	.00	.00	.00	.00	.00	.00	.00	.00	.00	Only safe driving limit
1	.05	.05	.04	.03	.03	.03	.02	.02	.02	Impairment begins
2	.10	.09	.08	.07	.06	.05	.05	.04	.04	Driving skills significantly affected; Possible criminal penalties
3	.15	.14	.11	.11	.09	.08	.07	.06	.06	
4	.20	.18	.15	.13	.11	.10	.09	.08	.08	
5	.25	.23	.19	.16	.14	.13	.11	.10	.09	
6	.30	.27	.23	.19	.17	.15	.14	.12	.11	Legally intoxicated†; Criminal penalties imposed
7	.35	.32	.27	.23	.20	.18	.16	.14	.13	
8	.40	.36	.30	.26	.23	.20	.18	.17	.15	
9	.45	.41	.34	.29	.26	.23	.20	.19	.17	
10	.51	.45	.38	.32	.28	.25	.23	.21	.19	

Subtract .01 for each 30 to 40 minutes of drinking.

* One drink is equal to 1½ oz. of 80 proof liquor, 12 oz. of beer, 4–5 oz. of unfortified table wine, or 4 oz. liqueur.

† In some states, the limit for legal intoxication is .08.

With the modified equation, researchers can better determine how to assess child or adolescent binge drinking. NIAAA defines binge drinking as a pattern of alcohol consumption that brings BAC to .08 grams percent or above, the legal limit for driving in all 50 states. For the typical adult male, this pattern corresponds to consuming five or more drinks in about two hours (four or more drinks for adult females).

The study determined that girls aged 9–17 can be legally intoxicated after having as few as three drinks in a two-hour period. Similarly, the study's authors estimate that a BAC of .08 or higher would also result among boys aged 9–13 who consume three drinks within two hours.

According to the study's author, John E. Donovan, PhD, the findings suggest that children may experience physical and psychological effects after drinking less than a full drink. Research has shown that the expectation of experiencing such effects increases the likelihood of starting to drink and of involvement in problem drinking in adolescence.

Table 18.3. Blood Alcohol Impairment Chart for Males

Approximate Blood Alcohol Percentage									
Drinks*	Body Weight in Pounds								Effect on Person
	100	120	140	160	180	200	220	240	
0	.00	.00	.00	.00	.00	.00	.00	.00	Only safe driving limit
1	.04	.03	.03	.02	.02	.02	.02	.02	Impairment begins
2	.08	.06	.05	.05	.04	.04	.03	.03	
3	.11	.09	.08	.07	.06	.06	.05	.05	Driving skills significantly affected; Possible criminal penalties
4	.15	.12	.11	.09	.08	.08	.07	.06	
5	.19	.16	.13	.12	.11	.09	.09	.08	
6	.23	.19	.16	.14	.13	.11	.10	.09	
7	.26	.22	.19	.16	.15	.13	.12	.11	Legally intoxicated†; Criminal penalties imposed
8	.30	.25	.21	.19	.17	.15	.14	.13	
9	.34	.28	.24	.21	.19	.17	.15	.14	
10	.38	.31	.27	.23	.21	.19	.17	.16	

Subtract .01 for each 30 to 40 minutes of drinking.

*One drink is equal to 1½ oz. of 80 proof liquor, 12 oz. of beer, 4–5 oz. of unfortified table wine, or 4 oz. liqueur.

†In some states, the limit for legal intoxication is .08.

Section 18.2

Alcohol Poisoning

"Facts about Alcohol Poisoning," National Institute on Alcohol Abuse and Alcoholism (NIAAA), July 11, 2007.

Excessive drinking can be hazardous to everyone's health. It can be particularly stressful if you are the sober one taking care of your drunk roommate, who is vomiting while you are trying to study for an exam.

Some people laugh at the behavior of others who are drunk. Some think it's even funnier when they pass out. But there is nothing funny about the aspiration of vomit leading to asphyxiation or the poisoning of the respiratory center in the brain, both of which can result in death.

Do you know about the dangers of alcohol poisoning? When should you seek professional help for a friend? Sadly enough, too many college students say they wish they would have sought medical treatment for a friend. Many end up feeling responsible for alcohol-related tragedies that could have easily been prevented.

Common myths about sobering up include drinking black coffee, taking a cold bath or shower, sleeping it off, or walking it off. But these are just myths, and they don't work. The only thing that reverses the effects of alcohol is time—something you may not have if you are suffering from alcohol poisoning. And many different factors affect the level of intoxication of an individual, so it's difficult to gauge exactly how much is too much (BAC calculators).

What happens to your body when you get alcohol poisoning?

Alcohol depresses nerves that control involuntary actions such as breathing and the gag reflex (which prevents choking). A fatal dose of alcohol will eventually stop these functions.

It is common for someone who drank excessive alcohol to vomit since alcohol is an irritant to the stomach. There is then the danger of choking on vomit, which could cause death by asphyxiation in a person who is not conscious because of intoxication.

You should also know that a person's blood alcohol concentration (BAC) can continue to rise even while he or she is passed out. Even after a person stops drinking, alcohol in the stomach and intestine continues to enter the bloodstream and circulate throughout the body. It is dangerous to assume the person will be fine by sleeping it off.

What are the critical signs and symptoms of alcohol poisoning?

- Mental confusion, stupor, coma, or person cannot be roused
- Vomiting
- Seizures
- Slow breathing (fewer than eight breaths per minute)
- Irregular breathing (10 seconds or more between breaths)
- Hypothermia (low body temperature), bluish skin color, paleness

What should I do if I suspect someone has alcohol poisoning?

- Know the danger signals.
- Do not wait for all symptoms to be present.
- Be aware that a person who has passed out may die.
- If there is any suspicion of an alcohol overdose, call 911 for help. Don't try to guess the level of drunkenness.

What can happen to someone with alcohol poisoning that goes untreated?

- Victim chokes on his or her own vomit.
- Breathing slows, becomes irregular, or stops.
- Heart beats irregularly or stops.
- Hypothermia (low body temperature).
- Hypoglycemia (too little blood sugar) leads to seizures.
- Untreated severe dehydration from vomiting can cause seizures, permanent brain damage, or death.

Even if the victim lives, an alcohol overdose can lead to irreversible brain damage. Rapid binge drinking (which often happens on a bet or a dare) is especially dangerous because the victim can ingest a fatal dose before becoming unconscious.

Don't be afraid to seek medical help for a friend who has had too much to drink. Don't worry that your friend may become angry or embarrassed—remember, you cared enough to help. Always be safe, not sorry.

Chapter 19

Alcohol Hangover

Despite its long history, however, hangover has received relatively scant formal attention from researchers. Little is known about the physiology underlying the hangover condition. For example, it is unclear whether hangover signs and symptoms are attributable to alcohol's direct effects on the body, its after effects, or a combination of both. Similarly, investigators are uncertain about the degree to which hangover affects a person's thinking and mentally controlled motor functions, a question with serious implications for activities such as job performance and driving. In addition, researchers know little about hangover prevention and treatment.

Although folk remedies for hangovers abound, their efficacy in reducing the intensity and duration of a hangover has not received systematic study. In fact, some researchers and clinicians question whether finding an effective treatment for hangovers is desirable, given that the hangover experience may deter some people from engaging in subsequent episodes of heavy drinking.

Although gaps clearly remain in scientific knowledge about hangovers, research has elucidated several aspects. This chapter describes what is known about the hangover condition, the possible physiological factors contributing to it, and treatment options.

Excerpted from "Alcohol Hangover," *Alcohol Health & Research World* Vol. 22, No. 1, 1998, National Institute on Alcohol Abuse and Alcoholism (NIAAA). The complete document with references is available at http://pubs.niaaa.nih.gov/publications/arh22-1/54-60.pdf. Reviewed in May 2010, by Dr. David A. Cooke, MD, FACP, Diplomate, American Board of Internal Medicine.

Understanding What a Hangover Is

A hangover is characterized by the constellation of unpleasant physical and mental symptoms that occur after a bout of heavy alcohol drinking. Physical symptoms of a hangover include fatigue, headache, increased sensitivity to light and sound, redness of the eyes, muscle aches, and thirst. Signs of increased sympathetic nervous system activity can accompany a hangover, including increased systolic blood pressure, rapid heartbeat (tachycardia), tremor, and sweating. Mental symptoms include dizziness; a sense of the room spinning (vertigo); and possible cognitive and mood disturbances, especially depression, anxiety, and irritability. The particular set of symptoms experienced and their intensity may vary from person to person and from occasion to occasion. In addition, hangover characteristics may depend on the type of alcoholic beverage consumed and the amount a person drinks. Typically, a hangover begins within several hours after the cessation of drinking, when a person's blood alcohol concentration (BAC) is falling. Symptoms usually peak about the time BAC is zero and may continue for up to 24 hours thereafter.

Overlap exists between hangover and the symptoms of mild alcohol withdrawal (AW), leading to the assertion that hangover is a manifestation of mild withdrawal. Hangovers, however, may occur after a single bout of drinking, whereas withdrawal occurs usually after multiple, repeated bouts. Other differences between hangover and AW include a shorter period of impairment (for example, hours for hangover versus several days for withdrawal) and a lack of hallucinations and seizures in hangover.

People experiencing a hangover feel ill and impaired. Although a hangover may impair task performance and thereby increase the risk of injury, equivocal data exist on whether hangover actually impairs complex mental tasks. When subjects with a BAC of zero were tested following alcohol intoxication with peak BAC in the range of 50 to 100 milligrams per deciliter (mg/dL), most of them did not show significant impairments in the performance of simple mental tasks, such as reaction time. Similarly, several studies that investigated the hangover effects on a more complex mental task (simulated automobile driving) did not report impaired performance. In contrast, a study of military pilots completing a simulated flying task revealed significant decrements in some performance measures (particularly among older pilots) 8–14 hours after they had consumed enough alcohol to be considered legally drunk.

Prevalence of hangover: Generally, the greater the amount and duration of alcohol consumption, the more prevalent is the hangover, although some people report experiencing a hangover after drinking low levels of alcohol (one to three alcoholic drinks), and some heavy drinkers do not report experiencing hangovers at all.

Physiological factors contributing to hangover: Hangover symptoms have been attributed to several causes, including the direct physiological effects of alcohol on the brain and other organs; the effects of the removal of alcohol from these organs after alcohol exposure (withdrawal); the physiological effects of compounds produced as a result of alcohol's metabolism (metabolites), especially acetaldehyde; and non-alcohol factors, such as the toxic effects of other biologically active chemicals (congeners) in the beverage, behaviors associated with the alcohol-drinking bout (other drug use, restricted food intake, and disruption of normal sleep time), and certain personal characteristics (temperament, personality, and family history of alcoholism).

Direct Alcohol Effects

Dehydration and electrolyte imbalance: Alcohol causes the body to increase urinary output (it is a diuretic). The consumption of 50 grams of alcohol in 250 milliliters (mL) of water (approximately four drinks) causes the elimination of 600 to 1,000 milliliters (mL) (or up to one quart) of water over several hours. Additional mechanisms must be at work to increase urine production, however, because antidiuretic hormone levels increase as BAC levels decline to zero during hangover. Sweating, vomiting, and diarrhea also commonly occur during a hangover, and these conditions can result in additional fluid loss and electrolyte imbalances. Symptoms of mild to moderate dehydration include thirst, weakness, dryness of mucous membranes, dizziness, and lightheadedness—all commonly observed during a hangover.

Gastrointestinal disturbances: Alcohol directly irritates the stomach and intestines, causing inflammation of the stomach lining (gastritis) and delayed stomach emptying, especially when beverages with a high alcohol concentration (greater than 15%) are consumed. High levels of alcohol consumption also can produce fatty liver, an accumulation of fat compounds called triglycerides and their components (free fatty acids) in liver cells. In addition, alcohol increases the production of gastric acid as well as pancreatic and intestinal secretions. Any or all of these factors can result in the upper abdominal pain, nausea, and vomiting experienced during a hangover.

Low blood sugar: Several alterations in the metabolic state of the liver and other organs occur in response to the presence of alcohol in the body and can result in low blood sugar levels (low glucose levels, or hypoglycemia). Alcohol metabolism leads to fatty liver and a buildup of an intermediate metabolic product, lactic acid, in body fluids (lactic acidosis). Both of these effects can inhibit glucose production.

Alcohol-induced hypoglycemia generally occurs after binge drinking over several days in alcoholics who have not been eating. In such a situation, prolonged alcohol consumption, coupled with poor nutritional intake, not only decreases glucose production but also exhausts the reserves of glucose stored in the liver in the form of glycogen, thereby leading to hypoglycemia. Because glucose is the primary energy source of the brain, hypoglycemia can contribute to hangover symptoms such as fatigue, weakness, and mood disturbances. Diabetics are particularly sensitive to the alcohol-induced alterations in blood glucose. However, it has not been documented whether low blood sugar concentrations contribute to hangover symptomatically.

Disruption of sleep and other biological rhythms: Although alcohol has sedative effects that can promote sleep onset, the fatigue experienced during a hangover results from alcohol's disruptive effects on sleep. Alcohol-induced sleep may be of shorter duration and poorer quality because of rebound excitation after BAC falls, leading to insomnia. Furthermore, when drinking behavior takes place in the evening or at night (as it often does), it can compete with sleep time, thereby reducing the length of time a person sleeps. Alcohol also disrupts the normal sleep pattern, decreasing the time spent in the dreaming state (rapid eye movement [REM] sleep) and increasing the time spent in deep (slow-wave) sleep. In addition, alcohol relaxes the throat muscles, resulting in increased snoring and, possibly, periodic cessation of breathing (sleep apnea). Alcohol interferes with other biological rhythms as well, and these effects persist into the hangover period. For example, alcohol disrupts the normal 24-hour (circadian) rhythm in body temperature, inducing a body temperature that is abnormally low during intoxication and abnormally high during a hangover. Alcohol intoxication also interferes with the circadian nighttime secretion of growth hormone, which is important in bone growth and protein synthesis. In contrast, alcohol induces the release of adrenocorticotropic hormone from the pituitary gland, which in turn stimulates the release of cortisol, a hormone that plays a role in carbohydrate metabolism and stress response; alcohol thereby disrupts the normal circadian rise and fall of cortisol levels. Overall, alcohol's disruption of circadian rhythms induces a jet lag that is hypothesized to account for some of the deleterious effects of a hangover.

Alcohol and headache: In a large epidemiological survey of headache in Danish 25- to 64-year-olds, the lifetime prevalence of hangover headache was 72%, making it the most common type of headache reported. Alcohol intoxication results in vasodilatation, which may induce headaches. Alcohol has effects on several neurotransmitters and hormones that are implicated in the pathogenesis of headaches, including histamine, serotonin, and prostaglandins. However, the etiology of hangover headache remains unknown.

Effects of alcohol metabolites: Alcohol undergoes a two-step process in its metabolism. First, an enzyme (alcohol dehydrogenase) metabolizes alcohol to an intermediate product, acetaldehyde; then a second enzyme (aldehyde dehydrogenase [ALDH]) metabolizes acetaldehyde to acetate. Acetaldehyde is a chemically reactive substance that binds to proteins and other biologically important compounds. At higher concentrations, it causes toxic effects, such as a rapid pulse, sweating, skin flushing, nausea, and vomiting. In most people, ALDH metabolizes acetaldehyde quickly and efficiently, so that this intermediate metabolite does not accumulate in high concentrations, although small amounts are present in the blood during alcohol intoxication. In some people, however, genetic variants of the ALDH enzyme permit acetaldehyde to accumulate. Those people routinely flush, sweat, and become ill after consuming small amounts of alcohol. Because of the similarity between the acetaldehyde reaction and a hangover, some investigators have suggested that acetaldehyde causes hangovers. Although free acetaldehyde is not present in the blood after BAC reaches zero, the toxic effects of acetaldehyde produced during alcohol metabolism may persist into the hangover period.

Treatments for Hangover

Many treatments are described to prevent hangover, shorten its duration, and reduce the severity of its symptoms, including innumerable folk remedies and recommendations. Few treatments have undergone rigorous investigation, however. Conservative management offers the best course of treatment. Time is the most important component, because hangover symptoms will usually abate over 8–24 hours.

Attentiveness to the quantity and quality of alcohol consumed can have a significant effect on preventing hangover. Hangover symptoms are less likely to occur if a person drinks only small, nonintoxicating amounts. Even among people who drink to intoxication, those who consume lower amounts of alcohol appear less likely to develop a hangover than those who drink higher amounts. Hangovers have not been associated with drinking beverages with a low alcohol content or with drinking nonalcoholic beverages.

The type of alcohol consumed also may have a significant effect on reducing hangover. Alcoholic beverages that contain few congeners (for example, pure ethanol, vodka, and gin) are associated with a lower incidence of hangover than are beverages that contain a number of congeners (such as brandy, whiskey, and red wine).

Other interventions may reduce the intensity of a hangover but have not been systematically studied. Consumption of fruits, fruit juices, or other fructose-containing foods, is reported to decrease hangover intensity. Also, bland foods containing complex carbohydrates, such as toast or crackers, can counter low blood sugar levels in people subject to hypoglycemia and can possibly relieve nausea. In addition, adequate sleep may ease the fatigue associated with sleep deprivation, and drinking nonalcoholic beverages during and after alcohol consumption may reduce alcohol-induced dehydration.

Certain medications may provide symptomatic relief for hangover symptoms. For example, antacids may alleviate nausea and gastritis. Aspirin and other nonsteroidal anti-inflammatory medications (such as ibuprofen or naproxen) may reduce the headache and muscle aches associated with a hangover but should be used cautiously, particularly if upper abdominal pain or nausea is present. Anti-inflammatory medications are themselves gastric irritants and will compound alcohol-induced gastritis. Although acetaminophen is a common alternative to aspirin, its use should be avoided during the hangover period, because alcohol metabolism enhances acetaminophen's toxicity to the liver.

Caffeine (often taken as coffee) is commonly used to counteract the fatigue and malaise associated with the hangover condition.

Readministration of alcohol reportedly cures a hangover, but people experiencing a hangover should avoid further alcohol use. Additional drinking will only enhance the existing toxicity of the alcohol consumed during the previous bout and may increase the likelihood of even further drinking.

Chapter 20

Alcohol Changes the Brain

Chapter Contents

Section 20.1

Alcohol Tolerance and Withdrawal

Text in this section is excerpted from "Neuroscience: Pathways to Alcohol
Dependence," *Alcohol Alert, Number 77*, National Institute on Alcohol
Abuse and Alcoholism (NIAAA), April 2009.

To function normally, the brain must maintain a careful balance
of chemicals called neurotransmitters—small molecules involved in
the brain's communication system that ultimately help regulate the
body's function and behavior. Just as a heavy weight can tip a scale,
alcohol intoxication can alter the delicate balance among different
types of neurotransmitter chemicals and can lead to drowsiness, loss
of coordination, and euphoria—hallmarks of alcohol intoxication.

Remarkably, with ongoing exposure to alcohol, the brain starts to
adapt to these chemical changes. When alcohol is present in the brain
for long periods as with long-term heavy drinking, the brain seeks to
compensate for its effects. To restore a balanced state, the function
of certain neurotransmitters begins to change so that the brain can
perform more normally in the presence of alcohol. These long-term
chemical changes are believed to be responsible for the harmful effects
of alcohol, such as alcohol dependence.

How Alcohol Changes the Brain

As the brain adapts to alcohol's presence over time, a heavy drinker
may begin to respond to alcohol differently than someone who drinks
only moderately. Some of these changes may be behind alcohol's effects,
including alcohol tolerance (having to drink more in order to become
intoxicated) and alcohol withdrawal symptoms. These effects are associated with alcohol dependence.

When the brain is exposed to alcohol, it may become tolerant or
insensitive to alcohol's effects. Thus, as a person continues to drink
heavily, he or she may need more alcohol than before to become intoxicated. As tolerance increases, drinking may escalate, putting a heavy
drinker at risk for a number of health problems including alcohol
dependence.

Even as the brain becomes tolerant to alcohol, other changes in the brain may increase some people's sensitivity to alcohol. Desire for alcohol may transition into a pathological craving for these effects. This craving is strongly associated with alcohol dependence.

Other changes in the brain increase a heavy drinker's risk for experiencing alcohol withdrawal—a collection of symptoms that can appear when a person with alcohol dependence suddenly stops drinking. Withdrawal symptoms can be severe, especially during the 48 hours immediately following a bout of drinking. Typical symptoms include profuse sweating, racing heart rate, and feelings of restlessness and anxiety. Research shows that alcohol-dependent people may continue drinking to avoid experiencing withdrawal. Feelings of anxiety associated with alcohol withdrawal can persist long after the initial withdrawal symptoms have ceased, and some researchers believe that over the long term this anxiety is a driving force behind alcohol-use relapse. Tolerance and withdrawal are tangible evidence of alcohol's influence on the brain. Scientists now understand some of the mechanisms that lead to these changes—changes that begin with the brain's unique communication system.

Under normal circumstances, the brain's balance of neurotransmitters allows the body and brain to function unimpaired. Alcohol can cause changes that upset this balance, impairing brain function. Alcohol can slow signal transmission in the brain, contributing to some of the effects associated with alcohol intoxication, including sleepiness and sedation.

As the brain grows used to alcohol, it compensates for alcohol's slowing effects by increasing the activity of excitatory neurotransmitters, speeding up signal transmission. In this way, the brain attempts to restore itself to a normal state in the presence of alcohol. If the influence of alcohol is suddenly removed (that is, if a long-term heavy drinker stops drinking suddenly), the brain may have to readjust once again: this may lead to the unpleasant feelings associated with alcohol withdrawal, such as experiencing the shakes or increased anxiety.

Section 20.2

Drinking and Cognitive Function

Text in this section is excerpted from "IACP Health Briefing: Drinking and Cognitive Function," © 2008 International Center for Alcohol Policies. Reprinted with permission. Reference numbers are retained in this excerpt. The complete document, including references, is available online at http://www.icap.org/PolicyTools/ICAPHealth Briefings.

What Is the Evidence?

Alcohol consumption has been shown to have both beneficial and harmful effects on cognitive and neurological functioning. The nature of this relationship depends on the pattern of drinking and follows a U-shaped curve.

- Heavy drinking, particularly chronic heavy drinking, is related to brain damage and cognitive decline.

- Moderate drinking may have a protective role against dementia,[1] especially among older adults.

Harmful Outcomes

Heavy drinking patterns (both chronic and episodic) can result in severe impairments of the nervous system, including brain function. Impairment of cognitive function, learning and memory, as well as personality changes have been described among heavy chronic drinkers and alcohol-dependent individuals.[15, 24]

- Chronic heavy drinking can also result in brain damage, including atrophy of nerve cells and brain shrinkage[25] in cortical and subcortical regions and the hippocampus.[26-28]

- Cognitive decline may result in serious irreversible neurological impairment.[29]

Cognitive deficits have also been described for episodic heavy drinkers.

194

- Impairments have been reported among nondependent individuals who are heavy episodic drinkers.[29]

- Among social binge or extreme drinkers, impairment of executive-type cognitive function and particularly memory has been described.[30]

There is evidence that brain atrophy among heavy chronic drinkers may be partially reversible once drinking has ceased.[31]

Various lifestyle and environmental factors may modulate cognitive deficits associated with heavy drinking. These factors include:

- family history, which may affect susceptibility to the effects of alcohol;

- nutritional factors, which have a mediating role—for example, among alcohol-dependent patients with Wernicke-Korsakoff syndrome or alcohol dementia, cognitive deficits are linked with thiamine deficiency and can be improved by a supplemented diet;[32, 33]

- long-term cigarette smoking with an impact on the dynamics of structural and cognitive changes in the brains of alcoholics;[34]

- family history of heavy drinking, which has been shown to correlate with smaller brain volume among alcohol-dependent individuals, suggesting a role in the onset of alcoholism and cognitive impairment;[35] and

- head trauma and other injuries.

Cognitive impairment from heavy drinking is cumulative throughout life; however, even among young heavy drinkers, there is evidence of early impairment.[36]

- Reduced cognitive function may be present without any associated structural brain abnormalities.[37]

Beneficial Outcomes

Research evidence shows that moderate drinking may slow cognitive decline. The relationship has been documented among those who drink little (less than one drink per week), as well as those who drink over two drinks per day.[5]

- Improved cognitive function in light-to-moderate drinkers is based on comparisons with abstainers, who are used as the baseline measure.

Protective effects for cognitive function are seen with light-to-moderate drinking patterns and have been described primarily for older individuals.

- Reduced risk of dementia is seen in individuals aged 55 and older.[6]

Moderate drinking patterns correlate with reduced prevalence of brain abnormalities, such as those seen in Alzheimer patients.[7] Both cognitive decline with aging and Alzheimer disease are related to vascular disease. The effect is independent of the type of alcohol beverage consumed.[3]

- The relationship between drinking and cognitive function, therefore, appears to be mediated through similar mechanisms as those involved in cardiovascular disease (CVD).[2]

- The relationship is modulated by other possible environmental and intrinsic factors.

Beneficial effects on cognition have been demonstrated in light-to-moderate drinkers as compared with abstainers.

- Compared with abstainers, light-to-moderate drinkers have been shown to have improved cognition and subjective wellbeing, as well as fewer symptoms of depression.[5, 8-14]

- The association applies to both men and women and is borne out across cultures and ethnic groups.

- Elderly women may benefit more than men from the protective effects of moderate drinking on cognitive function.[15] Among elderly women, moderate alcohol consumption has been found to be one of the predictors of maintaining optimal cognitive function into old age.[16]

- Improved cognitive skills among drinkers over abstainers may not be limited to the elderly. Benefits have been described in samples of young,[17, 18] and middle-aged adults.[19]

Effects on cognitive function seem to be better for current drinkers than for lifetime abstainers or former drinkers.[10] Those who drank in midlife showed enhanced cognitive function later in life as compared to abstainers.[20, 21]

- The relationship was found for both infrequent and frequent drinkers.

- An optimal level of drinking has not been determined.

While the relationship between drinking and cognitive function is robust, it may be confounded by various other factors. Abstainers' overall health and personality traits, as well as their demographics,[22] may account for some of the observed differences.

- The progression of some health conditions, notably type II diabetes mellitus, can have an impact on brain function, resulting in gradual cognitive impairment.[23]

- Lifestyle factors such as smoking and diet are associated with age-related changes in cognitive function, pre-dementia syndrome, and cognitive decline associated with neurodegenerative disease (such as Alzheimer disease).

- The relationship may also be influenced by differences in educational level between drinkers and abstainers.[22]

Section 20.3

Adolescent Brain Is Vulnerable to Alcohol Exposure

Text in this section is excerpted from "Alcohol and the Developing Adolescent Brain," National Institute on Alcohol Abuse and Alcoholism (NIAAA), 2007.

New Understanding of Adolescent Brain Development

Those who interact with children and adolescents are often struck by the ease with which they are able to learn a wide range of skills from speaking a foreign language to playing a musical instrument to mastering a sport to programming a computer. This facility for learning is due in large part to the tremendous adaptability (plasticity) of the developing brain. Imaging studies of normal brain development show an inverted U-shaped trajectory of change in gray matter volume; for girls, volume peaks at around age 8.5 years, while for boys it peaks at around age 10.5. It has been postulated that the initial increase reflects an overproduction of synapses and that the subsequent thinning of cortical gray matter during adolescence may be due to a use it or lose it phenomenon—synapses that are not used are lost, whereas those that are used are reinforced. This may help explain the increase in processing efficiency as the brain matures, although more research will be needed to confirm this hypothesis.

Research has also shown that the brain is not fully physiologically mature until a person's mid-twenties, and that maturational processes in the brain do not occur uniformly throughout it. These differences in maturational timing can have important implications for behavior. Perhaps most important for understanding adolescent behavior is the maturational gap between the limbic system and the prefrontal cortex. Early in adolescence, developmental changes in the limbic system result in alterations in the control of emotions and motivation. This occurs well before the cognitive systems involving the prefrontal cortex that are responsible for self-regulation, planning, and reasoning become sufficiently mature to exert control over the impulsive and emotional reactions generated in the limbic system. The emotional intensity characteristic of adolescence may in part be explained by the uneven timing in development across these regions of the brain.

Potential Vulnerabilities Arising from Alcohol Exposure to the Developing Adolescent Brain

The remarkable plasticity of the brain during adolescence, which confers significant advantages in terms of learning, may also make the teen brain particularly vulnerable to the effects of alcohol and other drugs. Research indicates that adolescent alcohol consumption may affect cognitive functioning and/or change the developing brain in ways that increase the risk for future dependence.

Cognitive functioning: A study in humans showed that a single, moderate dose of alcohol can disrupt learning more powerfully in people in their early twenties, compared with those in their late twenties. The effects of repeated alcohol consumption during adolescence may also be long-lasting. Studies in humans have detected cognitive impairments in adolescent alcohol abusers weeks after they stopped drinking, and a different pattern of brain response to tests of memory than among non-abusers. Research using imaging techniques to study brain structure in humans has found adolescent-onset alcohol abuse to be associated with a reduction in the size of the hippocampus, a part of the brain involved in memory and spatial navigation.

Future dependence: Early alcohol use in humans is correlated with future alcohol dependence. Forty percent of people who report drinking before the age of 15 also describe their drinking behavior at some point in their lives in a manner consistent with a diagnosis of alcohol dependence. In addition, in rats bred to voluntarily drink high levels of alcohol, repeated intake of alcohol during adolescence increases alcohol intake in adulthood, results in craving-like behavior, and increases potential for alcohol relapse.

Section 20.4

Wernicke-Korsakoff Syndrome (Alcoholic Encephalopathy)

"Wernicke-Korsakoff Syndrome," © 2010 A.D.A.M., Inc. Reprinted with permission.

Wernicke-Korsakoff syndrome is a brain disorder due to thiamine deficiency.

Causes: Wernicke's encephalopathy and Korsakoff syndrome are believed to be two stages of the same condition. Wernicke's encephalopathy is caused by damaging changes in the brain, usually due to a lack of vitamin B1 (thiamine). A lack of vitamin B1 is common in people with alcoholism. Heavy alcohol use affects the breakdown of thiamine in the body. Even if someone who drinks alcohol heavily follows a well-balanced diet, most of the thiamine is not absorbed. Korsakoff syndrome, or Korsakoff psychosis, tends to develop as Wernicke's symptoms go away. Korsakoff psychosis involves damage to areas of the brain involved with memory.

Symptoms:

* Inability to form new memories

* Loss of memory, can be severe

* Loss of muscle coordination (ataxia)—unsteady, uncoordinated walking

- Making up stories (confabulation)
- Seeing or hearing things that aren't really there (hallucinations)
- Vision changes—abnormal eye movements, double vision, eyelid drooping

Note: There may also be symptoms of alcohol withdrawal.

Exams and tests: Examination of the nervous/muscular system may show damage to many nerve systems including the following:

- Decreased or abnormal reflexes
- Problems with walk (gait) and coordination
- Muscle weakness and atrophy (loss of tissue mass)
- Abnormal eye movement
- Low blood pressure
- Low body temperature
- Fast pulse (heart rate)

The person may appear poorly nourished. The following tests are used to check a person's nutrition level:

- Pyruvate
- Serum B1 levels
- Transketolase activity

Blood or urine alcohol levels and liver enzymes may be high in people with a history of long-term alcohol abuse. Other conditions that may cause thiamine deficiency include:

- acquired immunodeficiency syndrome (AIDS),
- cancers that have spread throughout the body,
- extreme nausea and vomiting during pregnancy (hyperemesis gravidarum),
- heart failure (when treated with long-term diuretic therapy),
- long periods of intravenous (IV) therapy without receiving thiamine supplements,
- long-term dialysis,
- very high thyroid hormone levels (thyrotoxicosis).

A brain magnetic resonance image (MRI) in rare cases shows changes in the tissue of the brain.

Treatment: The goals of treatment are to control symptoms as much as possible and to prevent the disorder from getting worse. Some people may need to stay in the hospital early in the condition to help control symptoms. Monitoring and special care may be needed if the person is comatose, lethargic, or unconscious.

Thiamine (vitamin B1) may be given by injection into a vein or a muscle, or by mouth. It may improve symptoms of confusion or delirium, difficulties with vision and eye movement, and lack of muscle coordination. Thiamine does not usually improve loss of memory and intellect that occur with Korsakoff psychosis. Stopping alcohol use can prevent loss of brain function and damage to nerves. Eat a well-balanced, nourishing diet.

Support groups: You can often ease the stress of illness by joining a support group where members share common experiences and problems.

Outlook (prognosis): Without treatment, Wernicke-Korsakoff syndrome gets steadily worse and can be life threatening. With treatment, you can control symptoms (such as uncoordinated movement and vision difficulties), and slow or stop the disorder from getting worse. Some symptoms—especially the loss of memory and thinking skills—may be permanent. Other disorders related to alcohol abuse may also occur.

Possible complications:

- Alcohol withdrawal
- Difficulty with personal or social interaction
- Injury caused by falls
- Permanent alcoholic neuropathy
- Permanent loss of thinking skills
- Permanent loss of memory
- Shortened life span

In people at risk, Wernicke's encephalopathy may be caused by carbohydrate loading or glucose infusion. Always supplement with thiamine before glucose infusion to prevent this.

When to contact a medical professional: Call your health care provider if you have symptoms of Wernicke-Korsakoff syndrome, or if you have been diagnosed with the condition and your symptoms get worse or return.

Also, call if new symptoms develop, especially symptoms of alcohol withdrawal. Alcohol withdrawal can be fatal, so call the local emergency number (such as 911) or go to the emergency room if any severe symptoms occur.

Symptoms of alcohol withdrawal include the following:

- Agitation
- Delirium or confusion
- Fast heart rate
- Hallucinations
- Insomnia
- Jumpiness or nervousness
- Palpitations

Prevention: Not drinking alcohol or drinking in moderation and getting enough nutrition reduce the risk of developing Wernicke-Korsakoff syndrome. If a heavy drinker will not quit, thiamine supplements and a good diet may help prevent this condition, but not if damage has already occurred.

Alternative names: Korsakoff psychosis; alcoholic encephalopathy; encephalopathy–alcoholic; Wernicke's disease

Chapter 21

Alcohol-Induced Liver Disease

Chapter Contents

Section 21.1

Overview and Progression of Liver Disease

This section includes "Alcohol-Induced Liver Disease," and "Progression of Liver Disease," © 2007 American Liver Foundation (www.liver foundation.org). Reprinted with permission.

Alcohol-Induced Liver Disease

What is the liver's role in processing alcohol?

The liver breaks down alcohol so it can be eliminated from your body. If you consume more alcohol than the liver can process, the resulting imbalance can injure the liver by interfering with its normal breakdown of protein, fats, and carbohydrates.

What are the types of alcohol-induced liver disease?

There are three kinds of liver disease related to alcohol consumption:

Fatty liver is marked by a build-up of fat cells in the liver. Usually there are no symptoms, although the liver may be enlarged and you may experience discomfort in your upper abdomen. Fatty liver occurs in almost all people who drink heavily. The condition will improve after you stop drinking.

Alcoholic hepatitis is an inflammation of the liver. Up to 35% of heavy drinkers develop alcoholic hepatitis. Symptoms may include loss of appetite, nausea, vomiting, abdominal pain and tenderness, fever, and jaundice. In its mild form, alcoholic hepatitis can last for years and will cause progressive liver damage. The damage may be reversible if you stop drinking. In its severe form, the disease may occur suddenly, after binge drinking, and it can quickly lead to life-threatening complications.

Alcoholic cirrhosis is the most serious type of alcohol-induced liver disease. Cirrhosis refers to the replacement of normal liver tissue with scar tissue. Between 10% and 20% of heavy drinkers develop cirrhosis, usually after ten or more years of drinking. Symptoms of cirrhosis are similar to those of alcoholic hepatitis. The damage from cirrhosis is not reversible, and it is a life-threatening disease. Your condition may stabilize if you stop drinking.

Many heavy drinkers will progress from fatty liver to alcoholic hepatitis and finally to alcoholic cirrhosis, though the progression may vary from patient to patient. The risk of developing cirrhosis is particularly high for people who drink heavily and have another chronic liver disease such as viral hepatitis C.

What are the complications of alcohol-induced liver disease?

Serious complications from alcohol-induced liver disease typically occur after many years of heavy drinking. Once they do occur, the complications can be serious and life-threatening. They may include the following:

- Accumulation of fluid in the abdomen
- Bleeding from veins in the esophagus
- Enlarged spleen
- High blood pressure in the liver
- Changes in mental function, and coma
- Kidney failure
- Liver cancer

How is alcohol-induced liver disease diagnosed?

Alcohol-induced liver disease may be suspected based on other medical and lifestyle issues related to alcohol abuse. Blood tests and imaging tests (magnetic resonance imaging [MRI], computed tomography [CT] scan, or ultrasound) may help in diagnosis and to rule out other causes of liver disease. Proof is best established by liver biopsy.

How is alcohol-induced liver disease treated?

First, you must stop drinking. Your doctor may suggest changes in your diet and certain vitamin supplements to help your liver recover from the alcohol-related damage. Medications may be needed to manage the complications caused by your liver damage. In advanced cases of alcoholic cirrhosis, the only treatment option may be a liver transplant. However, active alcoholics will usually not qualify as suitable organ recipients.

In order to stop drinking, you may need to participate in an alcohol recovery program. The best resource is likely to be an alcoholic support group, because you must stay sober to recover from your liver disease.

What is the outlook for people with alcohol-induced liver disease?

Anyone with alcohol-induced liver disease will improve their health and life expectancy if they stop drinking. For patients who do not stop drinking, the outlook is poor; they are likely to suffer a variety of life-threatening health problems caused by alcohol-related liver damage.

Is there a safe level of drinking?

For most people, moderate drinking will not lead to alcohol-induced liver disease. Moderate drinking means no more than one drink a day for women and two drinks a day for men. (A standard drink is one 12-ounce beer, one 5-ounce glass of wine or one 1.5-ounce shot of distilled spirits.) However, for people with chronic liver disease, especially alcohol-induced liver disease, even small amounts of alcohol can make the liver disease worse. Patients with alcohol-induced liver disease and those with cirrhosis from any cause should stop using alcohol completely.

Women are more likely to be affected by alcohol-induced liver disease because women can be affected by smaller amounts of alcohol than men.

Even small amounts of alcohol can be dangerous when taken with medications containing acetaminophen, found in many over-the-counter pain relievers. The combination of alcohol and acetaminophen can be very harmful to the liver for anyone who drinks. Never take acetaminophen with alcohol, or immediately after a period of heavy drinking.

The Progression of Liver Disease

There are many different types of liver disease. But no matter what type you have, the damage to your liver is likely to progress in a similar way. Whether your liver is infected with a virus, injured by chemicals, or under attack from your own immune system, the basic danger is the same—that your liver will become so damaged that it can no longer work to keep you alive. Anything that keeps your liver from doing its job may put your life in danger.

The Healthy Liver

Your liver helps fight infections and cleans your blood. It also helps digest food and stores energy for when you need it. A healthy liver has the amazing ability to grow back, or regenerate, when it is damaged. Anything that keeps your liver from doing its job—or from growing back after injury—may put your life in danger.

Inflammation: In the early stage of any liver disease, your liver may become inflamed. It may become tender and enlarged. Inflammation shows that your body is trying to fight an infection or heal an injury. But if the inflammation continues over time, it can start to hurt your liver permanently.

When most other parts of your body become inflamed, you can feel it—the area becomes hot and painful. But an inflamed liver may cause you no discomfort at all. If your liver disease is diagnosed and treated successfully at this stage, the inflammation may go away.

Fibrosis: If left untreated, the inflamed liver will start to scar. As excess scar tissue grows, it replaces healthy liver tissue. This process is called fibrosis. Scar tissue is a kind of fibrous tissue. Scar tissue cannot do the work that healthy liver tissue can. Moreover, scar tissue can keep blood from flowing through your liver. As more scar tissue builds up, your liver may not work as well as it once did. Or, the healthy part of your liver has to work harder to make up for the scarred part. If your liver disease is diagnosed and treated successfully at this stage, there's still a chance that your liver can heal itself over time.

Cirrhosis: But if left untreated, your liver may become so seriously scarred that it can no longer heal itself. This stage—when the damage cannot be reversed—is called cirrhosis. Cirrhosis can lead to a number of complications, including liver cancer. In some people, the symptoms of cirrhosis may be the first signs of liver disease.

- You may bleed or bruise easily.
- Water may build up in your legs and/or abdomen.
- Your skin and eyes may take on a yellow color, a condition called jaundice.
- Your skin may itch intensely.
- In blood vessels leading to your liver, the blood may back up because of blockage; these blood vessels may burst.
- You may become more sensitive to medications and their side effects.

- You may develop insulin resistance and type 2 diabetes.

- Toxins may build up in your brain, causing problems with concentration, memory, sleeping, or other mental functions.

Once you've been diagnosed with cirrhosis, treatment will focus on keeping your condition from getting worse. It may be possible to stop or slow the liver damage. It is important to protect the healthy liver tissue you have left.

Liver cancer: Cancer that starts in the liver is called primary liver cancer. Cirrhosis and hepatitis B are leading risk factors for primary liver cancer. But cancer can develop in the liver at any stage in the progression of liver disease.

Liver failure: Liver failure means that your liver is losing or has lost all of its function. It is a life-threatening condition that demands urgent medical care. The first symptoms of liver failure are often nausea, loss of appetite, fatigue, and diarrhea. Because these symptoms can have any number of causes, it may be hard to tell that the liver is failing. Liver failure is a life-threatening condition that demands urgent medical care.

As liver failure progresses, the symptoms become more serious. The patient may become confused and disoriented, and extremely sleepy. There is a risk of coma and death. Immediate treatment is needed. The medical team will try to save whatever part of the liver that still works. If this is not possible, the only option may be a liver transplant.

When liver failure occurs as a result of cirrhosis, it usually means that the liver has been failing gradually for some time, possibly for years. This is called chronic liver failure. Chronic liver failure can also be caused by malnutrition. More rarely, liver failure can occur suddenly, in as little as 48 hours. This is called acute liver failure and is usually a reaction to poisoning or a medication overdose.

Cirrhosis, liver cancer, and liver failure are serious conditions that can threaten your life. Once you have reached these stages of liver disease, your treatment options may be very limited. That's why it's important to catch liver disease early, in the inflammation and fibrosis stages. If you are treated successfully at these stages, your liver may have a chance to heal itself and recover. Talk to your doctor about liver disease. Find out if you are at risk or if you should undergo any tests or vaccinations.

Section 21.2

Cirrhosis

This section begins with an excerpt from "Liver Cirrhosis Mortality in the United States, 1970–2005," National Institute on Alcohol Abuse and Alcoholism (NIAAA), August 2008; and continues with information excerpted from "Cirrhosis," National Institute of Diabetes and Digestive and Kidney Diseases (NIDDK), December 2008.

Liver Cirrhosis Mortality in the United States

- In 2005 liver cirrhosis was the 12th leading cause of death in the United States, with a total of 28,175 deaths, 621 more than in 2004.

- The crude death rate from all cirrhosis increased by 1.1% from 2004 to 2005, whereas the rate from alcohol-related cirrhosis increased by 2.3%.

- Among all cirrhosis deaths in 2005, 45.9% were alcohol-related. The proportion of alcohol-related cirrhosis was highest (65.0%) among decedents aged 35 to 44.

- The age-adjusted death rate from all cirrhosis for White Hispanic males was 1.8 times the rate for White non-Hispanic and Black non-Hispanic males. The rate for White Hispanic females was 1.4 times the rate for White non-Hispanic females and 1.7 times the rate for Black non-Hispanic females.

- Wide variations existed across Hispanic subgroups; the annual average of age-adjusted death rates from all cirrhosis was highest for Puerto Ricans and Mexicans and lowest for Cubans, among both males and females.

Cirrhosis Mortality Trends

- While the age-adjusted all-cause mortality rate declined by 34.7% from 1970 to 2005, the age-adjusted death rate from all liver cirrhosis declined for the same period by 48.3%, from 17.8

to 9.2 deaths per 100,000 population. Rates for White males, Black males, White females, and Black females declined by 44.4%, 69.1%, 42.1%, and 75.5%, respectively.

- The age-adjusted death rate from all liver cirrhosis for males was consistently more than twice the rate for females, regardless of race.

- The age-adjusted death rate from alcohol-related liver cirrhosis declined by 33.3%, from 6.3 deaths per 100,000 population in 1970 to 4.2 deaths per 100,000 population in 2005. Rates for White males, Black males, White females, and Black females declined by 22.4%, 68.2%, 29.0%, and 74.7%, respectively.

Cirrhosis Information from the National Institute on Alcohol Abuse and Alcoholism

Cirrhosis is a condition in which the liver slowly deteriorates and malfunctions due to chronic injury. Scar tissue replaces healthy liver tissue, partially blocking the flow of blood through the liver. Scarring also impairs the liver's ability to:

- control infections;

- remove bacteria and toxins from the blood;

- process nutrients, hormones, and drugs;

- make proteins that regulate blood clotting; and

- produce bile to help absorb fats—including cholesterol—and fat-soluble vitamins.

A healthy liver is able to regenerate most of its own cells when they become damaged. With end-stage cirrhosis, the liver can no longer effectively replace damaged cells. A healthy liver is necessary for survival.

Cirrhosis has various causes: In the United States, heavy alcohol consumption and chronic hepatitis C have been the most common causes of cirrhosis. Obesity is becoming a common cause of cirrhosis, either as the sole cause or in combination with alcohol, hepatitis C, or both. Many people with cirrhosis have more than one cause of liver damage. Cirrhosis is not caused by trauma to the liver or other acute, or short-term, causes of damage. Usually years of chronic injury are required to cause cirrhosis.

Symptoms of cirrhosis: Many people with cirrhosis have no symptoms in the early stages of the disease. However, as the disease progresses, a person may experience weakness, fatigue, loss of appetite, nausea, vomiting, weight loss, abdominal pain and bloating when fluid accumulates in the abdomen, itching, or spiderlike blood vessels on the skin.

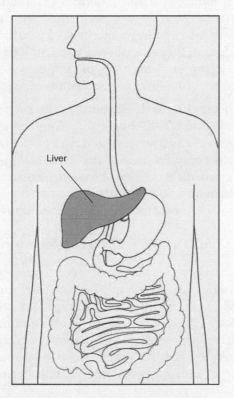

Figure 21.1. *The Liver and Digestive System*

Diagnosis of cirrhosis: The diagnosis of cirrhosis is usually based on the presence of a risk factor for cirrhosis, such as alcohol use or obesity, and is confirmed by physical examination, blood tests, and imaging. The doctor will ask about the person's medical history and symptoms and perform a thorough physical examination to observe for clinical signs of the disease. For example, on abdominal examination, the liver may feel hard or enlarged with signs of ascites. The doctor will order blood tests that may be helpful in evaluating the liver and increasing the suspicion of cirrhosis.

To view the liver for signs of enlargement, reduced blood flow, or ascites, the doctor may order a computerized tomography (CT) scan, ultrasound, magnetic resonance imaging (MRI), or liver scan. The doctor may look at the liver directly by inserting a laparoscope into the abdomen. A laparoscope is an instrument with a camera that relays pictures to a computer screen.

A liver biopsy can confirm the diagnosis of cirrhosis but is not always necessary. A biopsy is usually done if the result might have an impact on treatment. The biopsy is performed with a needle inserted between the ribs or into a vein in the neck. Precautions are taken to minimize discomfort. A tiny sample of liver tissue is examined with a microscope for scarring or other signs of cirrhosis. Sometimes a cause of liver damage other than cirrhosis is found during biopsy.

Treatment of cirrhosis: Treatment for cirrhosis depends on the cause of the disease and whether complications are present. The goals of treatment are to slow the progression of scar tissue in the liver and prevent or treat the complications of the disease. Hospitalization may be necessary for cirrhosis with complications. Eating a nutritious diet and avoiding alcohol and other substances is advised. The health care team will also provide treatment for specific complications

When is a liver transplant indicated for cirrhosis?

A liver transplant is considered when complications cannot be controlled by treatment. Liver transplantation is a major operation in which the diseased liver is removed and replaced with a healthy one from an organ donor. A team of health professionals determines the risks and benefits of the procedure for each patient. Survival rates have improved over the past several years because of drugs that suppress the immune system and keep it from attacking and damaging the new liver. Generally, organs are given to people with the best chance of living the longest after a transplant.

Section 21.3

Fatty Liver

"Fatty Liver," © 2007 American Liver Foundation (www.liver foundation.org). Reprinted with permission.

What is fatty liver?

Fatty liver is just what its name suggests: the build-up of excess fat in the liver cells. It is normal for your liver to contain some fat. But if fat accounts for more than 10% of your liver's weight, then you have fatty liver and you may develop more serious complications.

Fatty liver may cause no damage, but sometimes the excess fat leads to inflammation of the liver. This condition, called steatohepatitis, does cause liver damage. Sometimes, inflammation from a fatty liver is linked to alcohol abuse; this is known as alcoholic steatohepatitis. Otherwise the condition is called nonalcoholic steatohepatitis, or NASH.

An inflamed liver may become scarred and hardened over time. This condition, called cirrhosis, is serious and often leads to liver failure. NASH is one of the top three leading causes of cirrhosis.

What are the symptoms of fatty liver?

A fatty liver produces no symptoms on its own, so people often learn about their fatty liver when they have medical tests for other reasons. NASH can damage your liver for years or even decades without causing any symptoms. If the disease gets worse, you may experience fatigue, weight loss, abdominal discomfort, weakness, and confusion.

What causes fatty liver?

Eating excess calories causes fat to build up in the liver. When the liver does not process and break down fats as it normally should, too much fat will accumulate. People tend to develop fatty liver if they have certain other conditions, such as obesity, diabetes, or high triglycerides. Alcohol abuse, rapid weight loss and malnutrition may also lead to fatty liver. However, some people develop fatty liver even if they have none of these conditions—so everyone should know about it.

How is fatty liver diagnosed?

Your doctor may see something unusual in your blood test or notice that your liver is slightly enlarged during a routine checkup. These could be signs of a fatty liver. To make sure you don't have another liver disease, your doctor may ask for more blood tests, an ultrasound, a computed tomography (CT) scan or a magnetic resonance image (MRI). If other diseases are ruled out, you may be diagnosed with NASH. The only way to know for sure is to get a liver biopsy. Your doctor will remove a sample of liver tissue with a needle and check it under a microscope.

What new treatments for fatty liver are being studied?

Fatty liver is currently the focus of intense research to provide us with better tools for treatment in the future. Scientists are studying whether various medications can help reduce the inflammation on your liver, including new diabetes medications that may help you even if you don't have diabetes.

How is fatty liver treated?

There are no medical or surgical treatments for fatty liver, but there are some steps you can take that may help prevent or reverse some of the damage. In general, if you have fatty liver, and in particular if you have NASH, you should do the following:

- Lose weight safely. That usually means losing no more than one or two pounds a week.
- Lower your triglycerides through diet, medication or both.
- Avoid alcohol.
- Control your diabetes, if you have it.
- Eat a balanced, healthy diet.
- Increase your physical activity.
- Get regular checkups from a doctor who specializes in liver care.

If I've been diagnosed with fatty liver, what questions should I ask my doctor?

- What is the likely cause of my fatty liver?
- Do I have NASH? If not, how likely am I to develop NASH?

- Do I have cirrhosis? If not, how likely am I to develop cirrhosis?

- Do I need to lose weight? How can I do so safely?

- Should I be taking any medication to control my triglyceride levels?

- What medications or other substances should I avoid to protect my liver?

Who is at risk for fatty liver?

Most (but not all) fatty liver patients are middle-aged and overweight. The risk factors most commonly linked to fatty liver disease are:

- overweight (body mass index of 25–30),

- obesity (body mass index above 30),

- diabetes,

- elevated triglyceride levels.

What is the best way to prevent fatty liver?

The best way to reduce your risk of developing fatty liver is to maintain a healthy weight and normal triglyceride levels. You should also avoid excess alcohol and other substances that could harm your liver.

Section 21.4

Alcohol and Hepatitis C

Excerpted from "Alcohol and Hepatitis C," U.S. Department of Veterans Affairs, April 24, 2007.

Alcohol is one of the most widely used and abused substances in the world. It is a potent toxin to the liver, even in people without hepatitis C infection. Excessive alcohol use can lead to cirrhosis of the liver, even liver cancer. Regardless of alcohol use, people with hepatitis C are at risk for cirrhosis of the liver. Hepatitis C impairs the liver's natural function of breaking down alcohol and removing toxic by-products. As a result, the toxins in alcohol are not removed completely and remain within the body, creating a toxic environment.

For every 100 people infected with hepatitis C: Fifteen people get rid of the virus through their own immune system, and 85 will develop chronic, or long-term, infection. Of these 85 people, 66 will get only minor liver damage, 17 will develop cirrhosis and may have symptoms of advanced liver disease, and two will develop liver cancer. Which group you end up in (manageable liver disease, cirrhosis, or liver cancer) depends on many things, but it can be related to choices you make about your lifestyle.

Alcohol and fibrosis: Fibrosis is the medical term for scar tissue in the liver. Fibrosis is caused by infection, inflammation, or injury. It prevents the liver from working well. Alcohol damages the liver, causing more fibrosis. In a person with hepatitis C, the damage caused by alcohol is even greater. Fibrosis eventually can lead to severe scarring (cirrhosis), especially when a person drinks heavily.

Alcohol and cirrhosis: Cirrhosis is severe scarring of the liver and is the end result of damage to liver cells. Cirrhosis can be caused by many things, including viral hepatitis or alcohol, or both. Alcohol increases the damage done to the liver and speeds up the development of cirrhosis. Light drinkers or non-drinkers with hepatitis C (on average) have only moderate liver scarring, even up to 40 years after infection. Heavy drinkers—those who drink five or more drinks per day—develop

216

scar tissue in their liver much more quickly. After about 25 years of hepatitis C infection, heavy drinkers show more than twice the scarring of light drinkers or non-drinkers. After 40 years of infection and heavy drinking, most heavy drinkers have developed cirrhosis.

The chances of a person getting cirrhosis are increased by the combination of hepatitis C and alcohol. A heavy drinker with hepatitis C has 16 times the risk of cirrhosis that a non-drinker with hepatitis C has.

Alcohol use and viral load: The phrase viral load refers to the amount of a virus in the bloodstream. In this case, the virus is hepatitis C. The more drinks a person has per week, the more virus he or she will tend to have. Heavy alcohol use weakens the immune system, so the more you drink, the fewer resources you have to fight the hepatitis C virus. Alcohol is processed and broken down in the liver, so the harder the liver has to work to process alcohol, the more freedom the virus has to do damage.

Alcohol use and response to treatment: People who drink do not do as well on antiviral treatment as non-drinkers. A period of not drinking prior to treatment greatly increases the odds of treatment being effective. People who do not drink prior to starting antiviral treatment tend to have better response rates than people who do drink.

In one study, researchers found that people who drank infrequently or not at all responded to antiviral treatment three times more often than heavy drinkers. Of 20 people who drank heavily prior to treatment, only two people cleared the virus. Drinkers may be more likely to have trouble sticking with antiviral treatment as prescribed.

At present, no one knows if there is a safe level of alcohol for people with hepatitis C. The best advice is to not drink alcohol at all. This may be the hardest thing for you to do. If you drink more than two drinks in a day, or regularly drink six or seven days a week, it's important to take steps to reduce how much you drink, until you can give up alcohol altogether.

There are resources to help you stop such as change plans, an alcohol drinking diary, reducing alcohol availability and consumption levels, drinking slowly, and declining drinks. Also, staying active, getting support, and avoiding people, places, or times that make you drink will help you reduce or avoid alcohol.

Section 21.5

Nutrition Therapy in Alcoholic Liver Disease

Text in this section is excerpted from "The Role of Nutritional Therapy
in Alcoholic Liver Disease," National Institute on Alcohol Abuse and
Alcoholism (NIAAA), 2006.

The study of malnutrition in patients with alcoholic liver disease
(ALD) is based on several general concepts and observations. Researchers and clinicians previously believed that malnutrition was the primary
cause of liver injury in ALD rather than the consequence of excessive
alcohol consumption. This view was based on the prevalence of malnutrition in alcoholics and those with clinical evidence of liver (hepatic) dysfunction resulting from alcohol consumption. It now is widely accepted
that the quantity and duration of alcohol consumption are the principal
agents in the development of alcoholic liver injury. This is based on animal and human data showing that ALD can develop in well-nourished
individuals who consume large amounts of alcohol. However, a great deal
of variability exists regarding the individual development of progressive
alcoholic liver injury. Although more than 90% of people with excessive
alcohol consumption will develop fatty liver (defined as greater than
5% fat in the liver), only up to 35% will develop inflammation of the
liver caused by alcohol (alcoholic hepatitis) and only 20% will progress
to scarring of the liver (cirrhosis). Clearly, other risk factors, including
genetic predisposition, obesity, concomitant viral hepatitis infection, and
poor nutrition, may contribute variably to the development of ALD.

Indeed, in a large study of hospitalized patients with varying severity of ALD, malnutrition (especially the type caused by deficient protein
and calories) was closely associated (although not necessarily causal)
with the severity of liver injury. All patients with clinical evidence of
ALD (regardless of severity) exhibited some features of malnutrition.
With regard to the possible value of nutritional therapy, it would seem
logical that patients with more severe deficits would benefit more,
although convincing proof of this, to our knowledge, is not available.

Basis for malnutrition in ALD: The signs and symptoms of nutritional deficits in ALD patients have been well characterized and
include muscle wasting, decreased lean body mass, various vitamin

deficiencies, and decreased measurable serum proteins. A complete description of specific nutritional deficits is beyond the scope of this review; however, it is important to consider the factors that contribute to malnutrition in individuals with ALD, as they may have an influence on the administration of nutritional therapy. There are many reasons for the deficits and abnormalities that occur as a result of malnutrition. These include decreased dietary intake and poor absorption and digestion of nutrients.

Role of malnutrition in ALD: It is not precisely known how alcohol causes liver damage. The net effect of nutrition on the development of ALD may involve multiple factors, including free-radical damage and increased risk of infection.

Conclusion: It is obvious that nutrition plays some part in ALD given the prevalence of malnutrition, especially of the protein-calorie type. The malnutrition usually is associated with disease seen in hospitalized patients and correlates with the severity of ALD. The primary, established therapy for ALD consists of abstinence from alcohol. Good nutrition improves nitrogen balance, may improve liver tests, and may decrease hepatic fat accumulation, but generally it does not enhance survival. This suggests that adequate nutrition is beneficial when administered with other forms of treatment but is not sufficient therapy by itself. It has been suggested that sufficient nutritional repletion coupled with other treatment modalities may be effective in reducing complications associated with ALD—particularly infection.

Optimal nutrition requires adequate protein calories and vitamins. Ideally, the patient should receive adequate nutrition orally or through a feeding tube. This may require a feeding tube that goes through the nose to the stomach (nasogastric) or, if that is not possible, intravenous nourishment. Administration of nutritional therapy (amino acids/nitrogen) is tolerated well with little adverse effect in patients with ALD. There apparently is no problem with the precipitation of hepatic encephalopathy. Specific nutrients, although generally innocuous and well tolerated, require further evaluation. Overall, nutrition is not a panacea in the treatment of ALD, but it makes a significant positive contribution, especially in selected malnourished patients.

Chapter 22

Alcohol and Cardiovascular Disease

Chapter Contents

Section 22.1

Alcohol, Wine, and Cardiovascular Disease

This section includes: "Alcohol, Wine, and Cardiovascular Disease" and "Women who drink moderately may have lower risk of cardiovascular disease," reprinted with permission. © 2009 American Heart Association, Inc. (www.americanheart.org).

Are there cardiovascular risks associated with drinking alcohol?

Drinking too much alcohol can raise the levels of some fats in the blood (triglycerides) (tri-GLIS'er-idz). It can also lead to high blood pressure, heart failure and an increased calorie intake. (Consuming too many calories can lead to obesity and a higher risk of developing diabetes.) Excessive drinking and binge drinking can lead to stroke. Other serious problems include fetal alcohol syndrome, cardiomyopathy (karde-o-mi-OP'ah-the), cardiac arrhythmia (ah-RITH'me-ah), and sudden cardiac death.

American Heart Association Recommendation

If you drink alcohol, do so in moderation. This means an average of one to two drinks per day for men and one drink per day for women. (A drink is one 12 ounce (oz.) beer, 4 oz. of wine, 1.5 oz. of 80-proof spirits, or 1 oz. of 100-proof spirits.) Drinking more alcohol increases such dangers as alcoholism, high blood pressure, obesity, stroke, breast cancer, suicide, and accidents. Also, it's not possible to predict in which people alcoholism will become a problem. Given these and other risks, the American Heart Association cautions people not to start drinking if they do not already drink alcohol. Consult your doctor on the benefits and risks of consuming alcohol in moderation.

What about red wine and heart disease?

Over the past several decades, many studies have been published in science journals about how drinking alcohol may be associated with reduced mortality due to heart disease in some populations. Some researchers have suggested that the benefit may be due to wine, especially red wine. Others are examining the potential benefits of components in red wine such as flavonoids (FLAV'oh-noidz) and other antioxidants (an'tih-OK'sih-dants) in reducing heart disease risk. Some of these components may be found in other foods such as grapes or red grape juice. The linkage reported in many of these studies may be due to other lifestyle factors rather than alcohol. Such factors may include increased physical activity, and a diet high in fruits and vegetables and lower in saturated fats. No direct comparison trials have been done to determine the specific effect of wine or other alcohol on the risk of developing heart disease or stroke.

Are there potential benefits of drinking wine or other alcoholic beverages?

Research is being done to find out what the apparent benefits of drinking wine or alcohol in some populations may be due to, including the role of antioxidants, an increase in high density lipoprotein (HDL) (good) cholesterol or anti-clotting properties. Clinical trials of other antioxidants such as vitamin E have not shown any cardio-protective effect. Also, even if they were protective, antioxidants can be obtained from many fruits and vegetables, including red grape juice.

The best-known effect of alcohol is a small increase in HDL cholesterol. However, regular physical activity is another effective way to raise HDL cholesterol, and niacin can be prescribed to raise it to a greater degree. Alcohol or some substances such as resveratrol (res-VAIR'ah-trol) found in alcoholic beverages may prevent platelets in the blood from sticking together. That may reduce clot formation and reduce the risk of heart attack or stroke. (Aspirin may help reduce blood clotting in a similar way.) How alcohol or wine affects cardiovascular risk merits further research, but right now the American Heart Association does not recommend drinking wine or any other form of alcohol to gain these potential benefits. The AHA does recommend that to reduce your risk you should talk to your doctor about lowering your cholesterol and blood pressure, controlling your weight, getting enough physical activity, and following a healthy diet. There is no scientific proof that drinking wine or any other alcoholic beverage can replace these conventional measures.

What about alcohol and pregnancy?

Pregnant women shouldn't drink alcohol in any form. It can harm the baby seriously, including causing birth defects.

What about alcohol and aspirin?

There is a risk of stomach problems, including stomach bleeding, for people who take aspirin regularly. Alcohol use can increase these stomach risks, so ask your doctor if it is safe for you to drink alcohol in moderation.

Women Who Drink Moderately May Have Lower Risk of Cardiovascular Disease

Study highlights:

- Half to one drink a day was associated with a 26% lower risk of cardiovascular disease in women.

- An increase in high-density lipoproteins (HDL), the good cholesterol, and improved glucose metabolism were the most significant contributors to lowering risk.

- Moderate drinking resulted in a 35% decrease in total death rate and a 51% decrease in cardiovascular death rate, but wasn't as easily explained by these factors.

Women who drink moderately may have a lower risk of cardiovascular disease (CVD) and death from CVD in part because of how alcohol affects the body's processing of fats and sugar in the blood, researchers report in *Circulation: Journal of the American Heart Association*.

In an analysis of data from the Women's Health Study, researchers compared non-drinkers to moderate drinkers and found that an intake of one-half to one drink a day was associated with:

- 26% lower risk of CVD;

- 35% decrease in total mortality; and

- 51% decrease in CVD mortality.

CVD is a term that encompasses all diseases of the heart and blood vessels, including stroke and was defined in this study as a presence of heart attack, coronary bypass or angioplasty, stroke, or death from any of these conditions.

Moderate drinking was defined as 5–14.9 grams of alcohol a day—one-half to one drink. However, the risk of CVD among women consuming 15–30 grams of alcohol a day (more than one but no more than two drinks a day) was not significantly different from the risk of CVD among non-drinkers.

"Our data show that beyond one drink a day there isn't any benefit," said Luc Djoussé, MD, DSc, lead author of the study, assistant professor of medicine at Harvard University and associate epidemiologist at Brigham and Women's Hospital and Veterans Affairs Healthcare System in Boston, Massachusetts.

The effect of alcohol on blood fat was the most significant contributor to lowering the risk of CVD. It explained almost 29% of the lowered risk. Alcohol's effects on glucose metabolism accounted for about 25% of the lowered risk.

The effects of moderate drinking on inflammatory/hemostatic factors and blood pressure had a negligible contribution to the reduction in CVD risk, accounting for 5% and 4.6% respectively. These mediating factors explained 86.3% of the lower risk of CVD, but only about 19% of total mortality and 22% of CVD mortality.

"The findings add to a large body of evidence showing that moderate drinking favorably affects lipids and glucose metabolism, and thus contributes to a lower risk of cardiovascular disease in women," Djoussé said.

"The American Heart Association suggests a limit of one drink per day for women who already drink alcohol," said Jennifer H. Mieres, MD, spokesperson for the association's Go Red For Women campaign and director of Nuclear Cardiology at New York University. "However, those who do not currently drink alcohol don't need to start drinking to prevent cardiovascular disease. As the study's authors point out, alcohol can raise the risk of breast cancer, high blood pressure, and alcohol abuse. There are many ways women can lower their risk of cardiovascular disease."

Alcohol intake was strongly related to higher levels of high-density lipoproteins (HDL), the good cholesterol, as seen in previous studies, Djoussé said. "It may be that moderate drinking improves fat and muscle cells' ability to absorb glucose and may improve the levels of adiponectin, a hormone known to lower the risk of diabetes."

The effects of moderate drinking on inflammatory and hemostatic factors as well as blood pressure were minimal in explaining the lower risk of CVD in moderate drinkers, he said. "Drinking alcohol can be a double-edged sword, as alcohol can raise blood pressure."

During follow-up of more than 12 years, 1,039 CVD events, 785 confirmed total deaths and 153 CVD deaths occurred. The lowest CVD risk was in women who consumed 5–14.9 grams—or about one-half to one drink of alcohol a day.

Similarly, researchers found a relationship between alcohol consumption and total and CVD mortality, with the largest effect observed in women consuming half to one drink a day. However, no single factor explained most of the reduction in mortality.

"Even when putting all the factors together, only about 20% of the reduction in mortality was explained by the effects of moderate drinking on lipids, glucose metabolism, blood pressure, and inflammation/hemostatic factors," Djoussé said. Besides limiting alcohol to no more than one drink a day—due to the potential increased risk of breast cancer—"women should also stop smoking, eat a healthy diet, maintain a normal weight, and exercise," he said.

Section 22.2

Blood Pressure and Alcohol

This section includes an excerpt from "High Blood Pressure and Kidney Disease," National Institute of Diabetes and Digestive and Kidney Diseases (NIDDK), July 2008; and an excerpt from "Your Guide to Lowering High Blood Pressure," National Heart, Lung, and Blood Institute (NHLBI), November 2008.

Blood Pressure

Blood pressure measures the force of blood against the walls of the blood vessels. Extra fluid in the body increases the amount of fluid in blood vessels and makes blood pressure higher. Narrow, stiff, or clogged blood vessels also raise blood pressure. Hypertension can result from too much fluid in normal blood vessels or from normal fluid in narrow, stiff, or clogged blood vessels.

Most people with high blood pressure have no symptoms. The only way to know whether a person's blood pressure is high is to have a health professional measure it with a blood pressure cuff. The result is expressed as two numbers. The top number, called the systolic pressure, represents the pressure when the heart is beating. The bottom number, called the diastolic pressure, shows the pressure when the heart is resting between beats. A person's blood pressure is considered normal if it stays at or below 120/80, which is commonly stated as 120 over 80. People with a systolic blood pressure of 120 to 139 or a diastolic blood pressure of 80 to 89 are considered prehypertensive and should adopt lifestyle changes to lower their blood pressure and prevent heart and blood vessel diseases. A person whose systolic blood pressure is consistently 140 or higher or whose diastolic pressure is 90 or higher is considered to have high blood pressure and should talk with a doctor about the best ways to lower it.

Limit Alcohol Intake

Drinking too much alcohol can raise blood pressure. It also can harm the liver, brain, and heart. Alcoholic drinks also contain calories, which matter if you are trying to lose weight. If you drink alcoholic beverages, have only a moderate amount—one drink a day for women; two drinks a day for men.

Section 22.3

Cardiomyopathy

"Cardiomyopathy," reprinted with permission. © 2009 American Heart Association, Inc. (www.americanheart.org).

Editor's note: Alcohol use is one cause of cardiomyopathy. Consult your healthcare provider for guidance concerning alcohol use.

What is cardiomyopathy?

Cardiomyopathy is a serious disease in which the heart muscle becomes inflamed and doesn't work as well as it should. There may be multiple causes including viral infections.

Cardiomyopathy can be classified as primary or secondary. Primary cardiomyopathy can't be attributed to a specific cause, such as high blood pressure, heart valve disease, artery diseases, or congenital heart defects. Secondary cardiomyopathy is due to specific causes. It's often associated with diseases involving other organs as well as the heart. There are three main types of cardiomyopathy: dilated, hypertrophic, and restrictive.

What is dilated (congestive) cardiomyopathy?

This is the most common form. In it, the heart cavity is enlarged and stretched (cardiac dilation). The heart is weak and doesn't pump normally, and most patients develop heart failure. Abnormal heart rhythms called arrhythmias and disturbances in the heart's electrical conduction also may occur.

Blood flows more slowly through an enlarged heart, so blood clots may form. A blood clot that forms in an artery or the heart is called a thrombus. A clot that breaks free, circulates in the bloodstream, and blocks a small blood vessel is called an embolus.

- Clots that stick to the inner lining of the heart are called mural thrombi.

- If the clot breaks off the right ventricle (pumping chamber), it can be carried into the pulmonary circulation in the lung, forming pulmonary emboli.

- Blood clots that form in the heart's left side may be dislodged and carried into the body's circulation to form cerebral emboli in the brain, renal emboli in the kidney, peripheral emboli, or even coronary artery emboli.

A condition known as Barth syndrome, a rare and relatively unknown genetically linked cardiac disease, can cause dilated cardiomyopathy. This syndrome affects male children, usually during their first year of life. It can also be diagnosed later. In these young patients the heart condition is often associated with changes in the skeletal muscles, short stature, and an increased likelihood of catching bacterial infections. They also have neutropenia, which is a decrease in the number of white blood cells known as neutrophils. There are clinical signs of the cardiomyopathy in the newborn child or within the first months of life. These children also have metabolic and mitochondrial abnormalities.

How is dilated (congestive) cardiomyopathy treated?

A person with cardiomyopathy may suffer an embolus before any other symptom of cardiomyopathy appears. That's why anti-clotting (anticoagulant) drug therapy may be needed. Arrhythmias may require antiarrhythmic drugs. Therapy for dilated cardiomyopathy is often aimed at treating the underlying cause, however. If the person is young and otherwise healthy, and if the disease gets worse, a heart transplant may be considered.

When cardiomyopathy results in a significantly enlarged heart, the mitral and tricuspid valves may not be able to close properly, resulting in murmurs. Blood pressure may increase because of increased sympathetic nerve activity. These nerves can also cause arteries to narrow. This mimics hypertensive heart disease (high blood pressure). That's why some people have high blood pressure readings. Because the blood pressure determines the heart's workload and oxygen needs, one treatment approach is to use vasodilators (drugs that "relax" the arteries). They lower blood pressure and thus the left ventricle's workload.

What is hypertrophic cardiomyopathy?

In this condition, the muscle mass of the left ventricle enlarges or "hypertrophies." In one form of the disease, the wall (septum) between the two ventricles (pumping chamber) becomes enlarged and obstructs the blood flow from the left ventricle. The syndrome is known as hypertrophic obstructive cardiomyopathy (HOCM) or asymmetric septal hypertrophy (ASH). It's also called idiopathic hypertrophic subaortic stenosis (IHSS).

Besides obstructing blood flow, the thickened wall sometimes distorts one leaflet of the mitral valve, causing it to leak. Hypertrophic cardiomyopathy is the most common inherited heart defect, occurring in one of 500 individuals. Close blood relatives (parents, children or siblings) of such persons often have enlarged septums, although they may have no symptoms. This disease is most common in young adults.

In the other form of the disease, non-obstructive hypertrophic cardiomyopathy, the enlarged muscle doesn't obstruct blood flow. The symptoms of hypertrophic cardiomyopathy include shortness of breath on exertion, dizziness, fainting, and angina pectoris. (Angina is chest pain or discomfort caused by reduced blood supply to the heart muscle.) Some people have cardiac arrhythmias. These are abnormal heart rhythms that in some cases can lead to sudden death. Often an implanted cardioverter defibrillator (ICD) is needed to shock the heart to restart a normal heart rhythm and prevent sudden death. The obstruction to blood flow from the left ventricle increases the ventricle's work, and a heart murmur may be heard.

How is hypertrophic cardiomyopathy treated?

The usual treatment involves taking a drug known as a beta blocker (such as propranolol) or a calcium channel blocker. If a person has an arrhythmia, an antiarrhythmic drug may also be used. Surgical treatment of the obstructive form is possible in some cases if the drug treatment fails.

Alcohol ablation is a type of nonsurgical treatment for hypertrophic obstructive cardiomyopathy. It involves injecting alcohol down a small branch of one of the heart arteries to deaden the extra heart muscle. This allows the extra heart muscle to thin out without having to cut it out surgically.

What is restrictive cardiomyopathy?

This is the least common type in the United States. The myocardium (heart muscle) of the ventricles becomes excessively "rigid," so it's harder for the ventricles to fill with blood between heartbeats. A person with restrictive cardiomyopathy often complains of being tired, may have swollen hands and feet, and may have difficulty breathing on exertion. This type of cardiomyopathy is usually seen in the elderly and may be due to another disease process.

Chapter 23

Alcoholic Neuropathy

Alcoholic neuropathy is damage to the nerves that results from excessive drinking of alcohol.

The cause of alcoholic neuropathy is debated. It probably includes both a direct poisoning of the nerve by the alcohol, and the effect of poor nutrition associated with alcoholism. In severe cases, the nerves that regulate internal body functions (autonomic nerves) may be involved. Risks for alcoholic neuropathy include long-term heavy alcohol use and alcoholism that is present for ten years or more.

Symptoms

- Numbness in the arms and legs
- Abnormal sensations—"pins and needles"
- Painful sensations in the arms and legs
- Muscle weakness
- Muscle cramps or muscle aches
- Heat intolerance, especially after exercise
- Impotence (in men)
- Problems urinating
  - Incontinence (leaking urine)
  - Feeling of incomplete bladder emptying

"Alcoholic Neuropathy," © 2010 A.D.A.M., Inc. Reprinted with permission.

- Difficulty beginning to urinate
- Constipation
- Diarrhea
- Nausea, vomiting

Additional symptoms that may occur with this disease:

- Swallowing difficulty
- Speech impairment
- Loss of muscle function or feeling
- Muscle contractions or spasm
- Muscle atrophy
- Problems with movements

Note: Changes in muscle strength or sensation usually occur on both sides of the body and are more common in the legs than in the arms. Symptoms usually develop gradually and slowly become worse over time.

Exams and Tests

Your doctor will get an extensive description of the problem and will perform a neurological exam. Signs may include weakness, numbness to touch, and loss of reflexes (such as the knee jerk). Neurological problems usually affect both sides of the body in this condition.

An eye exam may show decreased pupil response or other problem. Blood pressure may fall when you stand up.

Alcoholism often causes nutritional deficiency. This is because people drink excessively instead of eating properly, and because some vitamins and minerals are used up or lost due to the alcohol. Nutritional studies may show the following deficiencies:

- Thiamine (vitamin B1)
- Pyridoxine (vitamin B6)
- Pantothenic acid and biotin
- Vitamin B12
- Folic acid
- Niacin (vitamin B3)
- Vitamin A

Additional tests may be done to rule out other possible causes of neuropathy. Tests may include the following:

- Serum electrolyte levels
- Studies of kidney and liver function
- Thyroid function tests
- Levels of vitamins and minerals in the body
- Nerve conduction tests
- Electromyography (EMG)
- Nerve biopsy
- Upper GI and small bowel series
- Esophagogastroduodenoscopy (EGD)
- Isotope studies of gastrointestinal function
- Voiding cystourethrogram

Treatment

Once the immediate alcohol problem has been addressed, treatment goals include: controlling symptoms, maximizing ability to function independently, and preventing injury.

It is important to supplement the diet with vitamins, including thiamine and folic acid.

Physical therapy and orthopedic appliances (such as splints) may be needed to maximize muscle function and maintain limb position.

Patients may take medication, if necessary, to treat pain or uncomfortable sensations. The response to medications varies. Patients are advised to take the least amount of medication needed to reduce symptoms, to help prevent drug dependence and other side effects of chronic use.

Common medications may include over-the-counter analgesics such as aspirin, ibuprofen, or acetaminophen to reduce pain. Tricyclic antidepressants or anticonvulsant medications such as phenytoin, gabapentin, or carbamazepine may help stabbing pains.

Positioning, or the use of a bed frame that keeps the covers off the legs, may reduce pain for some people.

Some people may need to treat blood pressure problems, difficulty with urination, and slow gastrointestinal movement.

Light-headedness or dizziness when standing up (orthostatic hypotension) may require several different treatments before you find one that successfully reduces symptoms. Treatments that may help include:

- wearing elastic stockings,

- eating extra salt,

- sleeping with the head elevated, and

- using medications such as fludrocortisones.

Bladder dysfunction may be treated with:

- manual expression of urine,

- intermittent catheterization, and

- medications such as bethanechol.

Impotence, diarrhea, constipation, or other symptoms are treated when necessary. These symptoms often respond poorly to treatment in people with alcoholic neuropathy.

It is important to protect body parts with reduced sensation from injury. This may include these actions:

- Checking the temperature of bath water to prevent burns

- Changing footwear

- Frequently inspecting the feet and shoes to reduce injury caused by pressure or objects in the shoes

- Guarding the extremities to prevent injury from pressure

Stop using alcohol to prevent the damage from getting worse. Treatment for alcoholism may include psychiatric therapy social support such as Alcoholics Anonymous (AA), medications, and behavior modification.

Outlook (Prognosis)

Damage to nerves from alcoholic neuropathy is usually permanent and may get worse if you continue to use alcohol or do not correct nutritional problems. Symptoms vary from mild discomfort to severe disability. The disorder is usually not life-threatening, but it may severely affect your quality of life.

Possible complications:

- Disability

- Long-term (chronic) discomfort or pain

- Injury to extremities

When to contact a medical professional: Call for an appointment with your health care provider if you have symptoms of alcoholic neuropathy.

Prevention: Avoid or minimize alcohol use. Avoiding alcohol entirely is the safest treatment for persons with alcoholism.

Alternative names: Neuropathy–alcoholic; alcoholic polyneuropathy

Reference: Shy ME. Peripheral neuropathies. In: Goldman L, Ausiello D, eds. *Cecil Medicine. 23rd ed.* Philadelphia, Pa: Saunders Elsevier; 2007:chap 446.

Chapter 24

Alcoholic Lung Disease

Although alcohol abuse has been known for centuries to increase the risk for lung infection (pneumonia), it only recently has been recognized that alcohol increases the risk of acute lung injury following major trauma, such as a serious motor vehicle accident, gunshot, or other event requiring hospitalization, or the spread of bacteria attributed to infection (sepsis). Recent advances in the understanding of alcohol's effects on both structural and immunological aspects of the lung are bringing to light the precise mechanisms by which alcoholics are predisposed to both pneumonia and acute lung injury. The well-known acute intoxicating effects of alcohol and the attendant risk of secretions or foreign material entering into the trachea and lungs (aspiration) are components in the development of alcohol-associated lung (pulmonary) disease. In the past decade, clinical and experimental evidence has emerged that implicates a chronic damaging chemical imbalance in the cell (oxidative stress) and consequent cellular dysfunction within the layer of tissue lining the airway (airway epithelium) as well as pathogen-ingesting white blood cells (macrophages) in the airway. Moreover, now it is recognized that these disruptions in lung function can occur even in young and otherwise healthy individuals long before they develop clinically apparent signs of alcoholic liver disease and/or other end-stage manifestations of longstanding alcohol abuse. Based on these recent studies, the concept of the alcoholic lung is emerging,

---

Text in this chapter is excerpted from "Alcoholic Lung Disease," National Institute on Alcohol Abuse and Alcoholism (NIAAA), 2008.

which is characterized by severe oxidative stress that alone may not cause detectable lung impairment but may predispose those who are dependent on or abuse alcohol to severe lung injury if they are unfortunate enough to suffer serious trauma or other acute illnesses.

Alcohol Abuse and Pneumonia

For over a century, alcohol abuse has been well recognized as a significant risk factor for serious pulmonary infections. For example, alcoholic patients are at increased risk for infection with tissue-damaging gram-negative pathogens, such as *Klebsiella pneumoniae*, or for the spread of bacteria in the blood and shock from typical pathogens, most notably *Streptococcus pneumoniae*. Importantly, alcoholics also are at increased risk for infections with *Mycobacterium tuberculosis*.

The impact of alcohol abuse on morbidity and mortality among patients with community-acquired pneumonia is substantial. For example, a study examining the outcomes of alcoholic patients hospitalized for community-acquired pneumonia over a three-year period found that the mortality in this group of patients was 64.3%, which was much higher than the predicted death rate for hospitalized patients (approximately 20%). Another fatal association between alcohol abuse and pneumonia was identified in a retrospective review of patients admitted with pneumococcal bacteremia that examined a subset with alcoholism and low white blood cell count (leukopenia). Ninety-three patients with pneumococcal bacteremia were identified, 12 of whom had a history of alcohol abuse and a white blood cell count of less than 4,000 cells per cubic millimeter (mm^3) of blood. Ten of these 12 (83.3%) patients died, whereas the mortality in the rest of the cohort was only 22%. Overall, these and other studies demonstrate the association between alcohol abuse and community-acquired pneumonia, an association that results in more severe infections and higher mortality.

Alcohol Abuse and Acute Lung Injury

Alcohol abuse increases the risk for acute lung injury and acute respiratory distress syndrome (ARDS). ARDS is characterized by a severe deficiency of oxygen in the bloodstream caused by alveolar inflammation (the accumulation of fluid in the airspaces) in both lungs that cannot be explained by heart failure (noncardiogenic pulmonary edema). Until recently, ARDS was associated with a very high mortality, ranging from 31%–74% in various studies. Unfortunately, despite four decades of laboratory-based and clinical research, no effective pharmacological treatments have been identified.

Although there are a number of diseases and conditions that can lead to ARDS—pneumonia, sepsis, trauma, and aspiration can account for up to 85% of cases—only a minority (approximately 30%) of these at-risk individuals go on to develop ARDS. For decades there was no explanation as to why some at-risk patients develop the syndrome and others do not. Just over ten years ago, alcohol abuse emerged as the only independent risk factor known to increase the odds of any given at-risk individual developing ARDS. The first study to identify this association examined 351 critically ill patients at high risk for developing ARDS. The incidence of ARDS in patients with a history of alcohol abuse was 43%, compared with an incidence of 22% in nonalcoholic subjects. Further, the in-hospital mortality was 65% in alcoholic patients with ARDS, whereas the mortality among nonalcoholic patients was 36%. If these findings are extrapolated to the population at large, then alcohol abuse contributes to the development of ARDS in tens of thousands of patients in the United States each year.

In addition to increasing the risk for developing ARDS, alcohol abuse also makes it more likely that an individual will develop a critical illness that puts them at risk for ARDS in the first place. Alcoholics have increased incidences and death from trauma, an increased severity of nonpulmonary organ dysfunction in septic shock, and an increased risk for aspiration. Alcohol also is a risk factor for the development of scarring of the liver (cirrhosis), which can lead to increased pressure in the vein that carries blood to the liver (portal hypertension), and gastrointestinal hemorrhage, which may warrant multiple transfusions of blood products, another risk factor for developing ARDS.

Systems Biology and the Study of Alcoholic Lung Disease

Genetic analysis has helped to identify potential candidate genes involved in alcohol-induced lung dysfunction that might explain the newly identified association between alcohol abuse and acute lung injury in humans. Although several genes of interest were identified and pursued, the vast majority of the genes that displayed significantly altered expression in the alcohol-fed rat lung have not yet been evaluated. In fact, the full power of genomic and proteomic tools, which are used to study an organism's genes and/or proteins, only now are being applied to complex lung diseases. No known research has applied such approaches to the evaluation of the alcoholic lung in humans, but there is great promise that the rapidly evolving tools of systems biology will accelerate the pace at which researchers are discovering how alcohol abuse produces such devastating lung damage.

Chapter 25

Alcohol Abuse Affects Bone Health

Chapter Contents

Section 25.1

The Link between Alcohol and Osteoporosis

Text in this section is excerpted from "What People Recovering from Alcoholism Need to Know about Osteoporosis," National Institute of Arthritis and Musculoskeletal and Skin Diseases (NIAMS), January 2009.

Osteoporosis is a condition in which bones become less dense and more likely to fracture. Fractures from osteoporosis can result in significant pain and disability. Osteoporosis is a major health threat for an estimated 44 million Americans, 68% of whom are women.

Risk factors for developing osteoporosis include:

- thinness or small frame,
- family history of the disease,
- being postmenopausal and particularly having had early menopause,
- abnormal absence of menstrual periods (amenorrhea),
- prolonged use of certain medications, such as those used to treat lupus, asthma, thyroid deficiencies, and seizures,
- low calcium intake,
- lack of physical activity,
- smoking, and
- excessive alcohol intake.

Osteoporosis often can be prevented. It is known as a silent disease because, if undetected, bone loss can progress for many years without symptoms until a fracture occurs. Osteoporosis has been called a childhood disease with old age consequences because building healthy bones in one's youth helps prevent osteoporosis and fractures later in life. However, it is never too late to adopt new habits for healthy bones.

Alcohol negatively affects bone health for several reasons. To begin with, excessive alcohol interferes with the balance of calcium, an essential nutrient for healthy bones. It also increases parathyroid hormone levels, which in turn reduce the body's calcium reserves. Calcium balance is further disrupted by alcohol's ability to interfere with the production of vitamin D, a vitamin essential for calcium absorption.

In addition, chronic heavy drinking can cause hormone deficiencies in men and women. Men with alcoholism tend to produce less testosterone, a hormone linked to the production of osteoblasts (the cells that stimulate bone formation). In women, chronic alcohol exposure often produces irregular menstrual cycles, a factor that reduces estrogen levels, increasing the risk for osteoporosis. Also, cortisol levels tend to be elevated in people with alcoholism. Cortisol is known to decrease bone formation and increase bone breakdown.

Because of the effects of alcohol on balance and gait, people with alcoholism tend to fall more frequently than those without the disorder. Heavy alcohol consumption has been linked to an increase in the risk of fracture, including the most serious kind—hip fracture. Vertebral fractures are also more common in those who abuse alcohol.

Osteoporosis Management Strategies

The most effective strategy for alcohol-induced bone loss is abstinence. People with alcoholism who abstain from drinking tend to have a rapid recovery of osteoblastic (bone-building) activity. Some studies have even found that lost bone can be partially restored when alcohol abuse ends.

Nutrition: Because of the negative nutritional effects of chronic alcohol use, people recovering from alcoholism should make healthy nutritional habits a top priority. As far as bone health is concerned, a well-balanced diet rich in calcium and vitamin D is critical. Good sources of calcium include low-fat dairy products; dark green, leafy vegetables; and calcium-fortified foods and beverages. Supplements can help ensure that you get adequate amounts of calcium each day, especially in people with a proven milk allergy.

Vitamin D plays an important role in calcium absorption and bone health. It is synthesized in the skin through exposure to sunlight. Food sources of vitamin D include egg yolks, saltwater fish, and liver. Many people obtain enough vitamin D by getting about 15 minutes of sunlight each day; others, especially those who are older or housebound, may need vitamin D supplements.

Exercise: Like muscle, bone is living tissue that responds to exercise by becoming stronger. The best exercise for your bones is weight-bearing exercise that forces you to work against gravity. Regular exercise, such as walking, may help prevent bone loss and will provide many other health benefits.

Healthy lifestyle: Smoking is bad for bones as well as the heart and lungs. Women who smoke tend to go through menopause earlier, resulting in earlier reduction in levels of the bone-preserving hormone estrogen and triggering earlier bone loss. In addition, smokers may absorb less calcium from their diets. Studies suggest that in people recovering from alcoholism, smoking cessation may actually enhance abstinence from drinking. Many suspect that smokers who abuse alcohol tend to be more dependent on nicotine than those who don't; therefore, a formal smoking cessation program may be a worthwhile investment for individuals in recovery.

Bone density test: A bone mineral density (BMD) test measures bone density in various parts of the body. This safe and painless test can detect osteoporosis before a fracture occurs and can predict one's chances of fracturing in the future. The BMD test can help determine whether medication should be considered. Individuals in recovery are encouraged to talk to their health care providers about whether they might be candidates for a BMD test.

Medication: There is no cure for osteoporosis. However, medications are available to prevent and treat osteoporosis. The Food and Drug Administration has approved several medications for the prevention and/or treatment of osteoporosis.

Section 25.2

Excessive Alcohol Intake Is a Risk Factor for Osteonecrosis

Text in this section is excerpted from "Questions and Answers about Osteonecrosis (Avascular Necrosis)," National Institute of Arthritis and Musculoskeletal and Skin Diseases (NIAMS), June 2009.

Osteonecrosis is a disease resulting from the temporary or permanent loss of blood supply to the bones. Without blood, the bone tissue dies, and ultimately the bone may collapse. If the process involves the bones near a joint, it often leads to collapse of the joint surface. Osteonecrosis is also known as avascular necrosis, aseptic necrosis, and ischemic necrosis. According to the American Academy of Orthopaedic Surgeons, 10,000 to 20,000 people develop osteonecrosis each year.

Although it can happen in any bone, osteonecrosis most commonly affects the ends (epiphysis) of the femur, the bone extending from the knee joint to the hip joint. Other common sites include the upper arm bone, knees, shoulders, and ankles. The disease may affect just one bone, more than one bone at the same time, or more than one bone at different times. Osteonecrosis of the jaw (ONJ) is a rare condition that has recently been linked to the use of bisphosphonate medications. ONJ has different causes and treatments than osteonecrosis found in other parts of the skeleton.

The amount of disability that results from osteonecrosis depends on what part of the bone is affected, how large an area is involved, and how effectively the bone rebuilds itself. Normally, bone continuously breaks down and rebuilds—old bone is replaced with new bone. This process, which takes place after an injury as well as during normal growth, keeps the skeleton strong and helps it to maintain a balance of minerals. In the course of osteonecrosis, however, the healing process is usually ineffective and the bone tissues break down faster than the body can repair them. If left untreated, the disease progresses, the bone collapses, and the joint surface breaks down, leading to pain and arthritis.

Causes: Osteonecrosis is caused by impaired blood supply to the bone, but it is not always clear what causes that impairment.

245

Osteonecrosis often occurs in people with certain medical conditions or risk factors (such as high-dose corticosteroid use or excessive alcohol intake). However, it also affects people with no health problems and for no known reason. Following are some potential causes of osteonecrosis and other health conditions associated with its development.

Excessive alcohol use is common cause of osteonecrosis. People who drink alcohol in excess can develop fatty substances that may block blood vessels, causing a decreased blood supply to the bones. Also, steroid medications, injury, radiation therapy, chemotherapy, and organ transplantation (particularly kidney transplantation) can cause osteonecrosis.

Symptoms: In the early stages of osteonecrosis, people may not have any symptoms. As the disease progresses, however, most experience joint pain. At first, the pain occurs only when putting weight on the affected joint. Later, it occurs even when resting. Pain usually develops gradually, and may be mild or severe. If osteonecrosis progresses and the bone and surrounding joint surface collapse, pain may develop or increase dramatically. Pain may be severe enough to limit range of motion in the affected joint. In some cases, particularly those involving the hip, disabling osteoarthritis may develop. The period of time between the first symptoms and loss of joint function is different for each person, but it typically ranges from several months to more than a year.

Diagnosis: After performing a complete physical examination and asking about the patient's medical history, the doctor may use one or more bone imaging techniques to diagnose osteonecrosis. As with many other diseases, early diagnosis increases the chances of treatment success.

Treatments

Appropriate treatment for osteonecrosis is necessary to keep joints from breaking down. Without treatment, most people with the disease will experience severe pain and limitation in movement within two years. To determine the most appropriate treatment, the doctor considers the age of the patient, the stage of the disease (early or late), the location and whether bone is affected over a small or large area, the underlying cause of osteonecrosis. With an ongoing cause such as corticosteroid or alcohol use, treatment may not work unless use of the substance is stopped.

The goal in treating osteonecrosis is to improve the patient's use of the affected joint, stop further damage to the bone, and ensure bone and joint survival. To reach these goals, the doctor may use one or more of the following surgical or nonsurgical treatments.

Nonsurgical treatments: Usually, doctors will begin with non-surgical treatments, alone or in combination. Unfortunately, although these treatments may relieve pain or help in the short term, for most people they don't bring lasting improvement. Nonsurgical treatments include medications, reduced weight bearing, range-of-motion exercises, and electrical stimulation.

Surgical treatments: A number of different surgical procedures are used to treat osteonecrosis. Most people with osteonecrosis will eventually need surgery. Surgical treatments include core decompression, osteotomy, bone graft, and arthroplasty/total joint replacement.

For most people with osteonecrosis, treatment is an ongoing process. Depending upon the stage of the disease, doctors may first recommend the least complex or nonoperative treatment plans, such as medication or reduced weight bearing. If these modalities are unsuccessful, surgical treatments may be needed. It is important that patients carefully follow instructions about activity limitations and work closely with their doctors to ensure that appropriate treatments are used.

Chapter 26

Other Organs at Risk from Alcohol Abuse

Chapter Contents

Section 26.1

Alcohol and the Gastrointestinal Tract

Excerpted from "Alcohol's Role in Gastrointestinal Tract Disorders," *Alcohol Health & Research World*, Vol. 21, No. 1, 1997. National Institute on Alcohol Abuse and Alcoholism (NIAAA). The complete document with references is available at http://pubs.niaaa.nih.gov/publications/arh21-1/76 .pdf. Reviewed in May 2010, by Dr. David A. Cooke, MD, FACP, Diplomate, American Board of Internal Medicine.

Alcohol's Role in Gastrointestinal Tract Disorders

Among the many organ systems that mediate alcohol's effects on the human body and its health, the gastrointestinal (GI) tract plays a particularly important part. Several processes underlie this role. First, the GI tract is the site of alcohol absorption into the bloodstream and, to a lesser extent, of alcohol breakdown and production. Second, the direct contact of alcoholic beverages with the mucosa that lines the upper GI tract can induce numerous metabolic and functional changes. These alterations may lead to marked mucosal damage, which can result in a broad spectrum of acute and chronic diseases, such as acute gastrointestinal bleeding (from lesions in the stomach or small intestine) and diarrhea. Third, functional changes and mucosal damage in the gut disturb the digestion of other nutrients as well as their assimilation into the body, thereby contributing to the malnutrition and weight loss frequently observed in alcoholics. Fourth, alcohol-induced mucosal injuries—especially in the upper small intestine—allow large molecules, such as endotoxin and other bacterial toxins, to pass more easily into the blood or lymph. These toxic substances can have deleterious effects on the liver and other organs.

The Oral Cavity and the Esophagus

The oral cavity, pharynx, and esophagus are exposed to alcohol immediately after its ingestion. Thus, alcoholic beverages are almost undiluted when they come in contact with the mucosa of these structures. It is therefore not surprising that mucosal injuries (lesions) occur quite frequently in people who drink large amounts of alcohol.

Chronic alcohol abuse damages the salivary glands and thus interferes with saliva secretion. In alcoholics this damage commonly manifests itself as an enlargement of the parotid gland, although the mechanisms leading to this condition are unknown. Moreover, alcoholics may suffer from inflammation of the tongue and the mouth. It is unclear, however whether these changes result from poor nutrition or reflect alcohol's direct effect on the mucosa. Finally, chronic alcohol abuse increases the incidence of tooth decay, gum disease, and loss of teeth.

Alcohol consumption can affect the esophagus in several ways. For example, alcohol distinctly impairs esophageal motility, and even a single drinking episode (acute alcohol consumption) significantly weakens the lower esophageal sphincter. As a result, gastroesophageal reflux may occur, and the esophagus' ability to clear the refluxed gastric acid may be reduced. Both of these factors promote the occurrence of heartburn. Moreover, some alcoholics exhibit an abnormality of esophageal motility known as a nutcracker esophagus, which mimics symptoms of coronary heart disease.

Chronic alcohol abuse leads to an increased incidence not only of heartburn but also of esophageal mucosal inflammation (esophagitis) and other injuries that may induce mucosal defects (esophagitis with or without erosions). In addition, alcoholics make up a significant proportion of patients with Barrett's esophagus. This condition, which occurs in 10%–20% of patients with symptomatic gastroesophageal reflux disease, is characterized by changes in the cell layer lining the esophagus (the epithelium) that lead to abnormal acid production. A diagnosis of Barrett's esophagus is an important indicator of an increased risk of esophageal cancer, because in some patients the altered epithelial cells become cancerous.

Another condition affecting alcoholics is Mallory-Weiss syndrome, which is characterized by massive bleeding caused by tears in the mucosa at the junction of the esophagus and the stomach. The syndrome accounts for 5%–15% of all cases of bleeding in the upper GI tract. In 20%–50% of all patients, the disorder is caused by increased gastric pressure resulting from repeated retching and vomiting following excessive acute alcohol consumption.

The Stomach

Both acute and chronic alcohol consumption can interfere with stomach functioning in several ways. For example, alcohol—even in relatively small doses—can alter gastric acid secretion, induce acute gastric mucosal injury, and interfere with gastric and intestinal motility.

Alcoholic beverages with a low alcohol content (beer and wine) strongly increase gastric acid secretion and the release of gastrin, the gastric hormone that induces acid secretion. In contrast, beverages with a higher alcohol content (whisky and cognac) stimulate neither gastric acid secretion nor gastrin release. Chronic alcohol abuse also affects gastric function. Thus, alcoholics have a significantly higher incidence of shrinkage of the gastric mucosa and decreased gastric secretory capacity.

Acute gastric mucosal injury: Researchers have known for more than 100 years that alcohol abuse can cause mucosal inflammation. In addition, alcohol abuse is an important cause of bleeding gastric lesions that can destroy parts of the mucosa. Although low or moderate alcohol doses do not cause such damage in healthy subjects, even a single episode of heavy drinking can induce mucosal inflammation and hemorrhagic lesions. Nonsteroidal anti-inflammatory drugs (aspirin and ibuprofen) may aggravate the development of alcohol-induced acute gastric lesions.

Gastric and intestinal motility: Alcohol can interfere with the activity of the muscles surrounding the stomach and the small intestine and thus alter the transit time of food through these organs. In humans, alcohol's effect on gastric motility depends on the alcohol concentration and accompanying meals. In general, beverages with high alcohol concentrations (above 15%) appear to inhibit gastric motility and thus delay the emptying of the stomach.

In the small intestine, alcohol decreases the muscle movements that help retain the food for further digestion (the impeding wave motility). In contrast, alcohol does not affect the movements that propel food through the intestine (the propulsive wave motility) in either alcoholics or healthy subjects. These effects may contribute to the increased sensitivity to foods with a high sugar content (candy and sweetened juices), shortened transit time, and diarrhea frequently observed in alcoholics.

The Small Intestine

The small intestine is the organ in which most nutrients are absorbed into the bloodstream. Studies in humans and animals as well as in tissue culture have demonstrated that alcohol can interfere with the absorption of several nutrients. Alcohol itself, however, also is rapidly absorbed in the small intestine. In the human jejunum, for example, the alcohol concentration can drop from 10% to just 1.45% over a distance of only 30 centimeters (12 inches, about a quarter of the total length of the jejunum). Therefore, alcohol's effects on nutrient absorption may vary throughout the small intestine, and tissue-culture experiments with constant alcohol concentrations may not always reflect the conditions in the body.

Several studies in humans have analyzed the effects of chronic alcohol consumption with the following results:

- Both in healthy people and in alcoholics, chronic alcohol consumption led to markedly reduced water and sodium absorption in the jejunum and ileum.

- Alcoholics exhibited a reduced absorption of carbohydrates, proteins, and fats in the duodenum, but not in the jejunum.

- Alcoholics without confounding disorders, such as cirrhosis or impaired pancreatic function, exhibited malabsorption of fat and protein.

- Alcoholics showed malabsorption of xylose, a sugar frequently used to study the function of the digestive tract.

- After chronic alcohol consumption, the absorption of thiamine (vitamin B1), folic acid, and vitamin B12 was either unchanged or decreased. Folic acid deficiency, which frequently occurs in alcoholics, can result in various disorders of the GI tract as well as in anemia. However, this deficiency is more likely to result from a diet containing insufficient folic acid than from poor folic acid absorption.

Intestinal enzymes: Alcohol can interfere with the activity of many enzymes that are essential for intestinal functioning. One of these enzymes is lactase, which breaks down the milk sugar lactose; lactase deficiency results in lactose intolerance. Alcohol also interferes with some of the enzymes involved in transporting nutrients from the intestine into the bloodstream and inhibits important enzymes that participate in the metabolism of drugs and other foreign organic substances in the gut.

Intestinal mucosal injury: Excessive alcohol consumption frequently causes mucosal damage in the upper region of the duodenum. Even in healthy people, a single episode of heavy drinking can result in duodenal erosions and bleeding.

Intestinal permeability: Intestinal permeability was enhanced in non-intoxicated alcoholics. The enhanced permeability induced by acute and chronic alcohol ingestion could allow toxic compounds, such as endotoxin and other bacterial toxins, to enter the bloodstream and subsequently reach the liver.

Intestinal bacterial microflora: Certain bacteria that are a major source of endotoxin may overgrow the normal bacterial flora in the jejunum of alcoholics. Together with the altered permeability of the gut induced by alcohol, this process may allow an increased escape of endotoxin from the intestine into the blood vessels leading to the liver, thus increasing the liver's exposure to these toxins and, consequently, the risk of liver injury.

The large intestine: In healthy humans, alcohol administration significantly reduced the frequency and strength of the muscle contractions in a segment of the rectum. These effects could reduce the transit time—and thus the compaction—of the intestinal contents and thereby contribute to the diarrhea frequently observed in alcoholics.

Medical Consequences

Alcohol-induced digestive disorders and mucosal damage in the GI tract can cause a variety of medical problems. These include a loss of appetite and a multitude of abdominal complaints, such as nausea, vomiting, feelings of fullness, flatulence, and abdominal pain. Diseases of the liver and pancreas may contribute to and aggravate these complaints. Thus, about 50% of alcoholics with an initial stage of liver damage (fatty liver) and 30–80% of patients with an advanced stage of alcohol-induced liver injury (alcoholic hepatitis) report some symptoms of abdominal discomfort. These abdominal complaints can lead to reduced food intake, thereby causing the weight loss and malnutrition commonly observed in alcoholics.

In addition to causing abdominal complaints, alcohol plays a role in the development of cancers of the GI tract. It is likely, however, that alcohol does not cause GI-tract cancers by itself but acts in concert with other cancer-inducing agents. Alcohol abuse, like smoking, is associated with the development of cancers of the tongue, larynx (the organ of voice), and pharynx; both alcohol consumption and smoking independently increase the risk for these tumors. Epidemiological studies also strongly indicate that chronic alcohol consumption, especially of distilled spirits, markedly contributes to the development of esophageal cancer. Thus, after adjusting for smoking habits, heavy beer drinkers have a ten times greater risk and heavy whisky drinkers a 25 times greater risk of developing esophageal cancer, compared with people who consume less than 30 grams of alcohol (about two standard drinks) daily. The differences between beer and whisky drinkers remain even if they consume the same amount of pure alcohol. In drinkers who also smoke 20 cigarettes or more daily, the risk of esophageal cancer increases about 45-fold.

Heavy alcohol consumption also is associated with the development of tumors in the colon and rectum. However, the relative risk of cancer is higher for rectal cancer than for colon cancer. Moreover, the increased risk of rectal cancer appears to result mainly from heavy beer consumption, whereas distilled spirits appear to have no effect.

Section 26.2

Alcoholism: A Common Cause of Pancreatitis

Excerpted from "Pancreatitis," National Institute of Diabetes and Digestive and Kidney Diseases (NIDDK), July 2008.

Pancreatitis is inflammation of the pancreas. The pancreas is a large gland behind the stomach and close to the duodenum—the first part of the small intestine. The pancreas secretes digestive juices, or enzymes, into the duodenum through a tube called the pancreatic duct. Pancreatic enzymes join with bile—a liquid produced in the liver and stored in the gallbladder—to digest food. The pancreas also releases the hormones insulin and glucagon into the bloodstream. These hormones help the body regulate the glucose it takes from food for energy.

Normally, digestive enzymes secreted by the pancreas do not become active until they reach the small intestine. But when the pancreas is inflamed, the enzymes inside it attack and damage the tissues that produce them. Pancreatitis can be acute or chronic. Either form is serious and can lead to complications. In severe cases, bleeding, infection, and permanent tissue damage may occur. Both forms of pancreatitis occur more often in men than women.

Acute Pancreatitis

Acute pancreatitis is inflammation of the pancreas that occurs suddenly and usually resolves in a few days with treatment. Acute pancreatitis can be a life-threatening illness with severe complications. Each year, about 210,000 people in the United States are admitted to the hospital with acute pancreatitis. The most common cause of acute pancreatitis is the presence of gallstones—small, pebble-like substances made of hardened bile—that cause inflammation in the pancreas as they pass through the common bile duct. Chronic, heavy alcohol use is also a common cause. Acute pancreatitis can occur within hours or as long as two days after consuming alcohol. Other causes of acute pancreatitis include abdominal trauma, medications, infections, tumors, and genetic abnormalities of the pancreas.

Symptoms: Acute pancreatitis usually begins with gradual or sudden pain in the upper abdomen that sometimes extends through the back. The pain may be mild at first and feel worse after eating. But the pain is often severe and may become constant and last for several days. A person with acute pancreatitis usually looks and feels very ill and needs immediate medical attention. Other symptoms may include a swollen and tender abdomen, nausea and vomiting, fever, and a rapid pulse. Severe acute pancreatitis may cause dehydration and low blood pressure. The heart, lungs, or kidneys can fail. If bleeding occurs in the pancreas, shock and even death may follow.

Diagnosis: While asking about a person's medical history and conducting a thorough physical examination, the doctor will order a blood test to assist in the diagnosis. During acute pancreatitis, the blood contains at least three times the normal amount of amylase and lipase, digestive enzymes formed in the pancreas. Changes may also occur in other body chemicals such as glucose, calcium, magnesium, sodium, potassium, and bicarbonate. After the person's condition improves, the levels usually return to normal. Diagnosing acute pancreatitis is often difficult because of the deep location of the pancreas. The doctor will likely order an imaging test to create visual images of the pancreas.

Treatment: Treatment for acute pancreatitis requires a few days stay in the hospital for intravenous (IV) fluids, antibiotics, and medication to relieve pain. The person cannot eat or drink so the pancreas can rest. If vomiting occurs, a tube may be placed through the nose and into the stomach to remove fluid and air. Unless complications arise, acute pancreatitis usually resolves in a few days. In severe cases, the person may require nasogastric feeding—a special liquid given in a long, thin tube inserted through the nose and throat and into the stomach—for several weeks while the pancreas heals.

Chronic Pancreatitis

Chronic pancreatitis is inflammation of the pancreas that does not heal or improve—it gets worse over time and leads to permanent damage.

Chronic pancreatitis, like acute pancreatitis, occurs when digestive enzymes attack the pancreas and nearby tissues, causing episodes of pain. Chronic pancreatitis often develops in people who are between the ages of 30 and 40.

The most common cause of chronic pancreatitis is many years of heavy alcohol use. The chronic form of pancreatitis can be triggered by one acute attack that damages the pancreatic duct. The damaged duct causes the pancreas to become inflamed. Scar tissue develops and the pancreas is slowly destroyed.

Symptoms: Most people with chronic pancreatitis experience upper abdominal pain, although some people have no pain at all. The pain may spread to the back, feel worse when eating or drinking, and become constant and disabling. In some cases, abdominal pain goes away as the condition worsens, most likely because the pancreas is no longer making digestive enzymes. Other symptoms include nausea, vomiting, weight loss, diarrhea, and oily stools.

People with chronic pancreatitis often lose weight, even when their appetite and eating habits are normal. The weight loss occurs because the body does not secrete enough pancreatic enzymes to digest food, so nutrients are not absorbed normally. Poor digestion leads to malnutrition due to excretion of fat in the stool.

Diagnosis: Chronic pancreatitis is often confused with acute pancreatitis because the symptoms are similar. As with acute pancreatitis, the doctor will conduct a thorough medical history and physical examination. Blood tests may help the doctor know if the pancreas is still making enough digestive enzymes, but sometimes these enzymes appear normal even though the person has chronic pancreatitis.

In more advanced stages of pancreatitis, when malabsorption and diabetes can occur, the doctor may order blood, urine, and stool tests to help diagnose chronic pancreatitis and monitor its progression. After ordering x-rays of the abdomen, the doctor will conduct one or more of the tests used to diagnose acute pancreatitis.

Treatment: Treatment for chronic pancreatitis may require hospitalization for pain management, intravenous (IV) hydration, and nutritional support. Nasogastric feedings may be necessary for several weeks if the person continues to lose weight.

When a normal diet is resumed, the doctor may prescribe synthetic pancreatic enzymes if the pancreas does not secrete enough of its own. The enzymes should be taken with every meal to help the person digest food and regain some weight. The next step is to plan a nutritious diet that is low in fat and includes small, frequent meals. A dietitian can assist in developing a meal plan. Drinking plenty of fluids and limiting caffeinated beverages is also important.

People with chronic pancreatitis are strongly advised not to smoke or consume alcoholic beverages, even if the pancreatitis is mild or in the early stages.

Complications: People with chronic pancreatitis who continue to consume large amounts of alcohol may develop sudden bouts of severe abdominal pain.

Section 26.3

Alcohol and Kidney Function

Excerpted from "Alcohol's Impact on Kidney Function," *Alcohol Health & Research World*, Vol. 21, No.1, 1997, National Institute on Alcohol Abuse and Alcoholism (NIAAA). The complete document with references is available at http://pubs.niaaa.nih.gov/publications/arh21-1/84.pdf. Reviewed in May 2010, by Dr. David A. Cooke, MD, FACP, Diplomate, American Board of Internal Medicine.

A cell's function depends not only on receiving a continuous supply of nutrients and eliminating metabolic waste products but also on the existence of stable physical and chemical conditions in the extracellular fluid bathing it. Among the most important substances contributing to these conditions are water, sodium, potassium, calcium, and phosphate. Loss or retention of any one of these substances can influence the body's handling of the others. In addition, hydrogen ion concentration (acid-base balance) influences cell structure and permeability as well as the rate of metabolic reactions. The amounts of these substances must be held within very narrow limits, regardless of the large variations possible in their intake or loss. The kidneys are the organs primarily responsible for regulating the amounts and concentrations of these substances in the extracellular fluid.

In addition to their role in regulating the body's fluid composition, the kidneys produce hormones that influence a host of physiological processes, including blood pressure regulation, red blood cell production, and calcium metabolism. Besides producing hormones, the kidneys respond to the actions of regulatory hormones produced in the brain, the parathyroid glands in the neck, and the adrenal glands located atop the kidneys.

Because of the kidneys' important and varied role in the body, impairment of their function can result in a range of disorders, from mild variations in fluid balance to acute kidney failure and death. Alcohol, one of the numerous factors that can compromise kidney function, can interfere with kidney function directly, through acute or chronic consumption, or indirectly, as a consequence of liver disease.

Gross and Microscopic Changes

Clinicians long have noted significant kidney enlargement in direct proportion to liver enlargement among chronic alcoholic patients afflicted with liver cirrhosis. In alcoholic patients with cirrhosis, these investigators reported a 33% increase in kidney weight, whereas they observed no appreciable kidney enlargement in alcoholic patients without cirrhosis compared with control subjects.

Blood-Flow Changes

Normally the rate of blood flow, or perfusion, through the kidneys is tightly controlled, so that plasma can be filtered and substances the body needs can be reabsorbed under optimal circumstances. Established liver disease impairs this important balancing act, however, by either greatly augmenting or reducing the rates of plasma flow and filtration through the glomerulus.

Effects on Fluid and Electrolyte Balance

One of the main functions of the kidneys is to regulate both the volume and the composition of body fluid, including electrically charged particles (ions), such as sodium, potassium, and chloride ions (electrolytes). However, alcohol's ability to increase urine volume alters the body's fluid level and produces disturbances in electrolyte concentrations. These effects vary depending on factors such as the amount and duration of drinking, the presence of other diseases, and the drinker's nutritional status.

Fluid: Alcohol can produce urine flow within 20 minutes of consumption; as a result of urinary fluid losses, the concentration of electrolytes in blood serum increases. These changes can be profound in chronic alcoholic patients, who may demonstrate clinical evidence of dehydration.

As most investigators now agree, increased urine flow results from alcohol's acute inhibition of the release of antidiuretic hormone (ADH), a hormone also known as vasopressin, which normally promotes the formation of concentrated urine by inducing the kidneys to conserve fluids. In the absence of ADH, segments of the kidney's tubule system become impermeable to water, thus preventing it from being reabsorbed into the body. Under these conditions, the urine formed is dilute and electrolyte concentration in the blood simultaneously rises. Although increased serum electrolyte concentration normally activates secretion of ADH so that fluid balance can be restored, a rising blood alcohol level disrupts this regulatory response by suppressing ADH secretion into the blood.

Age makes a difference in how rapidly the body escapes alcohol's ADH-suppressive effect. People older than age 50 overcome suppression of ADH more quickly than their younger counterparts do, despite reaching similar serum electrolyte concentrations after alcohol consumption. In older people, ADH levels sharply increase following alcohol intake, perhaps in part because sensitivity to increased electrolyte concentration is enhanced with age.

Sodium: The serum sodium level is determined by the balance of fluid in relation to that of sodium: Not enough fluid in the body results in a sodium concentration that is too high, whereas excessive amounts of fluid produce a sodium concentration that is too low. In general, neither acute nor chronic alcohol consumption directly causes significant changes in serum sodium concentrations, although impaired sodium excretion is a frequent complication of advanced liver disease.

Potassium: Normally the kidneys are a major route of potassium ion excretion and serve as an important site of potassium regulation. Alcohol consumption historically has been found to reduce the amount of potassium excreted by the kidneys, although the body's hydration state may help determine whether potassium excretion will increase or decrease in response to alcohol. Levels of potassium, like those of sodium, also can affect the way the kidneys handle fluid elimination or retention.

Phosphate: Low blood levels of phosphate commonly occur acutely in hospitalized alcoholic patients, appearing in more than one-half of severe alcoholism cases. Indeed, when the condition does not appear, clinicians treating alcoholic patients should suspect that another problem is masking the recognition of low phosphate levels, such as ongoing muscle dissolution, excess blood acidity, inadequate blood volume, or kidney failure. Several mechanisms may contribute to abnormally low phosphate levels. Simply lacking an adequate amount of phosphate in the diet is one possible reason for phosphate deficiency. For severely alcoholic patients who eat poorly, such a nutritional deficit may be an important contributor to hypophosphatemia. Another potential cause of hypophosphatemia in alcoholic patients is hyperventilation, which can occur during alcohol withdrawal.

Insulin administration also can lead to mild hypophosphatemia, because it decreases cellular acidity. Although insulin more likely plays a contributory, rather than principal, role in producing hypophosphatemia in alcoholic patients, there are clinical implications to consider.

Alcoholic patients also may develop low blood levels of phosphate by excreting too much of this ion into their urine. Typically, chronic alcoholic patients are losing up to 1.5 g/d of phosphate through their urine when they have reached the point of being sick enough to accept hospitalization. (For comparison, a normal healthy person excretes 0.7 to 0.8 g/d.) Over the next several days of hospitalization, these patients often excrete virtually no phosphate in their urine; simultaneously, their blood phosphate levels dip to low levels before returning to normal. The combination of low phosphate excretion and low blood levels indicates that phosphate is simply being shifted from the bloodstream into body cells, implying that kidney dysfunction is not a likely cause of phosphate wasting in this case.

Alcohol can induce abnormally high phosphate levels as well as abnormally low levels. Alcohol consumption apparently leads to excessive phosphate levels by altering muscle cell integrity and causing the muscle cells to release phosphate. This transfer of phosphate out of muscle cells and into the bloodstream results in an increased amount of phosphate passing through the kidneys' filtering system. In response, reabsorption of phosphate diminishes and excretion in urine increases in an effort to return blood levels of this ion to normal.

Magnesium: Chronic alcoholism is the leading cause of low blood levels of magnesium in the United States. Often it occurs simultaneously with phosphate deficiencies, also frequently encountered among alcoholic patients. Hypomagnesemia responds readily to magnesium supplementation treatment, however.

Calcium: Early studies showed that alcohol consumption markedly increases calcium loss in urine. In severely ill alcoholic patients, low blood levels of calcium occur about as often as low blood levels of phosphate and can cause convulsions or potentially life-threatening muscle spasms when respiratory muscles are involved. Alcoholic patients with liver disease often have abnormally low levels of a calcium-binding protein, albumin, and also may have impaired vitamin D metabolism; either of these two factors could result in reduced blood levels of calcium. Muscle breakdown and magnesium deficiency are other potential causes of hypocalcemia in alcoholic patients.

Body Fluid Volume and Blood Pressure

Chronic alcohol consumption may cause both fluid and solutes to accumulate, thereby increasing the overall volume of body fluids. In turn, such expansion of body fluid volume can contribute to high blood pressure, a condition often seen among chronic alcoholic patients. Clinical studies of hypertensive patients have demonstrated that reducing alcohol intake lowers blood pressure and resuming consumption raises it.

Acid-Base Balance Effects

Most of the metabolic reactions essential to life are highly sensitive to the acidity of the surrounding fluid. The kidneys play an important role in regulating acidity, thereby helping determine the rate at which metabolic reactions proceed. Alcohol can hamper the regulation of acidity, thus affecting the body's metabolic balance.

Because alcohol is a central nervous system depressant, it may slow the rate of breathing as well as reduce the brain's respiratory center's sensitivity to carbon dioxide levels. As a result, excess carbon dioxide accumulates, and the body's acid level subsequently increases. Respiratory acidosis is rare but carries an ominous prognosis when it occurs.

Excess blood acidity in alcoholic patients more often results from severe elevations of a product of glucose metabolism (lactate), which can be induced by alcohol consumption as well as other factors. A potentially serious condition known as alcoholic ketoacidosis is another disorder associated with abnormally high blood acidity. Typically, alcoholic ketoacidosis occurs in chronic alcohol abusers following a severe binge in which they consume alcoholic beverages and nothing else over several days.

Additional causes of nonrespiratory acidosis include drinking nonbeverage alcohol (for example, antifreeze or wood alcohol), which alcoholics sometimes resort to consuming when beverage alcohol is unavailable; aspirin overdose; and administration of paraldehyde, a sedative used for alcohol withdrawal.

If an acute alcoholic binge induces extensive vomiting, potentially severe alkalosis may result from losses of fluid, salt, and stomach acid. Like the kidneys, the liver plays an important role in maintaining acid-base balance. Liver diseases—including alcohol-induced liver problems—disrupt this function and can contribute directly or indirectly to a wide range of acid-base disturbances.

Regulatory Effects

To keep the kidneys functioning optimally and to maintain functional stability (homeostasis) in the body, a variety of regulatory mechanisms exert their influence. Alcohol can perturb these controls, however, to a degree that varies with the amount of alcohol consumed and the particular mechanism's sensitivity.

Alcohol consumption also is known to induce a state of low blood sugar and activate the portion of the nervous system that coordinates the body's response to stress. Both of these factors affect hormones that regulate kidney function, just as changes in fluid volume and electrolyte balance do.

Indirect Effects

Physicians have recognized an interrelationship between kidney and liver disorders at least since the time of Hippocrates. Although a disorder in one organ can complicate a primary problem in the other (or a pathological process may involve both organs directly), kidney dysfunction complicating a primary disorder of the liver (cirrhosis) is the most clinically significant scenario. Frequently, such kidney dysfunction results from liver problems related to alcohol. In fact, most patients in the United States diagnosed with both liver disease and associated kidney dysfunction are alcohol dependent. Three of the most prominent kidney function disturbances that arise in the presence of established liver disease are impaired sodium handling, impaired fluid handling, and acute kidney failure unexplained by other causes.

Chapter 27

How Alcohol Interacts with Other Diseases and Disorders

Chapter Contents

Section 27.1

Influence of Alcohol and Gender on Immune Response

Excerpted from "Influence of Alcohol and Gender on Immune Response," National Institute on Alcohol Abuse and Alcoholism (NIAAA), June 2003. Reviewed in May 2010, by Dr. David A. Cooke, MD, FACP, Diplomate, American Board of Internal Medicine.

Alcohol and Immune Responses

An overwhelming amount of evidence reveals that both acute and chronic alcohol exposure suppresses all branches of the immune system, including early responses to infection and the tumor surveillance system. For example, there is a decrease in the ability to recruit and activate germ-killing white blood cells and an increase in the incidence of breast cancer in people who consume alcohol.

Some experts suspect that alcohol exerts an all-or-none effect on immune response—that is, the presence or absence of alcohol, rather than its amount, dictates the immune response. Other researchers believe that low doses of alcohol—the amount equivalent to a glass of wine—can confer health benefits, including protection against damage to the cardiovascular and immune systems. Such benefits, if they are present, may be attributable to antioxidants in alcoholic beverages such as red wine. In any case, health experts agree that the beneficial effects of antioxidants in some alcoholic beverages are lost if the level of alcohol consumption is elevated.

There are several mechanisms by which alcohol impedes immune function. First, alcohol impairs the ability of white blood cells known as neutrophils to migrate to sites of injury and infection, a process called chemotaxis. In addition, removing germ-fighting white blood cells (macrophages) and proteins that act as messengers between immune cells (cytokines) from an animal that has not been given alcohol and culturing them in the presence of alcohol, or isolating these cells from humans or animals after administering alcohol, has been shown to alter production of these macrophages and cytokines.

Gender Differences in Immune Response Following Alcohol Exposure

To date, only a handful of studies have directly examined gender differences in the effects of alcohol on inflammatory and immune responses In general, estrogen stimulates immune responses and testosterone is immunosuppressive. During their reproductive years, females have more vigorous cellular and humoral immune responses than do males. This heightened immunity in females is evidenced by a more developed thymus (a gland located in the upper chest that is involved in the maturation of immune cells), higher antibody concentrations, and a greater ability to reject tumors and transplanted tissues. Ironically, the enhanced immune function in women of reproductive age is associated with a higher prevalence of autoimmune disorders than is found in postmenopausal women or in men. (Although estrogen is present in males, its concentration is too low to affect immune response.)

The effects of alcohol on production of the gonadal steroid hormones are well documented. In women, chronic alcohol exposure causes an initial increase in estrogen levels, followed by a marked decrease. In men, chronic alcohol consumption causes a decrease in testosterone. The alcohol-induced decrease in testosterone levels is significant enough to cause shrinkage (atrophy) of the testes, impotence, and loss of secondary sex characteristics.

Estrogen and cytokines: From the limited information available, it is thought that fluctuations in estrogen may alter immune cell function, in part, by increasing or decreasing the production of cytokines. Evidence that estrogen affects immune cell function, in part, by altering production of cytokines comes from cell culture studies in which estrogen was added to a culture of white blood cells. The effects of estrogen on cytokine production by immune target cells may involve direct interaction (binding) of the hormone and hormone receptors within those cells. The idea of direct effects of estrogen on target cells is supported by the existence of estrogen receptors not only in reproductive tissues, including the uterus, ovaries, and testes, where one would expect the hormone's actions to occur, but also in white blood cells.

Alcohol, stress responses, and immunity: Like other stressors, alcohol stimulates a neuroendocrine network known as the hypothalamic-pituitary-adrenal (HPA) axis, resulting in a dampening of the immune response. This process begins with activation of the hypothalamus (near the base of the brain), which produces a molecule called corticotropin-releasing hormone (CRH). This triggers the pituitary gland (below the hypothalamus) to secrete adrenal corticotropic hormone (ACTH). Finally, ACTH stimulates the adrenal glands (above the kidneys) to release glucocorticoids (cortisol in humans and corticosterone in rodents). These steroid hormones, which direct the activity of many cell types, are transmitted throughout the body in the blood. At high levels, they suppress inflammatory and immune responses. Several studies have documented that under resting (baseline) conditions and in response to stress, females have higher levels of glucocorticoids than do men. Furthermore, estrogen stimulates glucocorticoid production in females, whereas testosterone suppresses its production in both male and female subjects. Alcohol exposure stimulates glucocorticoid production in both males and females. Thus, there are two possible pathways by which alcohol-induced changes in steroid hormones could suppress immune responses in females, whereas there is only one such potential pathway in males. Further study will be required to determine if and how the two pathways interact to mediate alcohol-induced effects on immune function in females.

Gender, alcohol, and liver damage: Epidemiologic evidence clearly indicates that the adverse consequences of alcohol consumption, including severe liver disease, such as alcoholic cirrhosis, develop more quickly and require lower levels of alcohol exposure for females than for males. At any given level of alcohol intake, women are at higher risk than men of developing liver disease. It has been shown that a daily alcohol ingestion of as low as two drinks per day increases the risk of developing cirrhosis in women, although at least four drinks per day are required to increase this risk in men. These observations were made taking into account differences in body weight, fat distribution, body water, and other potentially confounding variables.

Section 27.2

Alcohol Use Increases Likelihood of Acquiring Sexually Transmitted Diseases (STDs)

Excerpted from "Sexually Transmitted Diseases and
Substance Use," Substance Abuse and Mental Health Services
Administration (SAMHSA), March 30, 2007.

* In 2005, 0.8% of persons aged 12 or older and 2.1% of young
  adults aged 18 to 25 had a sexually transmitted disease (STD)
  in the past year

* Among young adults aged 18 to 25, 1.4% of those who did not
  drink alcohol in the past month had a past year STD compared
  with 2.5% of those who drank but did not binge on alcohol in
  the past month, 2.4% of those who engaged in past month binge
  alcohol use but not heavy use, and 3.1% of past month heavy alcohol users

* Having an STD in the past year was more common among persons aged 18 to 25 who used both alcohol and an illicit drug in
  the past month (3.9%) than those who used neither alcohol nor
  an illicit drug (1.3%), those who used alcohol but no illicit drugs
  (2.1%), and those who used an illicit drug but not alcohol (2.1%)

Sexually transmitted diseases (STDs) are infections transmitted
mainly through sexual activity, although some STDs can be transmitted
by sharing drug injection equipment. In the United States in 2005, there
were 976,445 new cases of chlamydia, 339,593 new cases of gonorrhea,
266,000 new cases of herpes, and 8,724 new cases of syphilis. Sexually
active adolescents and young adults may be at higher risk of acquiring
STDs than older adults. Recent estimates suggest that persons aged
15 to 24 represent about 25% of all persons who were ever sexually
active, but nearly half of all new STD cases. In addition, research has
documented the association between substance use and STDs.

The National Survey on Drug Use and Health (NSDUH) asks questions to examine health conditions, including STDs. It also asks persons aged 12 or older to report on their use of alcohol and illicit drugs in

the past month. Those who report having used alcohol are asked about binge and heavy use. Illicit drugs refer to marijuana/hashish, cocaine (including crack), inhalants, hallucinogens, heroin, or prescription-type drugs used nonmedically. All findings presented in this report are based on 2005 NSDUH data.

Rates of Past Year Sexually Transmitted Diseases, by Past Month Alcohol Use among Persons Aged 18 to 25

The likelihood of having an STD in the past year was related to the frequency of alcohol use during the past month. Among young adults aged 18 to 25, 1.4% of those who did not drink alcohol in the past month had a past year STD compared with 2.5% of those who drank but did not binge on alcohol in the past month, 2.4% of those who engaged in past month binge alcohol use but not heavy use, and 3.1% of past month heavy alcohol users. Similar patterns were found for males and females.

Table 27.1. Percentages Having Past Year Sexually Transmitted Diseases among Young Adults Aged 18 to 25, by Level of Past Month Alcohol Use and Gender: 2005

Alcohol Use	Total	Male	Female
No past month alcohol use	1.4	0.4	2.1
Past month alcohol use, but not binge use	2.5	0.8	3.6
Past month binge alcohol use, but not heavy use	2.4	1.0	4.2
Past month heavy alcohol use	3.1	1.3	7.3

Source: SAMHSA, 2005 NSDUH.

Table 27.2. Percentages Having Past Year Sexually Transmitted Diseases among Young Adults Aged 18 to 25, by Past Month Alcohol and Illicit Drug Use and Gender: 2005

Alcohol and Illicit Drug Use	Total	Male	Female
Neither alcohol nor illicit drug use	1.3	0.3	2.1
Alcohol use, but not illicit drug use	2.1	0.8	3.4
Illicit drug use, but not alcohol use	2.1	1.0	3.3
Both alcohol and illicit drug use	3.9	1.5	7.9

Source: SAMHSA, 2005 NSDUH.

Rates of Past Year Sexually Transmitted Diseases, by Past Month Alcohol and Illicit Drug Use among Persons Aged 18 to 25

Having an STD in the past year was more common among persons aged 18 to 25 who used both alcohol and an illicit drug in the past month (3.9%) than those who used neither alcohol nor an illicit drug (1.3%), those who used alcohol but no illicit drugs (2.1%), and those who used an illicit drug but not alcohol (2.1%). Similar patterns were found for both males and females.

Section 27.3

Human Immunodeficiency Virus (HIV) and Alcohol Use

Excerpted from "Drugs and Alcohol," U.S. Department of Veterans Affairs, May 2, 2008.

If you've just found out that you are human immunodeficiency virus (HIV) positive, you might be wondering what alcohol and other "recreational" drugs will do to your body. (Recreational drugs are drugs that aren't used for medical purposes, such as beer, cocaine, and pot.)

Nobody can say for sure whether using alcohol or other drugs is bad for you. Each person is different, and a lot depends on which drugs you use and how often you use them. However, most experts would agree that, in large amounts, drugs and alcohol are bad for your immune system and your overall health. Remember, if you have HIV, your immune system is already weakened.

Effects on your immune system: Drinking too much alcohol can weaken your immune system. A weaker immune system will have a harder time fighting off common infections (such as a cold), as well as acquired immunodeficiency syndrome (AIDS)-related infections. A weaker immune system also increases the chance that you will experience more side effects from your HIV medications.

271

The organ in your body that alcohol and other drugs affect most is your liver. The liver rounds up waste from chemicals that you put in your body. Those chemicals include recreational drugs as well as prescription drugs, such as your HIV medications. A weaker liver means less efficient "housekeeping" and, probably, a weaker you. If you also have hepatitis C (or any other kind of hepatitis), your liver is already working very hard to fight the disease itself and deal with the strong drugs that you may be taking for your hepatitis treatment.

Interactions with your HIV meds: HIV medications are hard on your body, so when you are taking these drugs, it is important that your liver works as well as possible. The liver is responsible for getting rid of waste products from the medications. Once you are HIV positive, your body may react differently to alcohol and drugs. Many people find that it takes longer to recover from using pot, alcohol, or other recreational drugs than it did before they had HIV. Remember that having HIV means a major change has taken place in your body. You may choose to use alcohol and drugs in moderation, but be sure to respect your body. Pay attention to what and how much you eat, drink, smoke, and take into your body.

Drugs, alcohol, and safer sex: Alcohol can affect the decisions you make about safer sex. For example, if you have too much to drink, you may not be able to remember where you put the condoms, and decide simply not to use them. These are decisions you probably would not make if you were sober. These actions put your partner at risk for HIV and put you at risk for other sexually transmitted diseases. Remember to keep condoms handy in places where you might have sex. Also, try to limit the amount of alcohol you drink if you know you are going to have sex.

Section 27.4

Alcohol Increases Cancer Risks

This section includes "The Facts about Alcohol," © 2010 American Institute for Cancer Research (www.aicr.org). Reprinted with permission. And, "Alcohol, The Forgotten Cancer Risk," by Karen Collins, MS, RD, CDN. © 2008 American Institute for Cancer Research (www.aicr.org). Reprinted with permission.

The Facts about Alcohol

Are alcoholic drinks linked to cancer? There is convincing evidence that alcoholic beverages increase risk of cancers of the mouth, pharynx, larynx, esophagus, breast (both pre- and post-menopausal), and colorectum (in men). Drinking alcoholic beverages probably increases risk of colorectal cancer in women and liver cancer.

Why does drinking alcoholic beverages increase cancer risk? Tissues of the body directly exposed to alcohol (such as the mouth and esophagus) may suffer cell damage that can spark the cancer process. Years of drinking can lead to liver damage that may eventually turn to liver cancer. Although an association between alcohol consumption and breast cancer keeps turning up in study after study, the precise reason for the link is not yet clear. More research is needed.

Should I avoid alcohol completely to lower my cancer risk? Even small amounts of alcohol increase your risk for certain cancers, so the American Institute for Cancer Research (AICR) does not recommend alcohol consumption. However, moderate alcohol consumption may help protect against coronary heart disease and type 2 diabetes. Moderate consumption means no more than one drink per day for women; no more than two drinks per day for men.

Heavier drinking raises the risk of cancer, heart disease, high blood pressure, stroke, osteoporosis, malnutrition, inflammation of the pancreas, damage to the brain, liver cirrhosis, accidents, violence, and suicide. Alcohol causes birth defects too. If you are pregnant or may become pregnant, do not drink any alcohol.

Why is moderate drinking different for men and women? Women metabolize alcohol more slowly than men, so alcohol stays in a woman's bloodstream longer. Also, men tend to have more muscle than women; alcohol can be diluted into water held in muscle tissue, but not in fat tissue. A woman's risk for breast cancer—the most frequently diagnosed cancer in women—increases with greater alcohol consumption. Women at high risk for breast cancer should consider not drinking.

Alcohol, the Forgotten Cancer Risk

According to the 2007 landmark report, *Food, Nutrition, Physical Activity, and the Prevention of Cancer: a Global Perspective*, the evidence linking alcohol and cancer risk is now stronger than it was a decade ago. In fact, after reviewing the evidence, a 21-member international panel of experts noted that alcohol consumption increases risk for cancers of the mouth, throat, esophagus, colon, breast and probably the liver as well. It's an association that raises many questions for the public.

How can alcohol increase cancer risk? Researchers suspect that alcohol enhances the ability of carcinogens to penetrate cells where they can then initiate deoxyribonucleic acid (DNA) damage and promote cancer development. In the case of alcohol consumption with concurrent tobacco use, alcohol appears to intensify the effect of the potent carcinogen by inhibiting DNA repair. Furthermore, alcohol is broken down in the body into a substance called acetaldehyde, which scientists believe may promote cancer development as well. In addition, excessive alcohol seems to reduce the availability of folate, a B vitamin that is essential to DNA repair and replication. Without adequate folate, cells may be more susceptible to DNA damage and, in turn, cancer. Lastly, alcohol can also raise estrogen levels, which may increase breast cancer risk.

How much alcohol does it take to raise cancer risk? Alcohol's effect on cancer risk varies according to cancer site. Analyses of the evidence presented in the American Institute for Cancer Research (AICR) report reveal that one drink a day can increase a woman's risk of breast cancer by 7% to 15%. In relation to colon cancer, while some research shows that one drink daily raises risk only slightly, another analysis found a 13% risk increase at similar intake levels. Mouth and throat cancers are likely promoted by even small amounts of alcohol, according to experts.

The figures cited in the AICR report reference a portion described as one standard drink, which is equivalent to five ounces of wine, 12 ounces of beer or 1.5-ounces of 80-proof liquor. Note, however, that drinks are often served in portions far larger than these amounts. It's quite possible that one glass of wine or one mixed drink ordered at a restaurant will actually count as two standard drinks.

For maximum protection from cancer, you are best advised to avoid alcohol altogether. For those who choose to drink alcohol, one standard drink per day for women and two for men appear to be reasonably safe amounts. Women are directed to consume less than men because alcohol becomes more concentrated in their bodies.

If you choose to drink, does it matter whether you spread your alcohol consumption throughout the week or consume the entire week's allotment over the span of one weekend? In relation to cancer risk, there is no available evidence to answer this question. However, in regard to overall health and safety, consuming large amounts of alcohol at one time clearly poses a risk. In fact, while some studies link moderate alcohol consumption with reduced risk of heart disease, these benefits appear only with low doses of daily alcohol consumption. Drinking larger amounts at one time can raise blood pressure and increase risk of stroke, abnormal heart rhythm and heart attack.

What about the heart health benefits of alcohol? The benefits ascribed to alcohol in relation to reduced heart disease risk occur within the context of one drink per day for women or two drinks per day for men. Remember, however, that if alcohol consumption leads to high blood pressure or if the concentrated calories make weight control more difficult, the benefits to heart health may be offset.

Section 27.5

Alcohol and Hypoglycemia in Diabetics

Reprinted with permission from *Go Ask Alice!* Columbia University's Health Q & A Internet Resource, at www.gaoaskalice.columbia.edu. Copyright © 2010 by The Trustees of Columbia University. Additional information about material from Columbia University can be found at the end of this section.

Are there different sugar levels in different alcoholic beverages? I am hypoglycemic and have noticed different hangover levels contingent on the sugar level of alcohol consumed. Some have told me that scotch has the least amount of sugar of all alcoholic beverages. Since I occasionally enjoy a drink, I would appreciate knowing the lowest sugar content.

Answer: As someone who is hypoglycemic (has low blood sugar), it is smart for you to be attentive to how foods and drinks can affect your condition. In some ways, all alcoholic beverages have the same effect: while your liver is processing the alcohol you drink, it stops releasing glucose, the sugar that floats around in your bloodstream. For the entire time the alcohol stays in your body—and it takes your body an hour to break down about one ounce of alcohol (the amount in a standard drink)—the only glucose circulating through your system will be from the food and drinks you consume at the same time. The American Diabetes Association explains that this glucose-lowering effect can last for as long as eight to twelve hours after drinking.

For people with diabetes who, like you, must also keep track of their blood sugar levels, almost all alcoholic beverages count for the same thing: two fats in their food exchange system. Only regular beer is counted as two fats, plus one starch. The American Dietetic Association states that wine, hard liquor, and light beers all have similar caloric contents for one drink: a 5 ounce (oz.) glass of wine, 1.5 oz. of hard liquor (including scotch), 12 oz. of light beer. Regular beer, wine coolers, and mixed drinks all pack a more powerful calorie and sugar content punch; wine coolers have almost twice as many calories as a glass of dry table wine. Liqueurs and sweet wines have higher than average sugar levels, too.

Keep in mind that many alcoholic drinks are not just alcohol—mixed drinks, spritzers, coolers, and frozen daiquiris all contain additional ingredients, such as juice and soda, which can add a significant amount more sugar and calories to your drink. If you're looking to keep sugar levels low, stick with diet (no-calorie) soda or tonic water, seltzer, club soda, or water to mix in drinks.

Sometimes alcohol can cause blood sugar levels to go up, instead of down. This usually happens if someone eats a meal shortly after, or while drinking, particularly if they consume drinks high in carbohydrates, like beer and juice-alcohol mixers. This is particularly of concern for people with diabetes.

Interestingly, the signs of intoxication and too low blood sugar are the same: feeling dizzy, lack of coordination, and confusion. Because of this, you might not realize that you need to eat something. The people surrounding you also might not know you have low blood sugar and assume your behavior is simply the result of drinking too much. It's important to inform someone you'll be hanging out with of your hypoglycemia, so that s/he can get you appropriate help and/or food if necessary. You may even want to wear identification that identifies you as hypoglycemic. Also, since low blood sugar, as well as alcohol, can affect your coordination, perceptions, and reflexes, you'll need to be doubly careful by not driving or doing anything else requiring quick thinking and reflexes.

Here are some strategies to try to make sure your blood sugar levels don't dip too low:

• Eat a meal before drinking. Never drink on an empty stomach.

• Sample plenty of finger foods throughout the night, particularly those high in carbohydrates, such as pretzels and crackers. Avoid foods high in simple sugars, such as candy.

• If possible, mix your own drink, avoiding high sugar juices and sodas. Always measure the amount of alcohol that goes into your drink.

• Sip your drinks slowly.

So, you're right, your hangover symptoms might be more or less intense depending on what kind of drink you've had the night before. In fact, you may even be waking up with extremely low blood sugar, while blaming your headache, drowsiness, and confusion on too many drinks. (Although it's a good idea to drink in moderation anyway.) If you're concerned about your blood sugar level dipping to uncomfortable levels while you sleep, you can have a snack before going to bed, or even wake up in the middle of the night to eat something.

Additional Information about This Material

The information in this section is copyright © 2010 by the Trustees of Columbia University in the City of New York.

The document to which this notice is attached is protected by copyright owned in whole or in principal part by The Trustees of Columbia University in the City of New York (Columbia). You may download the document for reference and research purposes only.

Columbia makes no representations or warranties, express or implied, with respect to the document, or any part thereof, including any warranties of title, noninfringement or copyright or patent rights of others, merchantability, or fitness or suitability for any purpose.

Distribution and/or alteration by not-for-profit research or educational institutions for their local use is permitted as long as this notice is kept intact and attached to the document.

Any other distribution of copies of the document or any altered version thereof is expressly prohibited without prior written consent of Columbia.

Section 27.6

Alcohol and Sleep Difficulties

This section includes excerpts from "Your Guide to Healthy Sleep," National Heart, Lung, and Blood Institute (NHLBI), November 2005. Reviewed in May 2010, by Dr. David A. Cooke, MD, FACP, Diplomate, American Board of Internal Medicine.

Jet lag and alcohol: To relieve the stress of travel, avoid alcohol and caffeine. Although it may be tempting to drink alcohol to relieve jet lag and make it easier to fall asleep, you're more likely to sleep lighter and wake up in the middle of the night when the effects of the alcohol wear off. Caffeine can help keep you awake longer, but caffeine can also make it harder for you to fall asleep if its effects haven't worn off by the time you are ready to go to bed.

Driving and sleep deprivation: Don't drink alcohol. Just one beer when you are sleep deprived will affect you as much as two or three beers when you are well rested. Although alcohol is a sedative that makes it easier to fall asleep, it prevents deep sleep and rapid eye movement (REM) sleep, allowing only the lighter stages of sleep. People who drink alcohol also tend to wake up in the middle of the night when the effects of an alcoholic nightcap wear off.

Snoring: Long the material for jokes, snoring is generally accepted as common and annoying in adults but as nothing to worry about. However, snoring is no laughing matter. Frequent, loud snoring is often a sign of sleep apnea and may increase your risk of developing cardiovascular disease and diabetes, as well as lead to daytime sleepiness and impaired performance.

Snoring is caused by a narrowing or partial blockage of your airways at the back of the mouth and upper throat. This type of obstruction results in increased air turbulence when breathing in causing the soft tissues in your throat to vibrate. The end result is a noisy snore that can disrupt the sleep of your bed partner. This narrowing of the airways is typically caused by the soft palate, tongue, and throat relaxing while you sleep, but allergies or sinus problems can also contribute to a narrowing of the airways, as can being overweight and having extra soft tissue around your upper airways The larger the tissues in your soft palate, the more likely you are to snore while sleeping. Alcohol or sedatives taken shortly before sleep also promote snoring. These drugs cause greater relaxation of the tissues in your throat and mouth. Surveys reveal that about one-half of all adults snore and 50% of these adults do so loudly and frequently. African Americans, Asians, and Hispanics are more likely to snore loudly and frequently compared to Caucasians, and snoring problems increase with age.

Snoring in older children and adults may be relieved by less invasive measures, however. These measures include losing weight, refraining from tobacco, sleeping on the side rather than on the back, or elevating the head while sleeping. Treating chronic congestion and refraining from alcohol or sedatives before sleeping can also stop snoring. In some adults, snoring can be relieved by dental appliances that reposition the soft tissues in the mouth. Although numerous over-the-counter nasal strips and sprays claim to relieve snoring, no scientific evidence supports those claims.

Chronic insomnia is often caused by sleep-disrupting behavior such as drinking alcohol, exercising shortly before bedtime, ingesting caffeine late in the day, watching television or reading while in bed, or irregular sleep schedules due to shift work or other causes.

Some people who have chronic insomnia that is not corrected by behavioral therapy or treatment of an underlying condition may need a prescription medication. You should talk to a doctor before trying to treat insomnia with alcohol, over-the-counter or prescribed short-acting sedatives, or sedating antihistamines that induce drowsiness. The benefits of these treatments are limited, and they have risks. Some may help you fall asleep but leave you feeling tired in the morning. Others have longer-lasting effects and leave you feeling still tired and groggy in the morning. Some also may lose their effectiveness over time. Doctors may prescribe sedating antidepressants for insomnia, but the effectiveness of these medicines in people who do not have depression is not established, and there are significant side effects.

To reduce sleep problem symptoms: Avoid alcohol, smoking, sleeping pills, herbal supplements, and any other medications that make you sleepy. They make it harder for your airway to stay open while you sleep, and sedatives can make the breathing pauses longer and more severe. Tobacco smoke irritates the airways and can help trigger the intermittent collapse of the upper airway.

Chapter 28

Use with Caution: Alcohol and Medications

Chapter Contents

Section 28.1

Harmful Interactions: Mixing Alcohol with Medicines

Text in this section is excerpted from "Harmful Interactions: Mixing Alcohol with Medicines," National Institute on Alcohol Abuse and Alcoholism (NIAAA), 2007.

Warning: May cause drowsiness.
Alcohol may intensify this effect.

You've probably seen this warning on medicines you've taken. The danger is real. Mixing alcohol with certain medications can cause nausea and vomiting, headaches, drowsiness, fainting, or loss of coordination. It also can put you at risk for internal bleeding, heart problems, and difficulties in breathing. In addition to these dangers, alcohol can make a medication less effective or even useless, or it may make the medication harmful or toxic to your body.

Some medicines that you might never have suspected can react with alcohol, including many medications which can be purchased over-the-counter—that is, without a prescription. Even some herbal remedies can have harmful effects when combined with alcohol.

Medications are safe and effective when used appropriately. Your pharmacist or other health care provider can help you determine which medications interact harmfully with alcohol.

Did You Know?

Mixing alcohol and medicines can be harmful. Alcohol, like some medicines, can make you sleepy, drowsy, or lightheaded. Drinking alcohol while taking medicines can intensify these effects. You may have trouble concentrating or performing mechanical skills. Small amounts of alcohol can make it dangerous to drive, and when you mix alcohol with certain medicines you put yourself at even greater risk. Combining alcohol with some medicines can lead to falls and serious injuries, especially among older people.

Medicines may have many ingredients: Some medications—including many popular painkillers and cough, cold, and allergy remedies—contain more than one ingredient that can react with alcohol. Read the label on the medication bottle to find out exactly what ingredients a medicine contains. Ask your pharmacist if you have any questions about how alcohol might interact with a drug you are taking.

Some medicines contain alcohol: Certain medicines contain up to 10% alcohol. Cough syrup and laxatives may have some of the highest alcohol concentrations.

Alcohol affects women differently: Women, in general, have a higher risk for problems than men. When a woman drinks, the alcohol in her bloodstream typically reaches a higher level than a man's even if both are drinking the same amount. This is because women's bodies generally have less water than men's bodies. Because alcohol mixes with body water, a given amount of alcohol is more concentrated in a woman's body than in a man's. As a result, women are more susceptible to alcohol-related damage to organs such as the liver.

Older people face greater risk: Older people are at particularly high risk for harmful alcohol-medication interactions. Aging slows the body's ability to break down alcohol, so alcohol remains in a person's system longer. Older people also are more likely to take a medication that interacts with alcohol—in fact, they often need to take more than one of these medications.

Timing is important: Alcohol and medicines can interact harmfully even if they are not taken at the same time.

Remember: Mixing alcohol and medicines puts you at risk for dangerous reactions. Protect yourself by avoiding alcohol if you are taking a medication and don't know its effect. To learn more about a medicine and whether it will interact with alcohol, talk to your pharmacist or other health care provider.

Section 28.2

Alcohol Abuse Makes Prescription Drug Abuse More Likely

Excerpted from "Alcohol Abuse Makes Prescription Drug Abuse More Likely," *NIDA Notes: Research Findings*, Vol. 21, No. 5, National Institute on Drug Abuse (NIDA), March 2008.

Men and women with alcohol use disorders (AUDs) are 18 times more likely to report nonmedical use of prescription drugs than people who don't drink at all, according to researchers at the University of Michigan. Dr. Sean Esteban McCabe and colleagues documented this link in two National Institute on Drug Abuse (NIDA)-funded studies; they also discovered that young adults were most at risk for concurrent or simultaneous abuse of both alcohol and prescription drugs.

"The message of these studies is that clinicians should conduct thorough drug use histories, particularly when working with young adults," says Dr. McCabe. "Clinicians should ask patients with alcohol use disorders about nonmedical use of prescription drugs [NMUPD] and in turn ask nonmedical users of prescription medications about their drinking behaviors." The authors also recommend that college staff educate students about the adverse health outcomes associated with using alcohol and prescription medications at the same time.

Two Studies

The authors' first study looked at the prevalence of AUDs and NMUPD in 43,093 individuals 18 and older who participated in the National Epidemiologic Survey on Alcohol and Related Conditions (NESARC) between 2001 and 2005. Participants lived across the United States in a broad spectrum of household arrangements and represented White, African-American, Asian, Hispanic, and Native American populations. Although people with AUDs constituted only 9% of NESARC's total sample, they accounted for more than a third of those who reported NMUPD.

Since the largest group of alcohol/prescription drug abusers were between the ages of 18 and 24, the team's second study focused entirely on this population and involved 4,580 young adults at a large, public,

Midwestern university. The participants completed a self-administered Web survey, which revealed that 12% of them had used both alcohol and prescription drugs nonmedically within the last year but at different times (concurrent use), and 7% had taken them at the same time (simultaneous use).

When alcohol and prescription drugs are used simultaneously, severe medical problems can result, including alcohol poisoning, unconsciousness, respiratory depression, and sometimes death. In addition, college students who drank and took prescription drugs simultaneously were more likely than those who did not to blackout, vomit, and engage in other risky behaviors such as drunk driving and unplanned sex.

Who, What, and When

The prescription drugs that were combined with alcohol in order of prevalence included prescription opiates (Vicodin, OxyContin, Tylenol 3 with codeine, Percocet), stimulant medication (Ritalin, Adderall, Concerta), sedative/anxiety medication (Ativan, Xanax, Valium), and sleeping medication (Ambien, Halcion, Restoril). The college study asked about the respondent's use of medications prescribed for other people while the NESARC explored both use of someone else's prescription medications as well as the use of one's own prescription medications in a manner not intended by the prescribing clinician (to get high).

The researchers found that the more alcohol a person drank and the younger he or she started drinking, the more likely he or she was to report NMUPD. Compared with people who did not drink at all, drinkers who did not binge were almost twice as likely to engage in NMUPD; binge drinkers with no AUDs were three times as likely; people who abused alcohol but were not dependent on alcohol were nearly seven times as likely; and people who were dependent on alcohol were 18 times as likely to report NMUPD.

While the majority of the respondents in both studies were White (71% in NESARC and 65% in the college group), an even higher percentage of the simultaneous polydrug users in the college study were White males who had started drinking in their early teens. The NESARC study also found that Whites in general were two to five times more likely than African-Americans to report NMUPD during the past year. Native Americans were at increased risk for NMUPD, and the authors indicated that this subpopulation should receive greater research attention in the future.

Dr. McCabe emphasizes that many people who simultaneously drink alcohol and use prescription medications have no idea how dangerous the interactions between these substances can be. "Passing out is a protective mechanism that stops people from drinking when they are approaching potentially dangerous blood alcohol concentrations," he explains. "But if you take stimulants when you drink, you can potentially override this mechanism and this could lead to life-threatening consequences."

Dr. James Colliver, formerly of NIDA's Division of Epidemiology, Services and Prevention Research, offers perspective on these studies. "Prescription sedatives, tranquilizers, painkillers, and stimulants are generally safe and effective medications for patients who take them as prescribed by a clinician," Dr. Colliver states. "They are used to treat acute and chronic pain, attention deficit hyperactivity disorder, anxiety disorders, and sleep disorders. The problem is that many people think that, because prescription drugs have been tested and approved by the Food and Drug Administration, they are always safe to use; but they are safe only when used under the direction of a physician for the purpose for which they are prescribed."

Sources

McCabe, S.E., et al. The relationship between past year drinking behaviors and nonmedical use of prescription drugs: Prevalence of co-occurrence in a national sample. *Drug and Alcohol Dependence* 84(3):281-288, 2006.

McCabe, S.E., et al. Simultaneous and concurrent polydrug use of alcohol and prescription drugs: Prevalence, correlates, and consequences. *Journal of Studies on Alcohol* 67(4):529-537, 2006.

Part Four

The Effects of Alcohol on Reproductive and Fetal Health

Chapter 29

Alcohol and the Reproductive System

Alcohol and Female Reproductive Function

Alcohol and puberty: Rapid hormonal changes occurring during puberty make females especially vulnerable to the deleterious effects of alcohol exposure during this time. Thus, the high incidence of alcohol consumption among middle school and high school students in the United States is a matter of great concern.

A study found that estrogen levels were depressed among adolescent girls ages 12–18 for as long as two weeks after drinking moderately. This finding suggests the possibility that alcohol alters the reproductive awakening and maturation that marks puberty. Also, estrogen's role in bone maturation raises the question of whether alcohol use during adolescence has long-term effects on bone health. Alcohol consumption during adolescence is known to affect growth and body composition, perhaps by altering food intake patterns while alcohol is being consumed.

Alcohol and the female reproductive system: Alcohol markedly disrupts normal menstrual cycling in female humans. Alcoholic women are known to have a variety of menstrual and reproductive

This chapter includes excerpts from "Alcohol's Effects on Female Reproductive Function," National Institute on Alcohol Abuse and Alcoholism (NIAAA), 2002; and excerpts from "Alcohol's Effects on Male Reproduction," NIAAA, 1998. The complete documents are available at: http://pubs.niaaa.nih.gov/publications/arh26-4/274-281 .pdf [Female] and http://pubs.niaaa.nih.gov/publications/arh22-3/195.pdf [Male]. Reviewed in May 2010, by Dr. David A. Cooke, MD, FACP, Diplomate, American Board of Internal Medicine.

disorders, from irregular menstrual cycles to complete cessation of menses, absence of ovulation, and infertility. Alcohol abuse has also been associated with early menopause. However, alcoholics often have other health problems such as liver disease and malnutrition, so reproductive deficits may not be directly related to alcohol use.

In human females, alcohol ingestion, even in amounts insufficient to cause major damage to the liver or other organs, may lead to menstrual irregularities. It is important to stress that alcohol ingestion at the wrong time, even in amounts insufficient to cause permanent tissue damage, can disrupt the delicate balance critical to maintaining human female reproductive hormonal cycles and result in infertility. A study of healthy nonalcoholic women found that a substantial portion who drank small amounts of alcohol stopped cycling normally and became at least temporarily infertile. This anovulation was associated with a reduced or absent pituitary luteinizing hormone (LH) secretion. All the affected women had reported normal menstrual cycles before the study. This finding is consistent with epidemiologic data from a representative national sample of 917 women, which showed increased rates of menstrual disturbances and infertility associated with increasing self-reported alcohol consumption. Thus, alcohol-induced disruption of female fertility is a clinical problem that merits further study.

Alcohol in the postmenopausal female: In reviews of the research on alcohol's effects on post-menopausal females, some evidence was found that acute alcohol exposure results in a temporary increase in estradiol levels in menopausal women on hormone replacement therapy (HRT). This increase may be attributed to impaired estradiol metabolism, with decreased conversion of estradiol to estrone. Interestingly, alcohol exposure had no effect on estradiol levels in women who were not receiving HRT, or on estrone levels in either group of women. In contrast, women receiving HRT had lower levels of estradiol when their alcohol consumption was high. Thus, the amount of alcohol consumed appears to be an important variable in studies of hormone levels in postmenopausal women who consume alcohol. Other studies have demonstrated that alcohol consumption after menopause is unrelated to levels of testosterone and androstenedione. Overall, the data suggest that alcohol does not affect estrone levels but may increase estradiol.

Effects of alcohol-induced reproductive dysfunction on the skeleton: Heavy alcohol use is a recognized risk factor for osteoporosis in humans. Human observational studies have not clearly indicated whether the osteoporosis seen in people who used alcohol was caused by alcohol itself or by attendant nutritional deficiencies. Well-controlled experiments, however, have demonstrated that alcohol itself can cause osteoporosis in growing and adult animals.

Osteoporosis has many negative consequences. It increases vulnerability to fractures, which can lead to immobilization and subsequent depression, markedly decreased quality of life, loss of productive work time, bed sores, sepsis, and more osteoporosis. Risk for osteoporosis is in part related to low peak bone mass: the lower the peak bone mass, the greater the risk for osteoporosis. Active bone growth occurs during puberty, and alcohol's disruption of bone development in animals may cause lifelong osteoporosis in animals exposed to alcohol at a young age.

Alcohol abuse contributes to bone weakness, increasing the risk of fracture. Alcoholics have reduced bone mass, which is evident in the loss of bone tissue in the spine and iliac crest. There is general agreement that alcohol consumption decreases bone formation through a decrease in the number of bone cells responsible for bone formation, which is accompanied by a reduction in bone cell function.

In some of the studies reviewed, heavy alcohol consumption has been found to increase estrogen production, which should protect bone from the development of osteoporosis. Yet, despite this increase in estrogen, alcohol consumption leads to accelerated bone loss. Alcohol does not accelerate the bone loss associated with gonadal insufficiency and may reduce the number of bone-resorbing cells (osteoclasts).

Alcohol's Effects on Male Reproduction

Alcohol's effects on the testes: Numerous studies have indicated that alcohol abuse in men can cause impaired testosterone production and shrinkage of the testes. Those changes can result in impotence, infertility, and reduced male secondary sexual characteristics (for example, reduced facial and chest hair, breast enlargement, and a shift in fat deposition from the abdomen to the hip area). For example, in a classic study by Lloyd and Williams (1948), 72% of men with advanced alcoholic cirrhosis exhibited decreased libido and sexual potency. Similarly, Van Thiel and colleagues (1974) noted that impotence was "prominent in the majority of subjects, but occurred more frequently among patients with greater liver damage." Testicular atrophy also appears to be common among alcoholics, occurring in up to 75% of men with advanced alcoholic cirrhosis. This atrophy likely is caused by several factors, including (1) alcohol's damaging effects on the testes; (2) alcohol's effects on LH and FSH, which, among other factors, stimulate testicular growth; and (3) various confounding factors, such as malnutrition, concomitant treatment with various medications, and abuse of drugs other than alcohol by the subjects. Testicular atrophy results primarily from the loss of sperm cells and decreased diameter of the seminiferous tubules. Studies have confirmed alcohol's deleterious effects on the testosterone-producing Leydig cells, the Sertoli cells, and even on the offspring of alcohol-ingesting males, independent of co-occurring liver disease or malnutrition.

Alcohol's effects on Leydig cells and testosterone metabolism: Alcohol's adverse effects on Leydig cell function and testosterone production were demonstrated in a study of young, healthy male volunteers with normal liver function who received alcohol over a four-week period. Since those initial studies were performed, numerous studies in humans and laboratory animals have confirmed the reduction in testosterone levels after both one-time (acute) and long-term (chronic) alcohol exposure.

Alcohol's effects on testosterone metabolism are somewhat different, however, in men with alcoholic liver disease compared with men without alcoholic liver disease. Thus, although the production rates and blood levels of testosterone are reduced in both groups of men, the metabolic clearance of testosterone increases only in men without alcoholic liver disease. In men with alcoholic liver disease, in contrast, the metabolic clearance is decreased.

Several studies found that some people with alcoholic liver disease have increased levels of estrogens in the blood. Clinical studies have demonstrated that alcohol not only alters testosterone metabolism but also diminishes testosterone production. Studies in humans and animals found that alcohol exposure increases adrenal hormone levels, thereby interfering with reproductive functions.

Alcohol's effects on Sertoli cells: Sertoli cells also may be an important target for alcohol's actions on the reproductive system. Researchers have observed sperm abnormalities in men with histories of moderate or heavy alcohol consumption. For example, in an autopsy study, men with a history of low alcohol consumption (for example, 10–40 grams, or approximately 1–3.5 standard drinks, four per day) generally showed no abnormal sperm forms. Moderate alcohol consumption (for example, 40–80 grams, or approximately 3.5–7 standard drinks, per day) was associated with a slight alteration in sperm maturation. Finally, a history of heavy alcohol consumption (more than 80 grams, or more than seven drinks, per day) led to arrested sperm development in 20% of the cases. Studies in alcoholics who had not yet developed severe liver damage (in whom liver damage itself had not affected testicular function) found that 40% of the men studied had reduced sperm counts, 45% showed abnormal sperm shapes, and 50% exhibited altered sperm motility.

Alcohol's Effects on the Anterior Pituitary Gland

Effects on luteinizing hormone (LH) production, secretion, and activity: With the development of sophisticated techniques that allow measuring even low hormone levels in the blood (radioimmunoassays), researchers now are able to assess changes in the levels of the pituitary hormones LH and follicle-stimulating hormone (FSH) after alcohol exposure. Those studies confirmed an alcohol-related fall in testosterone levels. Surprisingly, however, the levels of LH in the blood often did not increase and, in fact, declined in some studies. Those results were unexpected, because if alcohol exclusively affected the testes, the reduced testosterone levels should have evoked a rise in LH levels as a result of the feedback mechanism regulating the hypothalamic-pituitary-gonadal (HPG) axis. Accordingly, the lack of an increase in LH levels in many cases implied that alcohol acted not only on the testes but also on the hypothalamus and/or the pituitary gland. Subsequently, studies in alcohol-fed rats established that the decrease in LH blood levels resulted from impairments in both LH production and LH secretion.

A related concern is whether alcohol affects LH release at the level of the pituitary and/or the hypothalamus. The results of experiments suggest that alcohol can decrease LH secretion even from isolated pituitary glands, implying that alcohol lowers LH levels at least in part by acting directly on the pituitary. Alcohol has been shown to result in the production of less potent LH variants. Thus, alcohol's deleterious effects on LH function are qualitative as well as quantitative.

Effects on follicle-stimulating hormone (FSH) production and activity: Research also has indicated that alcohol reduces FSH levels in the blood, although this effect is not as consistent as its effect on LH levels. FSH influences the activity of the testicular Sertoli cells, which support sperm cell development and maturation. Both reduced numbers of sperm and abnormal sperm forms have been found in men with histories of heavy drinking. Those changes in sperm formation may be associated with the decreased fertility reported in alcohol-abusing men. Furthermore, in light of the alcohol-induced disruption of Sertoli cell function and reduction in testosterone levels, one would expect FSH levels to be elevated, because FSH is part of the same negative feedback mechanism as LH. Consequently, normal FSH levels actually should be considered too low for the accompanying testosterone levels.

Alcohol's Effects on the Hypothalamus

Alcohol may affect LH levels by acting not only directly on the pituitary gland but also on the hypothalamus. Evidence suggests that alcohol decreases gonadotropin-releasing hormone (GnRH) secretion by acting at a site outside the hypothalamus and/or that alcohol's breakdown products (acetaldehyde), rather than alcohol itself, reduces GnRH secretion. The former option appears highly likely, because GnRH secretion is controlled by a complex mechanism involving various nerve impulses generated outside the hypothalamus. Alcohol might act on any of those impulses.

Chapter 30

Alcohol Use among Pregnant Women and Recent Mothers

Alcohol Use

Prenatal alcohol exposure increases the risk of birth defects, including physical, cognitive, and behavioral disorders. Research also shows a link between alcohol use during pregnancy and increased risk of preterm birth. In 2005–2006, an estimated 11.8% of pregnant women aged 15 to 44 reported using alcohol in the past month. A recent paper based on data from the National Survey on Drug Use and Health (NSDUH) found that illicit drug, alcohol, and cigarette use was lower among pregnant women, particularly during their second and third trimesters, than among their parenting or nonpregnant counterparts. The study also found indirect evidence of resumption of substance use after pregnancy.

To guide the development of public health interventions regarding alcohol use during pregnancy, data from population-based studies such as NSDUH are needed to show the scope of the problem and to identify subgroups that may be at significant risk. NSDUH asks female respondents aged 12 to 44 whether they are currently pregnant, and it also asks persons aged 12 or older to report on their alcohol use during the month prior to the survey. Respondents who drank alcohol in the past 30 days (current drinkers) also are asked the number of days they

This chapter includes excerpts from "Alcohol Use among Pregnant Women and Recent Mothers: 2002 to 2007," Substance Abuse and Mental Health Services Administration (SAMHSA), September 11, 2008; and an excerpt from "Substance Use among Women during Pregnancy and Following Childbirth," SAMHSA, May 21, 2009.

consumed alcohol in the past month and the average number of drinks they consumed per day on the days they drank.

This report concentrates on alcohol use among women of childbearing age (those aged 15 to 44). Comparisons are made between the alcohol use of pregnant women, recent mothers, and women who were not pregnant and not recent mothers. Pregnant women are defined as women who were pregnant at the time of the survey. Recent mothers are defined as women who were not pregnant at the time of the survey, but who gave birth during the prior 12 months. Nonpregnant women who were not recent mothers are defined as women who were not pregnant at the time of the interview and who did not have a biological child under one year old in the household. Analyses include trends and patterns based on data from 2002 to 2007. Additional findings are based on annual averages for the combined 2006 and 2007 NSDUH data.

What percentage currently used alcohol?

Combined 2006 and 2007 data indicate that the rate of past month alcohol use among women aged 15 to 44 was lower for those who were pregnant (11.6%) than for recent mothers (42.1%), who in turn had a lower rate than women who were not pregnant and not recent mothers (54.0%).

Among pregnant women aged 15 to 44, those aged 15 to 17 had the highest rate of past month alcohol use (15.8%), followed by those aged 26 to 44 (12.5%), and those aged 18 to 25 (9.8%); however, these rates did not differ significantly. Conversely, among recent mothers and nonpregnant women who were not recent mothers, those aged 15 to 17 had lower rates of past month alcohol use than women in the older age groups. White women were more likely than Hispanic women to have drunk alcohol in the past month regardless of their pregnancy status.

Generally, higher education status and higher family income were associated with higher rates of past month alcohol use among all women of childbearing age regardless of their pregnancy status. Among women aged 18 to 44, those with a college education were nearly twice as likely as their counterparts with less than a high school education to have used alcohol in the past month in each pregnancy status category. Similarly, women aged 15 to 44 with annual family incomes of $75,000 or higher had the highest rates of alcohol use in the prior month compared with those with lower family incomes in all three pregnancy status categories.

How often did they drink?

Among past month female alcohol users aged 15 to 44, pregnant women and recent mothers drank on fewer days in the past month than nonpregnant women who were not recent mothers—an average of 4.9, 4.4, and 6.1 days, respectively. Among pregnant past month alcohol users, there was no difference by race/ethnicity in the average number of days they drank in the past month, with White pregnant women drinking on an average of 4.8 days, Black pregnant women on an average of 4.9 days, and Hispanic pregnant women on an average of 5.2 days.

How much did they drink?

Among women aged 15 to 44 who used alcohol in the past month, those who were pregnant consumed an average of 2.4 drinks per day on the days they drank in the past month, while those who were recent mothers drank an average of 2.5 drinks, and those who were not pregnant and not recent mothers consumed an average of 3.0 drinks. Among past month alcohol users, pregnant women aged 15 to 17 and those aged 18 to 25 drank an average of 3.6 drinks per day on the days they drank compared with pregnant women aged 26 to 44, who drank an average of 1.7 drinks per day on the days they drank. The average number of drinks consumed per day generally declined with higher education status and higher income.

Consequences

Alcohol use during pregnancy can cause physical and mental birth defects, preterm births, and miscarriages. Because a safe level of alcohol intake during pregnancy cannot be determined, both the U.S. Surgeon General and the March of Dimes Foundation recommend that pregnant women not consume any alcohol. Additionally, because small amounts of alcohol can be transmitted in breast milk, they recommend alcohol abstinence for women who are breast feeding. Findings in this report indicate that many women may not be getting this message.

Identifying specific subgroups of women who are at risk for drinking during pregnancy is especially critical, given the need for careful allocation of scarce resources for prevention, intervention, and treatment activities. Pregnant women aged 15 to 17 may be in particular need of alcohol prevention services tailored for their age group because nearly 16.0% of them used alcohol in the past month. Pregnant women in this age group consumed an average of 24 drinks in the past month (for example, they drank on an average of six days during the past month and an average of about four drinks on the days that they drank).

Substance Use among Pregnant Women and Recent Mothers

In the United States, substance use among pregnant and postpartum women is a public health issue. Previous studies based on data from the National Survey on Drug Use and Health (NSDUH) have consistently shown that a substantial proportion of pregnant women, particularly those in the first trimester, were past month alcohol, cigarette, or illicit drug users and that rates among recent mothers were much higher than those among pregnant women. A recent study of this relationship that controlled for women's age and other sociodemographic characteristics found indirect evidence of resumption of substance use following childbirth. This section examines past month use of alcohol, cigarettes, and marijuana among pregnant and parenting women aged 18 to 44 to shed light on how rapidly use of these substances resumes after childbirth. It differentiates pregnant women by trimester of pregnancy and recent mothers by age of the youngest child in the household.

Combined 2002 to 2007 data show that past month alcohol use among women aged 18 to 44 was highest for those who were not pregnant and did not have children living in the household (63.0%). The rate was comparatively low for those in the first trimester of pregnancy (19.0%) and even lower for those in the second (7.8%) or third (6.2%) trimester. There were similar patterns across these four subgroups of women for past month binge alcohol use, cigarette use, and marijuana use.

Resumption of Substance Use among Recent Mothers

When compared with women in the third trimester of pregnancy, nonpregnant women with children under three months old in the household had much higher rates of past month alcohol use (6.2% versus 31.9%), binge alcohol use (1.0% versus 10.0%), cigarette use (13.9% versus 20.4%), and marijuana use (1.4% versus 3.8%), suggesting resumption of use among mothers in the three months after childbirth.

The increase in rates of substance use among parenting women tended to level off as the age of the youngest child increased. For alcohol, past month use increased from 31.9% for women with children under three months old to 43.9% for those with 3–5 month olds and

52.1% for those with 9–11 month olds; thereafter, the rate ranged from 49.4 to 54.9%, not significantly different from the rate among women with 9–11 month olds. The rate of binge alcohol use was 15.5% among women whose youngest children were aged 3–5 months and 19.7% for those whose youngest children were aged 18 months or older. Cigarette use among parenting women increased to 30.3% for those whose youngest children were aged 18 months or older, but for marijuana, there was no significant increase in use among women who had children aged three months or older.

These data provide indirect evidence of dramatic increases in the prevalence of substance use among mothers with babies under three months old based on cross-sectional reports from pregnant, parenting, and nonpregnant women. This increase implies a resumption of substance use following childbirth because new initiation of substance use among postpartum women is too rare to account for the observed differences.

Table 30.1. Women's (Aged 18 to 44 Years) Past Month Alcohol Use Rate by Pregnancy Trimester and Age of the Youngest Child in Household: 2002 to 2007

Pregnancy Trimester and Age of the Youngest Child in Household	Percent
NP,* No child	63.0%
Trimester 1	19.0%
Trimester 2	19.0%
Trimester 3	7.8%
NP, child less than three months	31.9%
NP, child 3–5 months	43.9%
NP, child 6–8 months	46.4%
NP, child 9–11 months	52.1%
NP, child 12–14 months	49.4%
NP, child 15–17 months	54.9%
NP, child 18 months or older	52.1%

*NP = Nonpregnant

Source: 2002 to 2007 SAMHSA National Surveys on Drug Use and Health (NSDUHs).

Chapter 31

Preventing Fetal Alcohol Spectrum Disorders (FASD)

Alcohol abuse is a serious public health concern. Did you know that alcohol can harm a fetus at any point in its development, often before a woman knows she's pregnant?

Fetal alcohol spectrum disorders (FASD) is an umbrella term describing the range of effects that can occur in an individual whose mother drank alcohol during pregnancy. These effects may include physical, mental, behavioral, and learning disabilities with lifelong implications. The term FASD is not intended for use as a clinical diagnosis. It refers to conditions such as fetal alcohol syndrome (FAS), alcohol-related neurodevelopmental disorder (ARND), and alcohol-related birth defects (ARBD).

Understanding the Risk

Any pregnant woman who drinks alcohol is at risk of having a child with an FASD, regardless of her education, income, or ethnicity. Women who are at particularly high risk of drinking during pregnancy and having a child with an FASD include the following:

- Women with substance abuse or mental health problems
- Women who have already had a child with an FASD[1,2]
- Recent drug users

"Preventing FASD: Healthy Women, Healthy Babies," Substance Abuse and Mental Health Services Administration (SAMHSA), 2007.

301

- Smokers

- Women who have multiple sex partners

- Recent victims of abuse and violence

Alcohol is a potent teratogen, a substance that can damage a developing fetus. There is no known safe level of alcohol use during pregnancy, so pregnant women or women who may become pregnant should not drink any alcohol from conception to birth.

Treatment for Women

Many women who need alcohol treatment may not receive it due to lack of money or child care, fear of losing custody of their children, or other barriers. For successful recovery, women often need a continuum of care for an extended period of time, including the following:

- Comprehensive inpatient or outpatient treatment for alcohol and other drugs

- Case management

- Counseling and other mental health treatment

- Medical and prenatal care

- Child care

- Transportation

- Follow-up pediatric and early intervention services for children

- Services that respond to women's needs regarding reproductive health, sexuality, relationships, and victimization

- Other support services, such as housing, education and job training, financial support services, parenting education, legal services, and aftercare[3]

Research shows that residential substance abuse treatment designed specifically for pregnant women and women with children can have substantial benefits in terms of recovery, pregnancy outcomes, parenting skills, and women's ability to maintain or regain custody of their children.[4]

Surgeon General's Advisory on Alcohol Use in Pregnancy

- A pregnant woman should not drink alcohol during pregnancy.

- A pregnant woman who has already consumed alcohol during her pregnancy should stop in order to minimize further risk.

- A woman who is considering becoming pregnant should abstain from alcohol.

- Recognizing that nearly half of all births in the United States are unplanned, women of childbearing age should consult their physician and take steps to reduce the possibility of prenatal alcohol exposure.

- Health professionals should inquire routinely about alcohol consumption by women of childbearing age, inform them of the risks of alcohol consumption during pregnancy, and advise them not to drink alcoholic beverages during pregnancy.

Three Ways to Prevent FASD

There are three main approaches to preventing FASD:[5]

- Increase public knowledge about FASD through general education, public service announcements, media attention, alcohol warning labels, posters, pamphlets, and billboards.

- Target women at risk by screening pregnant women and women of childbearing age for alcohol use, and by providing interventions with pregnant women who drink and with women who drink and do not use birth control. Brief interventions such as motivational interviewing may be effective at reducing risk.[6]

- Target women at highest risk through treatment of alcohol problems and strategies to encourage pregnancy prevention. Women at risk include those who abuse alcohol while pregnant or who are at risk of becoming pregnant, particularly women who have already given birth to a child with an FASD.

All three strategies are important, but targeting women at increased or highest risk may be more effective in reducing alcohol use during pregnancy. Primary care providers, such as obstetricians, gynecologists, and family doctors, play a key role in preventing FASD. They should follow these guidelines for FASD prevention:

- Talk to their patients about the dangers of drinking alcohol during pregnancy

- Identify women who are at risk by using screening tools such as T-ACE and TWEAK, which ask specific questions about drinking habits[7,8]

- Refer to treatment and other support services women with drinking problems, pregnant women who drink, and women who are at risk of an alcohol-exposed pregnancy

A woman's partner, other family members, and friends can also help prevent FASD:

- Share information with her about FASD and the importance of not drinking during pregnancy

- Model safe behavior by not drinking themselves

- Encourage her to talk about problems in her life that may lead her to drink

- Help her find treatment if she cannot stop drinking

Conclusion

Drinking during pregnancy can cause permanent damage to a fetus. However, FASD is 100% preventable. The only cause of FASD is prenatal exposure to alcohol. If a woman does not drink alcohol while she is pregnant, her baby will not have an FASD. Health care providers, families, friends, and other community members all have a role in addressing FASD.

References

1. Project CHOICES Research Group. 2002. Alcohol-exposed pregnancy: Characteristics associated with risk. *American Journal of Preventive Medicine* 23(3):166–173.

2. Astley, S.J.; Bailey, D.; Talbot, C.; et al. 2000. Fetal alcohol syndrome (FAS) primary prevention through FAS diagnosis: I. Identification of high-risk birth mothers through the diagnosis of their children. *Alcohol and Alcoholism* 35(5):499–508.http://alcalc.oxfordjournals.org/cgi/content/full/35/5/499?ijkey=c42ab8b64760a79a7445ab6ef918dc01a3c78acb.

3. Astley, S.J.; Bailey, D.; Talbot, C.; et al. 2000. Fetal alcohol syndrome (FAS) primary prevention through FAS diagnosis: II.

A comprehensive profile of 80 birth mothers of children with FAS. *Alcohol & Alcoholism,* 35(5):509–519.

4. Center for Substance Abuse Treatment. 2001. *Benefits of Residential Substance Abuse Treatment for Pregnant and Parenting Women: Highlights from a Study of 50 Demonstration Programs of the Center for Substance Abuse Treatment.* Rockville, MD: SAMHSA.

5. Stratton, K.; Howe, C.; and Battaglia, F., eds. *Fetal Alcohol Syndrome: Diagnosis, Prevention, and Treatment.* Washington, DC: National Academy Press, 1996.

6. Handmaker, N.S.; Miller, W.R.; and Manicke, M. 1999. Findings of a pilot study of motivational interviewing with pregnant drinkers. *Journal of Studies on Alcohol* 60(2):285–287.

7. Alvik, A.; Haldorsen, T.; and Lindemann, R. 2005. Consistency of reported alcohol use by pregnant women: Anonymous versus confidential questionnaires with item nonresponse differences. *Alcoholism: Clinical and Experimental Research* 29(8):1444–1449.

8. Moraes, C.L.; Viellas, E.F.; and Reichenheim, M.E. 2005. Assessing alcohol misuse during pregnancy: Evaluating psychometric properties of the CAGE, T-ACE and TWEAK in a Brazilian setting. *Journal of Studies on Alcohol* 66(2):165–173.

Chapter 32

Effects of Alcohol on a Fetus

Chapter Contents

Section 32.1

Drinking When You Are Pregnant Can Hurt Your Baby

"Drinking and Your Pregnancy," National Institute on Alcohol Abuse and Alcoholism (NIAAA), 2009.

When you are pregnant, your baby grows inside you. Everything you eat and drink while you are pregnant affects your baby. If you drink alcohol, it can hurt your baby's growth. Your baby may have physical and behavioral problems that can last for the rest of his or her life. Children born with the most serious problems caused by alcohol have fetal alcohol syndrome.

Children with fetal alcohol syndrome may:

- be born small,
- have problems eating and sleeping,
- have problems seeing and hearing,
- have trouble following directions and learning how to do simple things,
- have trouble paying attention and learning in school,
- need special teachers and schools,
- have trouble getting along with others and controlling their behavior, or
- need medical care all their lives.

Can I drink alcohol if I am pregnant? No. Do not drink alcohol when you are pregnant. When you drink alcohol, so does your baby. Think about it. Everything you drink, your baby also drinks.

Is any kind of alcohol safe to drink during pregnancy? No. Drinking any kind of alcohol when you are pregnant can hurt your baby. Alcoholic drinks are beer, wine, wine coolers, liquor, or mixed drinks. A glass of wine, a can of beer, and a mixed drink all have about the same amount of alcohol.

What if I drank during my last pregnancy and my baby was fine? Every pregnancy is different. Drinking alcohol may hurt one baby more than another. You could have one child that is born healthy and another child that is born with problems.

Will these problems go away? No. These problems will last for a child's whole life. People with severe problems may not be able to take care of themselves as adults. They may never be able to work.

What if I am pregnant and have been drinking? If you drank alcohol before you knew you were pregnant, stop drinking now. You will feel better and your baby will have a good chance to be born healthy. If you want to get pregnant, do not drink alcohol. You may not know you are pregnant right away. Alcohol can hurt a baby even when you are only one or two months pregnant.

How can I stop drinking? There are many ways to help yourself stop drinking. You do not have to drink when other people drink. If someone gives you a drink, it is okay to say no. Stay away from people or places that make you drink. Do not keep alcohol at home.

If you cannot stop drinking, get help. You may have a disease called alcoholism. There are programs that can help you stop drinking. They are called alcohol treatment programs. Your doctor or nurse can find a program to help you. Even if you have been through a treatment program before, try it again. There are programs just for women.

Section 32.2

How Alcohol Can Damage a Fetus

This section is excerpted from "Effects of Alcohol on a Fetus," Substance Abuse and Mental Health Services Administration (SAMHSA), 2007.

Prenatal exposure to alcohol can damage a fetus at any time, causing problems that persist throughout the individual's life. There is no known safe level of alcohol use in pregnancy.

How does alcohol damage a fetus? Defects caused by prenatal exposure to alcohol have been identified in virtually every part of the body, including the brain, face, eyes, ears, heart, kidneys, and bones. No single mechanism can account for all the problems that alcohol causes. Rather, alcohol sets in motion many processes at different sites in the developing fetus:

- Alcohol can trigger cell death in a number of ways, causing different parts of the fetus to develop abnormally.

- Alcohol can disrupt the way nerve cells develop, travel to form different parts of the brain, and function.

- By constricting the blood vessels, alcohol interferes with blood flow in the placenta, which hinders the delivery of nutrients and oxygen to the fetus.

- Toxic byproducts of alcohol metabolism may become concentrated in the brain and contribute to the development of an FASD.

Drinking at any time during pregnancy can harm the fetus. Figure 32.2 depicts developing parts and systems in the body of a fetus. These body parts and systems represent some of the sites that may be affected by alcohol.

Prenatal exposure to alcohol can cause permanent brain damage. The fetal brain can be harmed at any time, because the brain develops throughout pregnancy. Magnetic resonance imaging (MRI) reveals that some individuals who were prenatally exposed to alcohol have smaller brains. Some parts of the brain may also be damaged or missing, such as

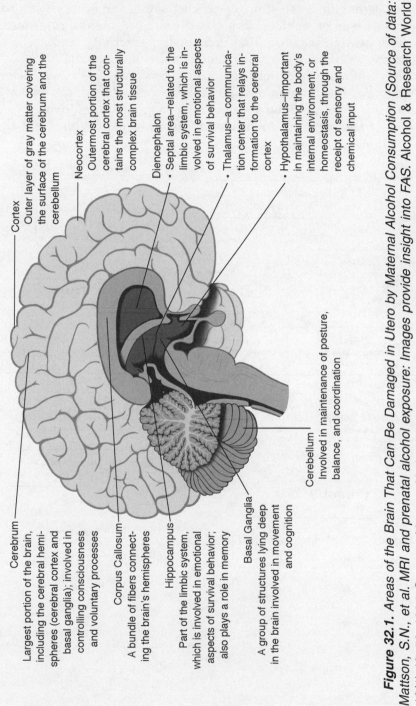

Cortex
Outer layer of gray matter covering the surface of the cerebrum and the cerebellum

Neocortex
Outermost portion of the cerebral cortex that contains the most structurally complex brain tissue

Diencephalon
· Septal area–related to the limbic system, which is involved in emotional aspects of survival behavior
· Thalamus–a communication center that relays information to the cerebral cortex
· Hypothalamus–important in maintaining the body's internal environment, or homeostasis, through the receipt of sensory and chemical input

Cerebrum
Largest portion of the brain, including the cerebral hemispheres (cerebral cortex and basal ganglia); involved in controlling consciousness and voluntary processes

Corpus Callosum
A bundle of fibers connecting the brain's hemispheres

Hippocampus
Part of the limbic system, which is involved in emotional aspects of survival behavior; also plays a role in memory

Basal Ganglia
A group of structures lying deep in the brain involved in movement and cognition

Cerebellum
Involved in maintenance of posture, balance, and coordination

Figure 32.1. *Areas of the Brain That Can Be Damaged in Utero by Maternal Alcohol Consumption (Source of data: Mattson, S.N., et al. MRI and prenatal alcohol exposure: Images provide insight into FAS. Alcohol & Research World 18(1):49–52, 1994. Source of Image: National Institute on Alcohol Abuse and Alcoholism, 2001.)*

the basal ganglia, cerebellum, corpus callosum, and others. Resulting impairments may include, but are not limited to, mental retardation, learning disabilities, attention deficits, hyperactivity, and problems with impulse control, language, memory, and social skills.

Although many questions remain unanswered, this much is clear: When a pregnant woman uses alcohol, her baby does, too. That's why abstaining from drinking throughout pregnancy and during breast feeding is the best gift a mother can give her child—it's a gift that lasts a lifetime.

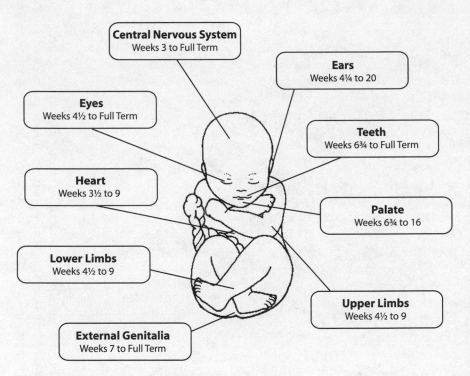

Figure 32.2. Periods of Fetal Development

Section 32.3

Alcohol Binges Linked to Increased Risk of Oral Clefts

"Alcohol Binges Early in Pregnancy Increase Risk of Infant Oral Clefts," National Institute of Environmental Health Sciences (NIEHS), July 31, 2008.

A study by researchers at the National Institute of Environmental Health Sciences (NIEHS), part of the National Institutes of Health, shows that pregnant women who binge drink early in their pregnancy increase the likelihood that their babies will be born with oral clefts.

The researchers found that women who consumed an average of five or more drinks per sitting were more than twice as likely than non-drinkers to have an infant with either of the two major infant oral clefts: cleft lip with or without cleft palate, or cleft palate alone. Women who drank at this level on three or more occasions during the first trimester were three times as likely to have infants born with oral clefts.

"These findings reinforce the fact that women should not drink alcohol during pregnancy," said Lisa A. DeRoo, PhD, an epidemiologist at NIEHS and author on the study. "Prenatal exposure to alcohol, especially excessive amounts at one time, can adversely affect the fetus and may increase the risk of infant clefts." The causes of clefts are largely unknown, but both genetic predisposition and environmental factors are believed to play a role in their development. The paper appeared in the *American Journal of Epidemiology*.

The population-based study was conducted in Norway, which has one of the highest rates of oral clefts in Europe. The investigators contacted all families of newborn infants born with clefts between 1996 and 2002. The study included 573 mothers who had babies born with cleft lip with or without cleft palate and cleft palate only; as well as 763 mothers randomly selected from all live births in Norway. The average age of the mostly married mothers was 29 years. Mothers completed a self-administered mailed questionnaire focused heavily on the mother's lifestyle and environmental exposures during her first three months of pregnancy when a baby's facial development takes place.

The researchers found increased risks of oral-facial clefts among infants whose mothers reported binge-level drinking of an average of five or more drinks per occasion during the first-trimester compared to non-drinkers. Risk was further increased among women who drank at this level most frequently.

Both animal and human data suggest that it is the dose of alcohol consumed at one time during pregnancy rather than the frequency or total amount over time that matters most. "The greater the blood alcohol concentration, the longer the fetus is exposed. A single binge during a critical period of an infant's development can be harmful," said DeRoo.

"Fortunately, heavy maternal drinking is uncommon in many populations, but the fact that it is happening at all tells us we need to do a better job of letting mothers know about the effects that alcohol can have on their baby's development," said Allen J. Wilcox, MD, PhD, NIEHS researcher and co-author on the paper. In Norway, a separate study found that 25% of Norwegian women reported at least one binge drinking episode early during pregnancy.

Alcohol is a recognized teratogen, or an environmental agent that can cause malformations of an embryo or fetus. One of the most severe outcomes of heavy maternal drinking is fetal alcohol syndrome, a life-long condition that causes physical and mental disabilities, including craniofacial malformations. There has been little research to determine if alcohol consumption is related to oral cleft risk.

Reference: DeRoo LA, Wilcox AJ, Drevon CA, Lie RT. First-trimester maternal alcohol consumption and the risk of infant oral clefts in Norway: a population-based case-control study. *American Journal of Epidemiology Advance Access* published July 30, 2008, doi: 10.1093/aje/kwn186.

Chapter 33

Fetal Alcohol Spectrum Disorders (FASD)

Chapter Contents

Section 33.1

Features and Symptoms of FASD

Excerpted from "The Language of Fetal Alcohol Spectrum Disorders," Substance Abuse and Mental Health Services Administration (SAMHSA), 2007.

Experts now know that the effects of prenatal alcohol exposure extend beyond fetal alcohol syndrome (FAS). Fetal alcohol spectrum disorders (FASD) is an umbrella term describing the range of effects that can occur in an individual whose mother drank alcohol during pregnancy. These effects may include physical, mental, behavioral, and learning disabilities with possible lifelong implications. FASD is not a diagnostic term used by clinicians. It refers to conditions such as:

- fetal alcohol syndrome, including partial FAS,

- fetal alcohol effects (FAE),

- alcohol-related neurodevelopmental disorder (ARND), and

- alcohol-related birth defects.

Fetal alcohol syndrome (FAS): FAS consists of a pattern of neurologic, behavioral, and cognitive deficits that can interfere with growth, learning, and socialization. FAS has four major components:

- a characteristic pattern of facial abnormalities (small eye openings, indistinct or flat philtrum, thin upper lip);

- growth deficiencies, such as low birth weight;

- brain damage, such as small skull at birth, structural defects, and neurologic signs, including impaired fine motor skills, poor eye-hand coordination, and tremors; and

- maternal alcohol use during pregnancy.

Behavioral or cognitive problems may include mental retardation, learning disabilities, attention deficits, hyperactivity, poor impulse control, and social, language, and memory deficits. Partial FAS describes persons with confirmed alcohol exposure, facial anomalies, and one other group of symptoms (growth retardation, central nervous system defects, or cognitive deficits).

Fetal alcohol effects: FAE describes children with prenatal alcohol exposure who do not have all the symptoms of FAS. Many have growth deficiencies, behavior problems, cognitive deficits, and other symptoms. However, they do not have the facial features of FAS. Although the term FAE is still used, the Institute of Medicine has coined more specific terms. These include alcohol-related neurodevelopmental disorder and alcohol-related birth defects.

Alcohol-related neurodevelopmental disorder: ARND refers to various neurologic abnormalities, such as problems with communication skills, memory, learning ability, visual and spatial skills, intelligence, and motor skills. Children with ARND have central nervous system deficits but not all the physical features of FAS. Their problems may include sleep disturbances, attention deficits, poor visual focus, increased activity, delayed speech, and learning disabilities.

Alcohol-related birth defects: Alcohol-related birth defects (ARBD) describe defects in the skeletal and major organ systems. Virtually every defect has been described in some patient with FAS. They may include abnormalities of the heart, eyes, ears, kidneys, and skeleton, such as holes in the heart, underdeveloped kidneys, and fused bones.

Origin and Impact of FASD

Cause of FASD: The only cause of FASD is alcohol use during pregnancy. When a pregnant woman drinks, the alcohol crosses the placenta into the fetal blood system. Thus, alcohol reaches the fetus, its developing tissues, and organs. This is how brain damage occurs, which can lead to mental retardation, social and emotional problems, learning disabilities, and other challenges. No alcohol consumption is safe during pregnancy. In addition, the type of alcohol (beer, wine, hard liquor, wine cooler, and so forth) does not appear to make a difference.

Prevalence of FASD: FASD occurs in about ten per 1,000 live births, or about 40,000 babies per year. FAS, the most recognized condition in the spectrum, is estimated to occur in 0.5–2 per 1,000 live births. It now outranks Down syndrome and autism in prevalence.

Assessment of FASD: It is extremely difficult to diagnose a fetal alcohol spectrum disorder. A team of professionals is needed, including a physician, psychologist, speech pathologist, and physical or occupational therapist. Diagnostic tests may include physical exams, intelligence tests, and occupational and physical therapy, psychological, speech, and neurologic evaluations. Diagnosis is easier if the birth mother confirms alcohol use during pregnancy. However, FAS can be diagnosed without confirming maternal alcohol use, if all the symptoms are present.

Impact of FASD: Children with FASD often grow up with social and emotional problems. They may have mental illness or substance abuse problems, struggle in school, and become involved with the corrections system. Costs of FAS alone are estimated at between 1–5 million dollars per child, not including incarceration. This estimate does not include cost to society, such as lost productivity, burden on families, and poor quality of life.

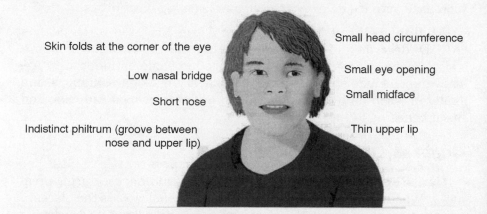

Figure 33.1. *Craniofacial Features Associated with Fetal Alcohol Syndrome: FAS has a characteristic pattern of mild facial anomalies, including small eye openings (for example, short palpebral fissures), a thin upper lip, or flattened ridges between the base of the nose and the upper lip (such as a flattened philtrum) associated with FAS (Source of data: Warren, K.R., and Foudin, L.L. Alcohol-related birth defects—The past, present, and future.* Alcohol Research & Health *25(3):153–158, 2001. Source of image: National Institute on Alcohol Abuse and Alcoholism [NIAAA], February 2005).*

Section 33.2

Diagnosing FASD

Text in this section is excerpted from "Fetal Alcohol Spectrum Disorders (FASD): Diagnosis," Centers for Disease Control and Prevention (CDC), August 24, 2009.

Fetal alcohol spectrum disorders (FASD) are a group of conditions that can occur in a person whose mother drank alcohol during pregnancy. These effects can range from mild to severe. They can affect each person in different ways and can include physical problems and problems with behavior and learning. The term FASD is not intended as a clinical diagnosis.

Guidelines for Diagnosing Fetal Alcohol Syndrome (FAS)

Deciding if a child has FAS takes several steps. There is no one test to diagnose FAS, and many other disorders can have similar symptoms. Following is an overview of the diagnostic guidelines for FAS. These criteria have been simplified for a general audience. They are listed here for information purposes and should be used only by trained healthcare professionals to diagnose or treat FAS.

Healthcare professionals look for the following signs and symptoms when diagnosing FAS:

1. **Abnormal facial features:** A person with FAS has three distinct facial features:

   - Smooth ridge between the nose and upper lip (smooth philtrum)

   - Thin upper lip

   - Short distance between the inner and outer corners of the eyes, giving the eyes a wide-spaced appearance

2. **Growth problems:** Children with FAS have height, weight, or both that are lower than normal (at or below the 10th percentile). These growth issues might occur even before birth. For some children with FAS, growth problems resolve themselves early in life.

3. **Central nervous system problems:** The central nervous system is made up of the brain and spinal cord. It controls all the workings of the body. When something goes wrong with a part of the nervous system, a person can have trouble moving, speaking, or learning. He or she can also have problems with memory, senses, or social skills. There are three categories of central nervous system problems:

I. Structural: FAS can cause differences in the structure of the brain. Signs of structural differences are: smaller-than-normal head size for the person's overall height and weight (at or below the 10th percentile); and significant changes in the structure of the brain as seen on brain scans.

II. Neurologic: There are problems with the nervous system that cannot be linked to another cause. Examples include poor coordination, poor muscle control, and problems with sucking as a baby.

III. Functional: The person's ability to function is well below what's expected for his or her age, schooling, or circumstances. To be diagnosed with FAS, a person must have: a) cognitive deficits (low intelligence quotient [IQ]), or significant developmental delay in children who are too young for an IQ assessment; or, b) problems in at least three of the following areas: cognitive deficits or developmental delays, executive functioning deficits, motor functioning delays, attention problems or hyperactivity, problems with social skills, or other problems (such as sensitivity to taste or touch, difficulty reading facial expression, or difficulty responding to common parenting practices).

4. **Mother's alcohol use during pregnancy:** Confirmed alcohol use during pregnancy can strengthen the case for FAS diagnosis. Confirmed absence of alcohol exposure would rule out the FAS diagnosis. It's helpful to know whether or not the person's mother drank alcohol during pregnancy. But confirmed alcohol use during pregnancy is not needed if the child meets the other criteria.

Summary: Criteria for FAS Diagnosis

A diagnosis of FAS requires the presence of all three of the following findings:

1. All three facial features.

2. Growth deficits.

3. Central nervous system problems. A person could meet the central nervous system criteria for FAS diagnosis if there is a problem with the brain structure, even if there are no signs of functional problems.

Chapter 34

FASD among Native Americans

Chapter Contents

Section 34.1

Scope of FASD among Native American Populations

This section is excerpted from "Fetal Alcohol Spectrum Disorders among Native Americans," Substance Abuse and Mental Health Services Administration (SAMHSA), 2007.

Native Americans have some of the highest rates of fetal alcohol syndrome (FAS) in the United States. Among some tribes the rates are as high as 1.5 to 2.5 per 1,000 live births. The prevalence of FAS in Alaska is 5.6 per 1,000 live births for American Indians/Alaska Natives, compared with 1.5 per 1,000 in the state overall. Among other tribes, the rate is comparable to that of the general population in the United States and ranges from 0.2 to 1.0 per 1,000 live births.

Why is fetal alcohol spectrum disorder (FASD) a problem among Native Americans?

The underlying causes of health disparities are complex. The history of Native Americans is filled with violence, oppression, displacement, and loss of self-determination. This legacy of trauma is believed to be a factor in many problems, including alcohol abuse.

Poverty and inadequate access to health care also play a role. About 32% of Native Americans live below the poverty level, compared with 13% of all Americans. In addition, Native American communities are very young, with a median age of 24. This is almost ten years younger than the overall population. This difference tends to magnify the impact of binge drinking and risky behaviors, which are more common among youth.

FASD, as well as alcoholism and alcohol abuse, are serious problems in some Native communities. However, the stereotype of the drunken Indian is misleading. In some tribes, alcohol use is similar to or lower than the general United States' population. On a typical day, abstinence is common.

Pregnancy is a sacred time for many Native Americans. Many tribes share the belief that individuals must consider the impact of their decisions on the next seven generations. Preventing alcohol abuse during pregnancy is a powerful way to protect future generations and ensure that all children have a healthy start, free of FASD.

Section 34.2

Tips for Native Men to Help Women Be Alcohol-Free

Text in this section is from "How to Help Your Family Member or Friend Be an Alcohol-Free Mother-to-Be: Tips for Native Men," Substance Abuse and Mental Health Services Administration (SAMHSA), 2007.

You could be a father-to-be or even a brother, a cousin, an uncle, or a grandfather. You could be a close friend or a co-worker. If you're close to a pregnant woman who drinks alcohol, you can help her in ways you might not realize. Alcohol hurts at least 40,000 babies born each year. Women of any age, income, or educational level who drink alcohol during pregnancy risk causing problems to their fetus, families, and futures. If you know someone who is (or may become) pregnant, don't be afraid to talk—and listen—to her. Some pregnant women who are careful not to smoke or use drugs during pregnancy may not know that even small amounts of alcohol can hurt their babies. Any information you can share will mean a lot. You'll show her that you care about her and her baby. Pregnant women and the people closest to them all want the same thing—strong, healthy babies. Help her make the safe choice to not drink alcohol during pregnancy.

Information to share: Drinking alcohol during pregnancy may cause mild to severe problems, called fetal alcohol spectrum disorders (FASD). These problems may include lifelong physical, mental, behavioral, and learning disabilities. Children whose mothers drank during pregnancy may need surgeries to fix physical problems. They may also have brain damage that can make it hard to remember things or solve problems. They may not be able to follow simple instructions or form friendships. These challenges may make it difficult to focus in school or follow everyday routines.

The following are important facts to remember and share about FASD:

- FASD is permanent. It cannot be cured.

- FASD is 100% preventable. If a woman doesn't drink when she's pregnant, her baby will not have an FASD.

325

- There is no known safe time, safe amount, or safe type of alcohol to drink while pregnant. Beer and wine are just as harmful as hard liquor.

- If a pregnant woman stops drinking as soon as possible, she can improve her chances of having a healthy baby.

People with an FASD can grow, improve, and succeed in life with the right support, but you can help prevent problems like those mentioned from even starting.

The role native men can play: Native men can have an important role in preventing FASD. They can encourage women not to drink alcohol during pregnancy. They also can support and respect a woman's decision not to drink. Native men can be role models for their significant others. By not drinking alcohol themselves, they are modeling the safest behavior for pregnant women. Native men can also help women get alcohol treatment and follow their treatment plans. These actions can help family members and friends remain alcohol free during their pregnancies.

Start the conversation: Sometimes it's tough to start the conversation with a pregnant friend or family member who is drinking alcohol. Find a quiet place to sit and talk about having a healthy baby. Use a gentle tone of voice, and let her know that you care about her and her child. Remember that your opinion means a lot. Here are some things you might want to talk about:

- Ask her how she is feeling, and remind her that pregnancy is a sacred time.

- Share some of the facts about the problems alcohol can cause and how to prevent FASD.

- Tell her that drinking alcohol during pregnancy can hurt the baby—the baby drinks whatever she drinks. Alcohol goes into the bloodstream and passes to the baby through the umbilical cord.

- Explain that a baby's body cannot get rid of alcohol the same way that adult bodies can.

- Ask her to talk about problems that may be causing her to drink alcohol.

- Remind her that she can talk to you whenever she wants, and be sure to check in on her occasionally.

- Help her connect with a counselor or support group for additional information.

What if your family member or friend says she drank during another pregnancy and the baby was okay? Remind her that every baby is different and that there is no known safe amount of alcohol to drink during pregnancy or even during breast feeding.

Suggest alcohol-free activities: The best time for a woman to stop drinking is before she gets pregnant, but helping your family member or friend stop now can still help her baby. If you stop drinking, this will help her stop drinking, too. You can still enjoy a good time together, engaging in the various activities:

- Go for a walk or treat yourselves to a movie and a pizza.

- With approval from her medical provider, exercise together— take a swim or ride bikes.

- Meet with friends and toast the baby-to-be with healthy drinks like milk, water, or juice. Everyone can have fun while the mother-to-be helps herself have a healthy baby.

If you need more ideas on alcohol-free activities, ask for advice from elders, family members, friends, and co-workers, and visit or call your local clinic or community center. By showing you care, you are helping a mother give her baby a healthy start in life.

Chapter 35

Adopting and Fostering Children with FASD

Parenting has been called the toughest but most fulfilling job in the world. Parenting children with special needs, such as fetal alcohol spectrum disorders (FASD), brings its own set of challenges. Many parents of children with an FASD are adoptive or foster parents. Some knew about FASD when they welcomed their children into their family, while others did not. In any case, information is the key to success in raising children with an FASD. Learning about FASD can help parents understand how their children are affected, which parenting strategies work best, and how to get services and support. For people who want to adopt or foster a child with an FASD, knowing the facts can help them make an informed decision.

FASD is an umbrella term describing the range of effects that can occur in an individual whose mother drank alcohol during pregnancy. These effects may include physical, mental, behavioral, and learning disabilities with possible lifelong implications. The term FASD is not intended for use as a clinical diagnosis. It refers to conditions such as fetal alcohol syndrome (FAS), alcohol-related neurodevelopmental disorder (ARND), and alcohol-related birth defects (ARBD). In the United States, FASD occurs in about ten per 1,000 live births, or about 40,000 babies per year. There is little information available about FASD and adoption or foster care. One study of children in foster care in Washington State revealed a rate

Excerpted from "Adopting and Fostering Children with Fetal Alcohol Spectrum Disorders," Substance Abuse and Mental Health Services Administration (SAMHSA), 2007.

of FAS 10–15 times higher than in the general population, suggesting that children in foster care are more likely to have an FASD. Estimates for international adoptions vary by country. In Russian orphanages, the rate of FAS alone has been estimated at 1–10 per 100.

Meeting the Challenges Associated with FASD

Brain damage and physical defects are the primary disabilities associated with FASD. Lifelong behavioral or cognitive problems may include the following:

- Mental retardation
- Learning disabilities
- Hyperactivity
- Attention deficits
- Problems with impulse control, social skills, language, and memory

These challenges can lead to other problems called secondary disabilities, which may include the following:

- Disrupted school experience
- Alcohol and substance abuse
- Mental illness
- Dependent living
- Problems with employment
- Inappropriate sexual behavior
- Involvement in the criminal or juvenile justice system
- Confinement (prison or inpatient treatment for mental health or substance abuse problems)

A child with an FASD is likely to need services throughout his or her life and may never be able to live independently. The lifetime cost for one child with FAS can be $2 million. Despite their challenges, children with an FASD have a number of strengths. For example, they tend to be caring, creative, determined, and eager to please. They also respond well to structure, consistency, concrete communication, and close supervision. With a supportive home, an early diagnosis, and appropriate services, many children with an FASD can avoid secondary disabilities and reach their full potential.

Gathering Information

Many children who have an FASD lack an accurate diagnosis and their problems may not be clear. Prospective parents may request a copy of a child's complete medical and family history. However, because records may not tell the whole story, prospective parents may also ask specific questions concerning:

- possible prenatal exposure to alcohol or drugs,
- the physical and mental health of the mother and any siblings,
- the developmental history of the child, including possible delays, and
- independent evaluations from a physician.

Most states require adoption and foster care agencies to share information with prospective parents about the health and social history of the child and birth parents. Some states require more information sharing than others, but few specifically address alcohol. Full investigation and disclosure is best for everyone so that placements are successful, parents are prepared, and children get the help they need.

Parenting offers many rewards, despite its hurdles. Those who choose to become a parent or caregiver to a child with an FASD experience great joy along with the challenges. The child can benefit from a stable, loving home with parents and caregivers who understand his or her needs. Ultimately, adoptive and foster parents can change the outlook for individuals with an FASD, one day at a time.

Tips for Adopting or Fostering Children Prenatally Exposed to Alcohol or Other Drugs

1. Work with informed professionals in quality adoption agencies.

2. Explore your feelings about alcohol and drug abuse, particularly among pregnant women.

3. Discuss the child's background with your social worker so that you have a realistic picture of the birth parents' substance use and related lifestyle.

4. Ask for written summaries of the child's diagnoses, medical complications, treatment services, and necessary follow-up care.

5. Ask for information on services and resources to meet the child's needs, including eligibility for adoption subsidies and Medicaid.

331

6. Find out how to reduce the impact of the child's biological risks by providing a nurturing, responsive, and healthy caregiving environment.

7. Recognize that you must be prepared for and able to tolerate the uncertainties that are part of adopting a child prenatally exposed to drugs or alcohol.

8. Resist negative stereotypes of children prenatally exposed to drugs or alcohol, which ignore the individuality of each child and the role of a healthy environment.

9. Recognize the importance of timely identification of problems and early intervention.

Source: Adapted from Edelstein, S. 1995. *Children with Prenatal Alcohol and / or Other Drug Exposure: Weighing the Risks of Adoption.* Washington, DC: CWLA Press.

Chapter 36

FASD May Co-Occur with Mental Illness

Often, a person with a co-occurring fetal alcohol spectrum disorder (FASD) and mental illness is not diagnosed with an FASD. This can cause pain, anger, and frustration. Failure to recognize co-occurring disorders can increase the risk of the following:

- Misdiagnosis and inappropriate or ineffective treatment
- Unemployment or underemployment
- Low self-esteem
- Psychiatric hospitalization
- Problems in school
- Family and relationship problems
- Homelessness
- Alcohol and drug abuse
- Legal problems
- Premature death (suicide, accident, murder, untreated physical illness)

Recognizing an FASD as a co-occurring disorder can help decrease anger and frustration among individuals, families, providers, and community members. Individuals may feel relieved to have an explanation

"How Fetal Alcohol Spectrum Disorders Co-Occur with Mental Illness," Substance Abuse and Mental Health Services Administration (SAMHSA), January 2006.

for their difficulties. Families and communities can understand the nature of the problems and provide support. Service providers can focus on ways to make treatment programs more effective.

What are fetal alcohol spectrum disorders?

Fetal alcohol spectrum disorders (FASD) is an umbrella term describing the range of effects that can occur in an individual who was prenatally exposed to alcohol. These effects may include physical, mental, behavioral, and/or learning disabilities with possible lifelong implications. FASD is not a diagnostic term used by clinicians.

Which disorders co-occur with FASD?

Prenatal alcohol exposure can cause behavioral, cognitive, and psychological problems. Signs and symptoms of FASD are similar to various mental health disorders. In many cases, the signs and symptoms of an FASD go unrecognized or are misdiagnosed as a mental illness or brain injury. Individuals with an FASD may also receive multiple diagnoses, such as attention deficit/hyperactivity disorder (ADHD), oppositional defiant disorder, and anxiety disorder. Therefore, it is important to determine if the signs and symptoms are a result of prenatal alcohol exposure. If an FASD is unrecognized, treatments may be ineffective. When the best possible diagnostic and treatment methods do not work, consider the possibility of an FASD. You may want to seek an FASD assessment, including neuropsychological tests, by a clinician familiar with FASD. FASD can co-occur with many disorders, such as these:

- Major depressive disorder
- Psychotic disorders
- Autism spectrum disorders, including Asperger disorder
- Bipolar disorder
- Personality disorders
- Substance use disorders
- Schizophrenia
- Conduct disorder
- Reactive attachment disorder
- Posttraumatic stress disorder
- Traumatic brain injury

Some conditions, such as reactive attachment disorder, may result from frequent changes in home placement and other environmental factors. In addition, FASD can lead to many of the psychosocial stressors noted in the *Diagnostic and Statistical Manual of Mental Disorders, 4th Edition (DSM-IV)*, such as the following:

- Educational problems

- Occupational problems

- Financial problems

- Legal problems

- Problems with relationships

The *DSM-IV* has no codes for fetal alcohol spectrum disorders. For insurance purposes, providers may list a co-occurring mental illness as the primary diagnosis. Regardless of which diagnostic code is used, an FASD must be seriously considered when developing an individual's treatment plan.

How can we recognize co-occurring conditions?

Co-occurring disorders among persons with an FASD may occur more often in those with a family history of mental health disorders. Some conditions, such as schizophrenia, mood disorders, and attention deficit/hyperactivity disorder (ADHD), have genetic vulnerability. Because persons with an FASD are likely to have co-occurring conditions, getting an accurate diagnosis is critical. A thorough diagnostic workup should be completed, including the following:

- Maternal alcohol history

- Medical and family history, including information such as head circumference and length of eye openings, illness, seizure disorders, and coordination problems

- Individual and family mental health history

- Evaluation of any developmental disabilities

- Thorough medical evaluation

- Neuropsychological tests

- Adaptive functioning tests

- Psychiatric evaluation

The cognitive impairments in FASD can hinder the ability to succeed in treatment. Such impairments include these:

- Difficulty following multiple directions at home, school, work, and treatment settings.

- Difficulty participating in treatment that requires receptive language skills, such as group therapy, 12-step programs, and motivational interviewing.

- Difficulty processing information outside sessions and applying what they have learned (for example, can recite rules but will repeatedly break them because they forget or cannot apply them).

- Tendency to process information very literally (for example, when told to take a cab home, one young man stole a cab).

- Difficulty grasping the concept of historic time and future time. Reward systems that involve earning points one week for rewards the next may be ineffective. Punishing people for things they did weeks ago may not produce positive change.

What can treatment personnel do?

To produce the best outcomes, it is necessary to diagnose and treat all conditions simultaneously. Treatment personnel should avoid over- or under-diagnosing. Communicating with families to get as much information as possible is key to an accurate diagnosis and an effective treatment plan.

Most importantly, treatment personnel can focus on positive outcomes for their clients. Instead of viewing individuals as failing if they do not do well in a program, staff need to view the program as not providing what the individual needs to succeed. Treatment personnel need to investigate the cause of any behavior, such as failure to understand instructions.

Understanding the individual's disorders, needs, and strengths will help in developing an effective approach that enables the person to succeed. Correctly identifying all co-occurring disorders and treating them appropriately can lead to improved outcomes for the individual, family, and service providers.

Part Five

Mental Health Problems Associated with Alcohol Abuse

Chapter 37

Anxiety Disorders and Alcohol Abuse

For many people, a glass of wine after a long day at work helps take the edge off, or a drink at a party helps them loosen up. But for those with an anxiety disorder, alcohol or other substances can make anxiety symptoms worse and may even trigger a panic attack. The risk and occurrence of alcohol abuse is high in people who have an anxiety disorder.

According to a 2004 study released on co-occurring alcohol abuse and mental health disorders (*National Epidemiologic Survey on Alcohol and Related Conditions,* conducted by the National Institute on Alcohol Abuse and Alcoholism), about 20% of American adults with an anxiety or mood disorder (such as depression) also have an alcohol or other substance abuse disorder; about 20% of those with an alcohol or substance abuse disorder also have an anxiety or mood disorder. Although having co-occurring alcohol abuse and anxiety disorders makes things complicated, the disorders are treatable—separately and together.

Are people with anxiety disorders more likely to suffer from alcohol abuse than the general population and vice versa?

People with anxiety disorders are two to three times more likely to have an alcohol or other substance abuse disorder at some point in their lives than the general population and vice versa. However the risk and prevalence of alcohol abuse is more common among people with some anxiety disorders.

Which occurs first, an anxiety disorder or alcohol abuse?

A great deal of variability exists in how people experience these conditions together. Following are possible courses of the co-occurring conditions:

- The alcohol abuse and anxiety disorders are independent, meaning that one does not cause the other. However, the symptoms of one can worsen the symptoms of the other.

- An anxiety disorder leads someone to use alcohol or another substance to self-medicate, or attempt to alleviate their anxiety symptoms. This usually exacerbates anxiety.

- An alcohol abuse problem causes heightened anxiety during specific periods of abuse, such as during drinking or withdrawal; some studies have shown the withdrawal from alcohol may activate the same neural pathways as anxiety. These anxiety symptoms may go away at other times and usually are eliminated completely after problem drinking stops.

- An alcohol or other substance abuse problem leads to development of a substance-induced anxiety disorder. This may happen because some substances change the way brain cells communicate, including affecting the neurotransmitters (or chemical messengers) in the nervous system; substance abuse can damage parts of the brain that keep anxiety in check. This type of anxiety disorder will last during a period of substance abuse and sometimes for a short period afterward.

According to the *National Epidemiologic Survey on Alcohol and Related Conditions*, most people with alcohol or substance abuse and anxiety disorders experience them independently, with none or only some anxiety episodes induced by alcohol or drugs. This is important for patients as well as therapists, who should not assume that treating substance abuse will solve an anxiety disorder. Treating the disorders together is often necessary.

Can other difficulties arise from alcohol abuse and having an anxiety disorder?

Having an anxiety disorder and alcohol abuse disorder can cause a vicious cycle. For example, someone with an anxiety disorder may alleviate anxiety symptoms with alcohol, which causes more anxiety as a side effect, and then leads to more drinking. Other complications may include the following:

* High risk for medical illnesses, hospitalizations, financial and family problems, and other issues

* Lower treatment compliance

* Increased risk of relapse into alcohol abuse

* Increased risk of dangerous interactions between prescription medication and alcohol

* May have more pronounced alcohol withdrawal symptoms

It is of the utmost importance to treat both types of disorders. Discuss the points above with your doctor when determining your treatment plan.

Are specific anxiety disorders more often associated with alcohol abuse? How does the relationship between anxiety and alcohol differ based on a person's anxiety disorder?

Research has found that co-occurrence is more common in people with social anxiety disorder and posttraumatic stress disorder (PTSD). And some research has shown the order in which the disorders develop may vary based on the type of anxiety disorder. For example, alcohol abuse in people with social anxiety disorder and agoraphobia usually develops after the onset of the anxiety disorder; people report drinking alcohol to control anxiety. Or alcohol abuse commonly begins before or at the same time as symptoms in people with generalized anxiety disorder (GAD) and panic disorder.

Some disorders also have noteworthy circumstances when co-occurring with alcohol abuse:

Panic disorder: Panic attacks can often be caused by use of alcohol or drugs, worsening or even inducing the course of the disorder. Panic disorder has also been singled out in research as a risk factor for a major substance abuse relapse among people with both disorders.

Posttraumatic stress disorder (PTSD): PTSD and alcohol abuse may commonly co-occur for a variety of reasons, including that alcohol abuse may increase the likelihood of being exposed to trauma (and developing PTSD), or people who have PTSD may use alcohol to self-medicate. Many characteristics of substance abuse can exacerbate symptoms of PTSD such as sleep disturbance and irritability. Many professionals now treat both disorders at the same time because symptoms of PTSD can drive relapse to substance abuse.

341

Social anxiety disorder: People with social anxiety disorder often report that alcohol helps lessen their symptoms. But substance use often makes anxiety worse. Certain treatment approaches commonly used for substance abuse, such as group therapy or 12-step programs (used by Alcoholics Anonymous or Narcotics Anonymous) may be difficult for a person very anxious in social situations. In this case, a more individualized treatment strategy is necessary.

Can an anxiety disorder and substance abuse be treated at the same time and by the same professional?

Many professionals or treatment teams can treat these disorders together for the best chance of successful recovery and the least chance of relapse, particularly when one disorder doesn't cause the other. Find out if your doctor can treat both conditions or if another professional will be part of your treatment team.

What treatments are available for people suffering from both conditions?

Many therapists prefer to use non-medication treatments because the risk for medication abuse increases. Therapists prescribe medications that have low potential for abuse and are safe if a person relapses into substance abuse. (Even when considered safe, medications for anxiety and substance abuse are less effective when used with alcohol or drugs.)

Many doctors prescribe SSRIs (selective serotonin reuptake inhibitors), which are a class of antidepressants commonly used in the treatment of anxiety disorders and often used in conjunction with therapy. They may avoid prescribing benzodiazepines, another class of medications, which carry an increased risk of abuse, tolerance, and physical dependence; this is not the best option for someone who has experienced substance abuse.

The choice of medication always depends on individual conditions, including the specific anxiety disorder, and appropriate options must be discussed with a doctor.

Other treatment options for anxiety disorders and substance abuse, which can be used alone or in combination with medication, include these:

- **Cognitive-behavioral therapy (CBT):** This short-term form of therapy teaches people how to replace negative and unproductive thought patterns with more realistic and useful ones.

- **Individual psychotherapy:** Patients explore areas of emotional and social conflict.

- **Group psychotherapy:** People meet in a group to discuss shared and individual experiences.

- **Self-help or other treatment groups:** People with similar needs or experiences join meetings that are facilitated by a consumer, survivor, or other layperson. Self-help groups for anxiety disorders can be found at the Anxiety Disorders Association of America (ADAA) website: http://www.adaa.org. Contact Alcoholics Anonymous or Narcotics Anonymous for meetings in your area.

Chapter 38

Depression and Alcohol Use

Chapter Contents

Section 38.1

Depression and Initiation of Alcohol Use among Youth

This section is excerpted from "Depression and the Initiation of Alcohol and Other Drug Use among Youths Aged 12 to 17," Substance Abuse and Mental Health Services Administration (SAMHSA), May 3, 2007. The complete report with references is available at http://www.oas.samhsa.gov/2k7/newUserDepression/newUserDepression.htm.

Research has shown that there is a strong association between mental health disorders and substance use disorders, but findings about the order of onset and direction of influence vary by substance and type of disorder. There is strong evidence, for example, that alcohol abuse can be a contributing factor to the development of depression, but more typically the mental condition occurs prior to the substance use disorder. Associations also exist between mental disorders and substance use behaviors that do not meet the criteria for substance use disorders. For example, research suggests that adults and adolescents with major depressive episode (MDE) in the past year were more likely than those without MDE to have used alcohol heavily or to have used an illicit drug in the past year.

The National Survey on Drug Use and Health (NSDUH) includes questions for youths aged 12 to 17 to assess lifetime and past year MDE. For these estimates, MDE is defined using the diagnostic criteria set forth in the fourth edition of the *Diagnostic and Statistical Manual of Mental Disorders (DSM-IV)*, which specifies a period of two weeks or longer during which there is either depressed mood or loss of interest or pleasure and at least four other symptoms that reflect a change in functioning, such as problems with sleep, eating, energy, concentration, and self-image.

NSDUH also asks youths aged 12 to 17 to report on their use of alcohol and illicit drugs in their lifetime and in the past year. Illicit drugs refer to marijuana/hashish, cocaine (including crack), inhalants, hallucinogens, heroin, or prescription-type drugs used nonmedically. Respondents who reported use of a given substance were asked when they first used it; responses to these questions were used to identify persons at risk for substance use initiation (persons who had not ever

346

used the substance prior to the 12 months preceding the survey) and to identify recent initiates (persons who used the substance for the first time in the 12 months prior to the survey). In 2005 among youths aged 12 to 17, past year initiates accounted for 29.8% of all past year illicit drug users and 32.5% of past year alcohol users.

Past Year Major Depressive Episode

In 2005, 8.8% of youths aged 12 to 17 (2.2 million persons) experienced at least one MDE in the past year. Females were three times as likely as males to have a past year MDE (13.3% versus 4.5%). Rates of past year MDE varied by age, with youths aged 17 having the highest rate of past year MDE (11.9%) and those aged 12 having the lowest rate (4.3%). Rates of past year MDE were relatively similar across racial/ethnic groups.

Initiation of Alcohol and Illicit Drug Use in the Past Year

The 2005 NSDUH indicates that 2.7 million youths aged 12 to 17 were past year initiates of alcohol use, representing 15.4% of youths who were at risk for initiation of alcohol use. An estimated 1.5 million youths were past year initiates of illicit drug use, which represents 7.6% of youths at risk for initiation of illicit drug use.

Major Depressive Episode and Substance Use Initiation in the Past Year

Past year MDE was associated with substance use initiation in the past year. Among youths aged 12 to 17 who had not previously used alcohol, those who experienced a past year MDE were twice as likely to have initiated alcohol use in the past year as those who had not experienced a past year MDE (29.2% versus 14.5%). Similarly, among youths who had not previously used an illicit drug, those who experienced a past year MDE were over twice as likely to have initiated use of an illicit drug in the past year as those who had not experienced a past year MDE (16.1% versus 6.9%).

Table 38.1. Percentages Reporting Past Year Substance Use Initiation among Persons Aged 12 to 17 Who Were at Risk for Substance Use Initiation,* by Past Year Major Depressive Episode (MDE): 2005

Substance Use	Past Year MDE	No Past Year MDE
Initiated Alcohol Use	29.2	14.5
Initiated Illicit Drug Use	16.1	6.9

Source: SAMHSA, 2005 NSDUH.
*Persons at risk for substance use initiation are defined as individuals who had not ever used the substance prior to the 12 months preceding the survey.

Section 38.2

Co-Occurring Major Depressive Episode (MDE) and Alcohol Use Disorder among Adults

This section is excerpted from "Co-Occurring Major Depressive Episode (MDE) and Alcohol Use Disorder among Adults," Substance Abuse and Mental Health Services Administration (SAMHSA), February 16, 2007. The complete report with references is available at http://www.oas.samhsa .gov/2k7/alcDual/alcDual.htm.

Depression and alcohol use problems can each impair a person's ability to carry out routine activities at home or work and negatively impact daily life. The occurrence of depression and alcohol use problems in the same individuals is a major public health concern.

The National Survey on Drug Use and Health (NSDUH) asks persons aged 12 or older questions to assess lifetime and past year major depressive episode (MDE). NSDUH defines MDE using the diagnostic criteria set forth by the fourth edition of the *Diagnostic and Statistical Manual of Mental Disorders* (*DSM-IV*), which specifies a period of two weeks or longer in which there is either depressed mood or loss of interest or pleasure and at least four other symptoms that reflect a change in functioning, such as problems with sleep, eating, energy, concentration, and self-image. Respondents with MDE were asked about their experiences with treatment for depression during the past year. Treatment for MDE is defined as seeing or talking to a medical doctor or other health professional or taking prescription medication for MDE.

NSDUH also asks respondents questions to assess their symptoms of alcohol dependence or abuse during the past year. NSDUH defines alcohol dependence or abuse using criteria specified in the *DSM-IV*, including symptoms such as withdrawal, tolerance, use in dangerous situations, trouble with the law, and interference in major obligations at work, school, or home during the past year. Individuals who meet the criteria for either alcohol dependence or abuse are said to have an alcohol use disorder. Respondents are also asked about treatment they received in the past year for alcohol problems. For these analyses, an individual is defined as having received treatment for an alcohol use disorder only if he or she reported receiving such treatment at a specialty facility in the past year.

This report examines past year MDE, alcohol use disorder, and co-occurring MDE and alcohol use disorder among adults aged 18 or older. For the purposes of this report, individuals with both MDE and alcohol use disorders in the past 12 months are said to have co-occurring MDE and alcohol use disorders. All findings presented in this report are based on combined 2004 and 2005 NSDUH data.

Past Year Major Depressive Episode

Combined data from 2004 and 2005 indicate that 7.6% of adults (an estimated 16.4 million persons) experienced at least one MDE in the past 12 months. Women were nearly twice as likely as men to have past year MDE (9.8% versus 5.4%). Persons aged 50 or older were less likely to have past year MDE than adults in other age groups (Figure 38.1). Adults aged 18 or older with a past year alcohol use disorder were more than twice as likely as those with no past year alcohol use disorder to have experienced MDE in the past year (Figure 38.2).

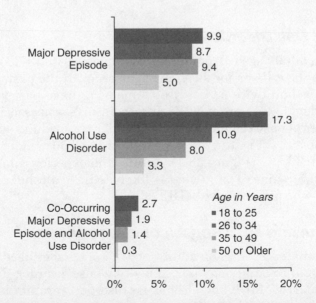

Figure 38.1. Percentages of Persons Aged 18 or Older with Past Year Major Depressive Episode, Alcohol Use Disorder, and Co-Occurring Major Depressive Episode and Alcohol Use Disorder, by Age Group: 2004–2005. Source of data: SAMHSA, 2004 and 2005 NSDUHs.

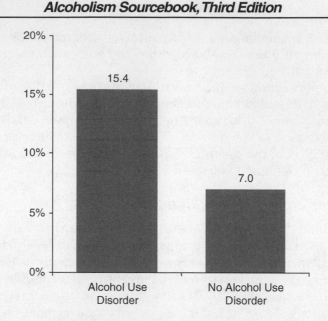

Figure 38.2. *Percentages of Past Year Major Depressive Episode among Persons Aged 18 or Older, by Past Year Alcohol Use Disorder: 2004–2005. Source of data: SAMHSA, 2004 and 2005 NSDUHs.*

Alcohol Use Disorder

Among adults aged 18 or older, 8.0% (an estimated 17.3 million persons) met the criteria for alcohol use disorder in the past year. Males were more than twice as likely as females to have past year alcohol use disorder (11.2% versus 5.0%). Increasing age was associated with a lower rates of past year alcohol use disorder, with adults aged 18 to 25 having the highest rate (17.3%) and adults aged 50 or older having the lowest rate (3.3%) (Figure 38.1). Adults who experienced MDE in the past year were more than twice as likely to have alcohol use disorder as adults who did not have MDE.

Co-Occurring MDE and Alcohol Use Disorder

An estimated 2.7 million adults, or 1.2% of persons aged 18 or older, had past year co-occurring MDE and alcohol use disorder. Rates of past year co-occurring MDE and alcohol use disorder were similar for males and females (1.3% and 1.1%, respectively). Increasing age was associated with lower rates of past year co-occurring MDE and alcohol use disorder, with adults aged 18 to 25 having the highest rate (2.7%) and adults aged 50 or older having the lowest rate (0.3%) (Figure 38.1).

Treatment of MDE and Alcohol Use Disorder

Adults with past year co-occurring MDE and alcohol use disorder may receive treatment for their MDE only, for their alcohol use disorder only, for both their MDE and alcohol use disorder, or for neither problem. Among adults with past year co-occurring MDE and alcohol use disorder, 40.7% did not receive treatment in the past year for either problem. Nearly half (48.6%) received treatment in the past year for MDE only, 1.9% received treatment at a specialty facility for alcohol use disorder only, and 8.8% received treatment for both problems.

Chapter 39

Post-Traumatic Stress Disorder (PTSD) and Problems with Alcohol Use

Post-traumatic stress disorder (PTSD) does not automatically cause problems with alcohol use; there are many people with PTSD who do not have problems with alcohol. However, PTSD and alcohol together can be serious trouble for the trauma survivor and his or her family.

How do PTSD and alcohol use affect each other and make problems worse?

PTSD and alcohol problems often occur together: People with PTSD are more likely than others with similar backgrounds to have alcohol use disorders both before and after being diagnosed with PTSD, and people with alcohol use disorders often also have PTSD. Being diagnosed with PTSD increases the risk of developing an alcohol use disorder.

Women exposed to trauma show an increased risk for an alcohol use disorder even if they are not experiencing PTSD. Women with problematic alcohol use are more likely than other women to have been sexually abused at some point in their lives.

Men and women reporting sexual abuse have higher rates of alcohol and drug use disorders than other men and women. Twenty-five to seventy-five percent of those who have survived abusive or violent trauma also report problems with alcohol use.

"PTSD and Problems with Alcohol Use," U.S. Veteran Affairs (VA) National Center for Posttraumatic Stress Disorder, May 22, 2007.

Ten to thirty-three percent of survivors of accidental, illness, or disaster trauma report problematic alcohol use, especially if they are troubled by persistent health problems or pain. Sixty to eighty percent of Vietnam veterans seeking PTSD treatment have alcohol use disorders. Veterans over the age of 65 with PTSD are at increased risk for attempted suicide if they also experience problematic alcohol use or depression. War veterans diagnosed with PTSD and alcohol use tend to be binge drinkers. Binges may be in reaction to memories or reminders of trauma.

Alcohol problems often lead to trauma and disrupt relationships: Persons with alcohol use disorders are more likely than others with similar backgrounds to experience psychological trauma. They also experience problems with conflict and intimacy in relationships. Problematic alcohol use is associated with a chaotic lifestyle, which reduces family emotional closeness, increases family conflict, and reduces parenting abilities.

PTSD symptoms often are worsened by alcohol use: Although alcohol can provide a temporary feeling of distraction and relief, it also reduces the ability to concentrate, enjoy life, and be productive. Excessive alcohol use can impair one's ability to sleep restfully and to cope with trauma memories and stress. Alcohol use and intoxication also increase emotional numbing, social isolation, anger and irritability, depression, and the feeling of needing to be on guard (hyper-vigilance). Alcohol use disorders reduce the effectiveness of PTSD treatment.

Many individuals with PTSD experience sleep disturbances (trouble falling asleep or problems with waking up frequently after falling asleep). When a person with PTSD experiences sleep disturbances, using alcohol as a way to self-medicate becomes a double-edged sword. Alcohol use may appear to help symptoms of PTSD because the alcohol may decrease the severity and number of frightening nightmares commonly experienced in PTSD. However, alcohol use may, on the other hand, continue the cycle of avoidance found in PTSD, making it ultimately much more difficult to treat PTSD because the client's avoidance behavior prolongs the problems being addressed in treatment. Also, when a person withdraws from alcohol, nightmares often increase.

Additional Mental Health Issues

Individuals with a combination of PTSD and alcohol use problems often have additional mental or physical health problems. As many as 10%–50% of adults with alcohol use disorders and PTSD also have one or more of the following serious disorders:

- Anxiety disorders (such as panic attacks, phobias, incapacitating worry, or compulsions)

- Mood disorders (such as major depression or a dysthymic disorder)

- Disruptive behavior disorders (such as attention deficit or anti-social personality disorder)

- Addictive disorders (such as addiction to or abuse of street or prescription drugs)

- Chronic physical pain due to physical injury/illness or due to no clear physical cause

What are the most effective treatment patterns?

Because the existence of both PTSD and an alcohol use disorder in an individual makes both problems worse, alcohol use problems often must be addressed in PTSD treatment. When alcohol use is (or has been) a problem in addition to PTSD, it is best to seek treatment from a PTSD specialist who also has expertise in treating alcohol (addictive) disorders. In any PTSD treatment, several precautions related to alcohol use and alcohol disorders are advised:

- The initial interview and questionnaire assessment should include questions that sensitively and thoroughly identify patterns of past and current alcohol and drug use.

- Treatment planning should include a discussion between the professional and the client about the possible effects of alcohol use problems on PTSD, sleep, anger and irritability, anxiety, depression, and work or relationship difficulties.

- Treatment should include education, therapy, and support groups that help the client address alcohol use problems in a manner acceptable to the client.

- Treatment for PTSD and alcohol use problems should be designed as a single consistent plan that addresses both sources of difficulty together. Although there may be separate meetings or clinicians devoted primarily to PTSD or to alcohol problems, PTSD issues should be included in alcohol treatment, and alcohol use (addiction or sobriety) issues should be included in PTSD treatment.

- Relapse prevention must prepare the newly sober individual to cope with PTSD symptoms, which often seem to worsen or become more pronounced with abstinence.

Where can you get help?

For a listing of professionals in the USA and Canada who treat alcohol disorders and PTSD, we suggest consulting the membership directories of the International Society for Traumatic Stress Studies or the Association of Traumatic Stress Specialists. For veterans experiencing problems with PTSD and alcohol use, the Department of Veterans Affairs has a network of specialized PTSD and substance use treatment programs. For information on these programs, contact the local VA Vet Center or the Psychiatry Service at a VA Medical Center. (For addresses and telephone numbers, look under the "United States Government" listings in the telephone directory.)

References

Evans, K. and Sullivan, J. M. (1995). *Treating addicted survivors of trauma*. New York: Guilford Press.

Kofoed, L., Friedman, M.J., and Peck, R. (Summer 1993). Alcoholism and drug abuse in patients with PTSD. *Psychiatric Quarterly*, 64(2), 151-171.

Matsakis, A. (1992). *I can't get over it: A handbook for trauma survivors*. Oakland, CA: New Harbinger Publications.

Chapter 40

Attention Deficit/Hyperactivity Disorder (ADHD) with Conduct Disorder Raises Alcohol-Abuse Risk

Adolescents who were diagnosed with attention deficit/hyperactivity disorder (ADHD) as children face a higher risk of alcohol abuse and dependence, and problems indicating a conduct-disorder diagnosis appear to increase this risk further. Children with attention-deficit/ hyperactivity disorder (ADHD) may be at risk for alcohol-use disorders when they reach adolescence, according to new findings from University of Pittsburgh researchers.

"We found that once children diagnosed with ADHD became teenagers, they were more likely than those without ADHD to drink heavily or to have diagnosable alcohol use disorders," Brooke Molina, PhD, told *Psychiatric News*. The results of the study she and her colleagues conducted appear in the April Alcoholism: Clinical and Experimental Research.

The researchers wanted to test whether there was an association between childhood ADHD and later alcohol use and whether conduct problems in childhood could predict risk for alcohol problems among those who had been diagnosed with ADHD as children.

They interviewed 364 adolescents and young adults enrolled in the Pittsburgh ADHD Longitudinal Study, all of whom had been diagnosed with ADHD as children, and 240 age-matched controls who had never been diagnosed with ADHD. The 364 teenagers and young adults had initially been diagnosed with ADHD at the Western Psychiatric

Institute and Clinic in Pittsburgh between 1987 and 1996. Most were in elementary school at the time. Researchers recruited subjects in the control group from the Pittsburgh area between 1999 and 2001 through several large pediatric practices and advertisements placed in newspapers and at local colleges.

Molina and her colleagues evaluated these participants either as adolescents (11 to 17 years old) or young adults (18 to 25 years old) for the presence of alcohol use disorders as well as on a number of drinking measures, including the frequency and quantity of drinking. They also assessed whether those who had been diagnosed with ADHD as children had comorbid conduct disorder, and whether those who were adults at the time of the follow-up evaluation had comorbid antisocial personality disorder.

Researchers used the parent and teacher Disruptive Behavior Disorder Rating Scale to determine whether adolescents had conduct disorder. To determine whether young adults had antisocial personality disorder, parents and subjects completed the Antisocial Personality Disorder portion of the Structured Clinical Interview for *DSM-IV*.

Molina noted that for adolescents who had previously been diagnosed with ADHD, the risk for heavy drinking or drinking problems began at around age 15. For example, the teens aged 15 to 17 with childhood ADHD reported being drunk an average of 14 times in the previous year versus 1.8 times for those without an ADHD diagnosis. Approximately 14% of those who had been diagnosed with ADHD were diagnosed upon follow-up with alcohol abuse or dependence, and none of the 15- to 17-year-olds without childhood ADHD had alcohol problems.

The researchers also found that those with ADHD and co-existing conduct disorder as adolescents had significantly higher rates of alcohol abuse than did those with ADHD alone: for instance, 20.7% of those with ADHD and concurrent conduct disorder as adolescents were diagnosed with alcohol abuse, compared with 4.8% of those with ADHD alone. Molina also found that 10.3% of adolescents with ADHD and concurrent conduct disorder met criteria for alcohol dependence, compared with 1.6% of those with only ADHD.

For those assessed in early adulthood (aged 18 to 25), Molina found that 42% of those with ADHD and antisocial personality disorder met criteria for alcohol abuse or dependence as compared with less than 20% of those with only ADHD.

Molina pointed out that children with ADHD have a higher risk of developing both adolescent conduct disorder and alcohol problems, even when they don't have serious conduct problems in childhood. This means that all children with ADHD should be considered potentially at risk, especially if alcoholism runs in the family. The importance of familial alcoholism as a risk factor is described in the researchers' second paper in the same issue of *Alcoholism: Clinical and Experimental Research*.

Molina acknowledged that in general most people tend to drink most heavily between the ages of 18 and 25, so she and her collaborator William Pelham, PhD, hope to follow the sample into their 30s to examine whether drinking problems decline with age, as they do in the general population.

"The message to most of us in the ADHD field is that ADHD persists into adolescence for about two-thirds of youth, so parents and practitioners need to stay involved. Among other things, heavy drinking is a possible outcome for a substantial minority of these youth," Molina noted. "This seems to be a disorder that [even with treatment] stays in place. So we need more research on how to help these kids once they reach adolescence and adulthood."

Chapter 41

Alcohol and Other Addiction Disorders

Chapter Contents

Section 41.1

Alcohol and Tobacco

Text in this section is excerpted from "Alcohol and Tobacco," National Institute on Alcohol Abuse and Alcoholism (NIAAA), January 2007. The complete document with references is available at http://pubs.niaaa.nih.gov/publications/AA71/AA71.htm.

Alcohol and tobacco are among the top causes of preventable deaths in the United States. Moreover, these substances often are used together: Studies have found that people who smoke are much more likely to drink, and people who drink are much more likely to smoke. Dependence on alcohol and tobacco also is correlated: People who are dependent on alcohol are three times more likely than those in the general population to be smokers, and people who are dependent on tobacco are four times more likely than the general population to be dependent on alcohol.

The link between alcohol and tobacco has important implications for those in the alcohol treatment field. Many alcoholics smoke, putting them at high risk for tobacco-related complications including multiple cancers, lung disease, and heart disease (cardiovascular disease). In fact, statistics suggest that more alcoholics die of tobacco-related illness than die of alcohol-related problems. Also, questions remain as to the best way to treat these co-occurring addictions; some programs target alcoholism first and then address tobacco addiction, whereas others emphasize abstinence from drinking and smoking simultaneously. Effective treatment hinges on a better understanding of how these substances—and their addictions—interact.

Understanding just how alcohol and tobacco interact is challenging. Because co-use is so common, and because both substances work on similar mechanisms in the brain, it's proving difficult to tease apart individual and combined effects of these drugs. In this Alcohol Alert, we examine the latest research on the interactions between these two substances, including the prevalence of co-occurring tobacco and alcohol use disorders (AUDs), some of the health consequences of combined use, biological mechanisms and genetic vulnerabilities to co-use and dependence, barriers to the treatment of tobacco dependence in patients with alcohol and other drug (AOD) use disorders, therapies that are proving effective in treating co-occurring tobacco and alcohol dependence in depressed patients, and treatment interventions for adolescent patients with co-occurring tobacco and AOD use disorders.

How prevalent are alcohol and tobacco use?

The National Institute on Alcohol Abuse and Alcoholism's (NIAAA's) 2001–2002 National Epidemiologic Survey on Alcohol and Related Conditions (NESARC), which is one of the largest comorbidity studies ever conducted, included extensive questions about alcohol and tobacco use and related disorders. NESARC data confirmed the widespread use of alcohol with tobacco: Approximately 46 million adults used both alcohol and tobacco in the past year, and approximately 6.2 million adults reported both an AUD and dependence on nicotine.

Alcohol and tobacco use varied according to gender, age, and ethnicity, with men having higher rates of co-use than women. Younger people tended to have a higher prevalence of AUDs, nicotine dependence, and co-use. Although Whites were more likely to drink alcohol, American Indians/Alaskan Natives were most likely to smoke, or to smoke and drink concurrently. Asians/Native Hawaiians/Pacific Islanders were least likely to smoke or drink, or smoke and drink concurrently.

Comorbid mood or anxiety disorders are another risk factor for both alcoholism and nicotine dependence. NESARC data show that alcohol abuse is strongly correlated with a co-occurring mood or anxiety disorder. The presence of comorbid mental illness also raises risk for tobacco addiction. In another study, Williams and Ziedonis found that 50% to 90% of people with mental illness or addiction were dependent on nicotine.

What health risks are associated with alcohol and tobacco use?

Alcohol and tobacco use may lead to major health risks when used alone and together. In addition to contributing to traumatic death and injury (through car crashes), alcohol is associated with chronic liver disease, cancers, cardiovascular disease, acute alcohol poisoning (alcohol toxicity), and fetal alcohol syndrome. Smoking is associated with lung disease, cancers, and cardiovascular disease. Additionally, a growing body of evidence suggests that these substances might be especially dangerous when they are used together; when combined, alcohol and tobacco dramatically increase the risk of certain cancers.

Why do tobacco and alcohol use co-occur so frequently?

Clearly environmental factors contribute to the problem. Both drugs are legally available and easily obtained. Over the past two decades, however, it also has become clear that biological factors are at least partly responsible. Although tobacco and nicotine have very different effects and mechanisms of action, Funk and colleagues speculate that they might act on common mechanisms in the brain, creating complex interactions. These possible mechanisms are difficult to study because alcohol and nicotine can affect people differently depending on the amount of the drugs consumed and because numerous factors, including gender and age, influence the interaction between nicotine and alcohol. Still, a common mechanism might explain many of the interactions between tobacco and alcohol, as well as a possible genetic link between alcoholism and tobacco dependence.

Mutual craving: Studies show that consuming tobacco and alcohol together can augment the pleasure users experience from either drug alone. For example, in a study by Barrett and colleagues, subjects were given either nicotine-containing or nicotine-free cigarettes and asked to perform progressively more difficult tasks in order to earn alcoholic beverages. The subjects who smoked nicotine-containing cigarettes worked harder and drank more alcohol than those smoking nicotine-free cigarettes. Conversely, Rose and colleagues showed that drinking alcohol enhances the pleasure reported from smoking cigarettes. This research is supported by animal studies, which show that nicotine-treated animals consumed more alcohol than did control animals.

Common brain system: Evidence increasingly suggests that both alcohol and tobacco may act on the mesolimbic dopamine system, a part of the brain that is involved in reward, emotion, memory, and cognition. Brain cells (neurons) that release dopamine—a key brain chemical involved in addiction—have small docking molecules (receptors) to which nicotine binds. Evidence suggests that the interaction between alcohol and tobacco may take place at these nicotinic receptors. When nicotinic receptors are blocked, people not only tend to consume less nicotine but also less alcohol. This common mechanism of action may explain some of the interactions between alcohol and tobacco, including why alcohol and tobacco can cause users to crave the other drug and the phenomenon of cross-tolerance.

Tolerance and cross-tolerance: A decrease in a person's sensitivity to a drug's effects often is referred to as tolerance. This phenomenon occurs when a person must consume more of a substance in order to achieve the same rewarding effect. In the case of alcohol and tobacco, this puts him or her at greater risk for developing dependence. Cross-tolerance—that is, when tolerance to one drug confers tolerance to another—also has been documented in people who smoke and drink.

Genetic factors: Studies suggest that common genetic factors may make people vulnerable to both alcohol and tobacco addiction. Clearly, both alcohol and nicotine dependence runs in families. Identical twins (who share 100% of their deoxyribonucleic acid [DNA]) are twice as likely as fraternal twins (who, like all siblings, share 50% of their DNA) to be nicotine and alcohol dependent if the other twin is dependent. And recently, the Collaborative Study on the Genetics of Alcoholism—the first study to examine the human genetic makeup (or genome) for regions that involve both alcohol dependence and smoking—has identified genes and regions of genes that may be involved in both AUDs and nicotine dependence.

Conclusion

Because of the mortality and morbidity associated with both tobacco and alcohol abuse, it is important to address both addictions. Research is beginning to explain some of the reasons behind the frequent co-occurrence of these disorders. Treating co-occurring disorders remains a challenge; however, evidence suggests that combining treatments might be the most effective way to address concurrent addictions. Special populations, such as depressed patients and adolescents, present additional challenges, but research is exploring new strategies targeting these groups. Although more work needs to be done, it is clear that research already is helping to improve the lives of people with co-occurring addictions to alcohol and nicotine.

Section 41.2

Concurrent Alcohol and Illicit Drug Use

This section is excerpted from "Concurrent Illicit Drug and Alcohol Use," Substance Abuse and Mental Health Services Administration (SAMHSA), March 19, 2009. The complete document with references is available at http://oas.samhsa.gov/2k9/alcDrugs/alcDrugs.htm.

Concurrent use of illicit drugs and alcohol is a serious public health concern because of the potential additive or interactive effects of multiple substance use, which may lead to more severe adverse consequences than use of a single substance. Little is known about the prevalence of illicit drug use at the same time or within a few hours of alcohol use. The National Survey on Drug Use and Health (NSDUH) can help to address the need for information in this area. This section examines this topic using annual averages based on combined 2006 and 2007 NSDUH data.

Illicit Drug Use Concurrent with Last Alcohol Use

Illicit drug use concurrent with the respondent's last alcohol use was reported by 5.6% of past month alcohol users aged 12 or older; this is equivalent to an estimated 7.1 million persons. The illicit drug most frequently used with alcohol was marijuana (4.8%), followed by cocaine and pain relievers (0.6 and 0.4%, respectively) (Figure 41.1).

Concurrent Illicit Drug and Alcohol Use, by Demographic Characteristics

Among past month alcohol users, males were nearly twice as likely as females to report illicit drug use concurrent with last alcohol use (7.1% versus 3.9%). Rates were higher among adolescent and young adult past month drinkers than their older counterparts (14.2% among 12 to 17 year olds, 13.5% among 18 to 25 year olds, 7.7% among 26 to 34 year olds, 4.3% among 35 to 49 year olds, and 1.1% among those aged 50 or older) (Figure 41.2). American Indian or Alaska Native past month drinkers had the highest rate of illicit drug use concurrent with last alcohol use, and Asian drinkers had the lowest rate (11.7% and 2.1%, respectively).

Concurrent Illicit Drug Use and Level of Alcohol Use

The likelihood of using illicit drugs concurrently with last alcohol use varied with the number of drinks consumed. Among past month alcohol users, those who binged on alcohol during their last occasion of use (had five or more drinks within a couple of hours) were more likely than their counterparts who did not binge (had four or fewer drinks) to have used illicit drugs concurrently with their last alcohol use (13.9% versus 3.8%, respectively).

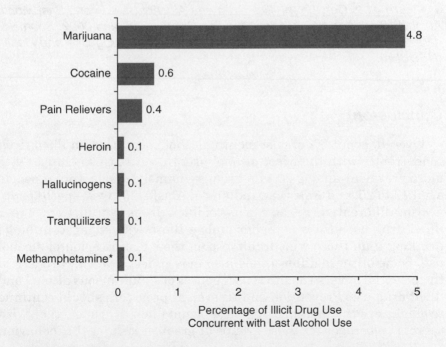

Figure 41.1. *Illicit Drug Use Concurrent with Last Alcohol Use among Past Month Alcohol Users Aged 12 or Older, by Type of Illicit Drug: 2006 and 2007. Source of data: 2006 and 2007 SAMHSA National Surveys on Drug Use and Health (NSDUHs).*

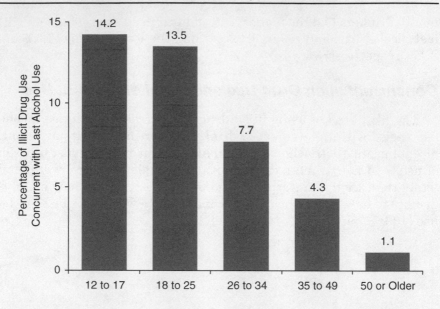

Figure 41.2. *Concurrent Illicit Drug and Alcohol Use among Past Month Alcohol Users Aged 12 or Older, by Age Group: 2006 and 2007. Source of data: 2006 and 2007 SAMHSA National Surveys on Drug Use and Health (NSDUHs).*

Conclusion

Overall, about 6% of past month alcohol users used an illicit drug concurrently with their last alcohol use. However, this behavior was more prevalent among certain groups—namely, males, young people aged 12 to 25, and American Indians or Alaska Natives—perhaps reflecting differentials in rates of use of illicit drugs overall. Concurrent illicit drug use also was higher among those who engaged in binge drinking than those who drank less on their last occasion of alcohol use. Some of these differentials also may reflect lower awareness of the potential adverse health consequences of simultaneous alcohol and illicit drug use. Prevention and treatment providers should continue to emphasize the risks of using alcohol and illicit drugs together, with targeted messages for those groups at greatest risk for this behavior.

Section 41.3

Alcohol and Risks for Other Drug Dependence

Excerpted from "Alcohol and Other Drugs," *Alcohol Alert,* Number 76, July 2008, National Institute of Alcohol Abuse and Alcoholism (NIAAA). The complete document with references is available at http://pubs.niaaa.nih.gov/publications/AA76/AA76.htm.

Drug and alcohol dependence often go hand in hand. Research shows that people who are dependent on alcohol are much more likely than the general population to use drugs, and people with drug dependence are much more likely to drink alcohol. For example, Staines and colleagues found that, of 248 alcoholics seeking treatment, 64% met the criteria for a drug use disorder at some point in their lifetime.

Patients with co-occurring alcohol and other drug use disorders also are likely to have more severe dependence-related problems than those without combined disorders—that is, they meet a higher number of diagnostic criteria for each disorder (three out of seven criteria are required to meet the diagnosis of dependence). People with co-occurring alcohol and other drug use disorders are more likely to have psychiatric disorders such as personality, mood, and anxiety disorders; they are more likely to attempt suicide and to suffer health problems. People who use both alcohol and drugs also are at risk for dangerous interactions between these substances. For example, a person who uses alcohol with benzodiazepines, whether these drugs are prescribed or taken illegally, is at increased risk of fatal poisoning.

How common is alcohol and other drug use, and how often do alcohol and drug use disorders co-occur? To answer these questions, the National Institute on Alcohol Abuse and Alcoholism (NIAAA) conducted the National Epidemiologic Survey on Alcohol and Related Conditions (NESARC), one of the largest surveys of its kind ever performed. It examined the prevalence of alcohol and other drug use and abuse in the United States. According to NESARC, 8.5% of adults in the United States met the criteria for an alcohol use disorder, whereas 2% met the criteria for a drug use disorder and 1.1% met the

369

criteria for both. People who are dependent on drugs are more likely to have an alcohol use disorder than people with alcoholism are to have a drug use disorder. Young people ages 18–24 had the highest rates of co-occurring alcohol and other drug use disorders. Men were more likely than women to have problems with alcohol, drugs, or the two substances combined.

Genetics of Alcohol and Other Drug Use Disorders— Shared Risk Factors?

Research has established that some of the risk for addiction to both drugs and alcohol is inherited. Children of alcoholics are 50% to 60% more likely to develop alcohol use disorders than people in the general population. Similarly, children of parents who abuse illicit drugs may be 45% to 79% more likely to do so themselves than the general public. This suggests that some of the risk factors for alcohol and other drug use are rooted in genetics, though studies of specific families have not proven a genetic contribution.

Researchers believe that some of the same genes that increase a person's risk for problems with alcohol also might put him or her at greater risk for drug dependence. Moreover, those same genes might increase the risk for other psychiatric problems, such as conduct disorder and adult antisocial behavior (externalizing behaviors).

Diagnosing Substance Use Disorders: Barriers and Challenges

An accurate diagnosis is the first step toward treatment and recovery. However, diagnosing people with drug and alcohol disorders can be complicated, especially when these disorders occur concurrently. There are barriers to diagnosis: For example, patients may be unwilling to talk about their addiction, and clinicians may be unaware of the signs and symptoms of abuse and dependence.

Clinicians should screen patients for alcohol and other drug use disorders in a systematic, step-by-step fashion. Clinicians may screen patients for drug problems using instruments such as the Drug Abuse Screening Test (DAST) or the CAGE–Adapted to Include Drugs (CAGE–AID), or using a urine drug test. Clinicians should take a full history of any patient suspected of having a problem with drugs, asking, for example, about which drugs are used, age of first use, pattern of use, consequences of use, attempts to quit, and treatment history. It also is crucial to evaluate patients for signs of intoxication or withdrawal.

370

Clinicians should assess the patient's psychiatric history, medical history, family history, and social and developmental history.

Despite careful screening, however, some substance use disorders go undetected. Patients often misreport their substance use because of the stigma associated with an alcohol or other drug use disorder diagnosis, or they may fear legal reprisals. To address these fears, clinicians should make sure patients know the scope of confidentiality required by law. Clinicians also should make an effort to be empathic, accepting, and nonjudgmental; to ask questions in a direct and straightforward manner; and to deal with their own discomfort regarding drug use so as not to communicate their anxiety to their patients.

Although not as common, some patients over-report their substance use. For example, a patient suffering from untreated or inadequately treated pain may exaggerate his or her use of opiates in order to obtain methadone or buprenorphine (drugs used to treat opioid addiction) to alleviate that pain. Such patients would benefit from treatment by a pain specialist.

Additionally, clinicians may fail to recognize substance use disorders because they do not routinely screen for substance use, especially in patients who do not look like typical substance users. According to NESARC data, there is no typical substance user; problem alcohol and drug use occurs in people across genders, age-groups, and ethnic backgrounds. It is important that clinicians evaluate all patients for substance use disorders.

Treatment

Behavioral therapies: For most patients, the most effective treatment approaches combine behavioral treatments (motivation enhancement therapy [MET] and cognitive-behavioral therapy [CBT]) and pharmacological treatments. MET seeks to motivate patients who are resistant to treatment, and CBT gives people the skills to reduce their drinking or to abstain from drinking. Contingency management interventions are another tool. These interventions center on rewarding positive behavior. Behavioral therapy also is an important tool for helping patients comply with medication regimens.

Pharmacotherapies: In addition to behavioral therapy, pharmacotherapies can help patients to curb their use of alcohol and other drugs. This section explores traditional and new medications available to treat alcohol and drug dependence.

Disulfiram interferes with the breakdown of alcohol. When a person taking disulfiram drinks alcohol, it causes a buildup of acetaldehyde—a toxic byproduct of alcohol—in the body. This causes a variety of unpleasant effects, including reddening or flushing of the face and neck, nausea, and nervousness. The U.S. Food and Drug Administration (FDA) approved disulfiram in 1949 for the treatment of alcohol use disorders. In a study of 600 male veterans, overall, disulfiram had no effect on long-term abstinence. Among individuals who drank, however, the active dosage of the medication (250 mg/day) reduced the number of days the subjects spent drinking. Disulfiram can cause potentially serious effects when combined with alcohol, so the patient's goal must be abstinence. Patients who respond well to disulfiram tend to be older, with greater social stability and motivation for recovery; they tend to have a longer drinking history, attend Alcoholics Anonymous meetings, and be free of alcohol-related dementia and other cognitive problems.

Disulfiram may be useful in treating cocaine addiction, both by producing an adverse reaction similar to that produced with alcohol and by reducing the euphoria associated with the drug. Successful treatment with disulfiram requires strict adherence to the medication regimen—patients who take disulfiram must be highly motivated to continue treatment.

Naltrexone blocks the activity of a class of molecules (opiate receptors). These molecules are involved in relaying chemical messages in the brain that are involved in addiction. In addition to an oral form, the FDA has approved a long-acting, injectable form of naltrexone for the treatment of alcohol dependence. Research shows that naltrexone reduces the risk of relapse in heavy drinkers; however, there is less evidence that it reduces the number of drinking days or that it helps patients to maintain total abstinence.

Studies also have shown that naltrexone may be useful in treating drug use disorders, including opioid and cocaine dependence. Naltrexone has been approved by the FDA for the treatment of opioid dependence; however, because it can cause acute withdrawal from opiates (potentially making the patient feel very ill), patients should be drug-free for at least seven days before beginning treatment. Additionally, patients should be warned that if they return to using opiates heavily, they run the risk of death because naltrexone will reduce their tolerance to opiates and put them at risk for overdose.

Acamprosate also affects certain chemical messengers (neurotransmitters) in the brain. Although the FDA approved acamprosate for the treatment of alcohol dependence, research with this medication has produced mixed results. European studies have shown that acamprosate not only reduces the risk of heavy drinking, but nearly doubles the likelihood that patients will achieve abstinence. These studies suggest that acamprosate is most useful in patients who develop alcohol dependence later in life, who do not have a family history of alcohol dependence, and who display physical dependence and higher than usual levels of anxiety. It is important to note that other studies show that acamprosate is no more effective than placebo.

Anticonvulsant medications: Topiramate has been shown to be an effective treatment for alcohol dependence and may be beneficial for cocaine dependence treatment. Other anticonvulsants, including carbamazepine and valproate, also have shown some effectiveness in treating alcohol use disorders, and they may be especially useful in patients with co-occurring alcohol dependence and bipolar disorder.

Serotonergic and other medications: Although studies are scarce, some research has shown that medications which target other mechanisms in the brain (selective serotonin reuptake inhibitors [SSRIs], atypical antipsychotic medications, or lithium) may be useful in treating substance use disorders. The medications appear to be particularly useful for treating certain subgroups of alcohol-dependent patients, based on the age of onset of problem drinking.

Conclusion

Addictive disorders represent a major health issue both in the United States and worldwide. Because alcohol and drug dependence are likely to co-occur, exploring how alcohol addiction may relate to and interact with other addictions is important. Current research is exploring the underlying causes of addiction, and why alcohol and other drug use disorders co-occur so frequently, as well as how behavioral and drug therapies can best treat these disorders. There is no magic bullet for treating addiction—no treatment will work for everyone in every situation. More research is needed to identify effective treatments for different populations, especially youth, older people, and patients with co-occurring psychiatric disorders. Such research is vital to better understand the mechanisms and course of addiction as well as its diagnosis and treatment.

Section 41.4

Substance Use and Dependence Following Initiation of Alcohol Use

This section is excerpted from "Substance Use and Dependence Following Initiation of Alcohol or Illicit Drug Use," Substance Abuse and Mental Health Services Administration (SAMHSA), March 27, 2008. The complete document with references is available at http://www.oas.samhsa.gov/2i8/newUseDepend/newUseDepend.htm.

A series of recent research reports has examined the characteristics associated with the development of dependence soon after the initiation of alcohol, marijuana, cocaine, and hallucinogen use. These studies suggest that each drug class has a different trajectory from first use to cessation of use, continuation of use without dependence, or dependence upon the drug.

The National Survey on Drug Use and Health (NSDUH) asks persons aged 12 or older to report on their use of alcohol and illicit drugs during their lifetime and in the past year. Illicit drugs refer to marijuana/hashish, cocaine (including crack), inhalants, hallucinogens, heroin, or prescription-type drugs used non-medically. Respondents who reported use of a given substance were asked when they first used it; responses to these questions were used to determine the number of months since they initiated use of the substance.

NSDUH also asks questions to assess symptoms of substance dependence during the past year. NSDUH defines substance dependence using criteria specified by the fourth edition of the *Diagnostic and Statistical Manual of Mental Disorders* (*DSM-IV*). It includes such symptoms as withdrawal, tolerance, unsuccessful attempts to cut down on use, and continued use despite health and emotional problems caused by the substance.

This section examines the development of dependence upon a substance in the two years following substance use initiation (1–24 months after initiation). For the purposes of this report, persons who initiated use of a substance 13 to 24 months prior to the interview are referred to as year-before-last initiates. Year-before-last initiates were assigned to three mutually exclusive categories reflecting their substance use trajectories following initiation: those who had not used the substance in the past 12 months (past year), those who had used the substance during the past year but were not dependent on the substance during the past year, and those who had used the substance and were dependent on the substance during the past year.

Comparisons are made across substance classes in terms of the percentages of these year-before-last initiates classified in each of these three past year categories. All findings presented in this report are annual averages based on combined 2004, 2005, and 2006 NSDUH data.

Table 41.1. Percentages of Past Year Use and/or Dependence among Year-Before-Last Initiates Aged 12 or Older, by Substance: 2004–2006

Substance	No Use in Past 12 Months	Use in Past 12 Months but Not Dependent	Use in Past 12 Months and Dependent in Past 12 Months
Alcohol	25.7%	71.1%	3.2%
Marijuana	42.4%	51.8%	5.8%
Cocaine use			
Cocaine (not including Crack)*	57.5%	38.8%	3.7%
Crack*	75.6%	15.2%	9.2%
Heroin	69.4%	17.2%	13.4%
Hallucinogens	61.5%	36.6%	1.9%
Inhalants	72.6%	26.5%	0.9%
Nonmedical use of psycho-therapeutics*			
Pain relievers	56.6%	40.2%	3.1%
Tranquilizers	58.8%	40.0%	1.2%
Stimulants	59.1%	36.2%	4.7%
Sedatives	63.7%	33.9%	2.4%

*Dependence for cocaine not specific to form.

Source: SAMHSA, 2004–2006 NSDUHs

Noncontinuation of Substance Use Following Initiation

Among year-before-last initiates of specific substances, over two-thirds of crack cocaine, inhalant, and heroin initiates did not use the drug in the past year. Alcohol and marijuana were the only substances for which the majority of year-before-last initiates used the substance in the past year.

Risk for Developing Alcohol Dependence Following Initiation

Among year-before-last initiates of alcohol, one-fourth (25.7%) had not used alcohol during the past year, 71.1% had used alcohol in the past year but were not dependent on alcohol, and 3.2% were both using and dependent on alcohol during the past year.

Chapter 42

Alcohol's Association with Suicide

Chapter Contents

Section 42.1

Excessive Alcohol Use Increases Risk of Suicidal Thoughts and Suicide Attempts

Excerpted from "Suicidal Thoughts, Suicide Attempts, Major Depressive Episode, and Substance Use among Adults" Substance Abuse and Mental Health Services Administration (SAMHSA), December 30, 2008. The complete document with references is available at http://oas.samhsa.gov/2k6/suicide/suicide.htm.

Suicidal Thoughts, Suicide Attempts, Major Depressive Episode, and Substance Use among Adults

Suicide is a major public health problem in the United States. In 2003, suicide was the 11th leading cause of death among adults and accounted for 30,559 deaths among people aged 18 or older. Suicide rates vary across demographic groups, with some of the highest rates occurring among males, Whites, and the older population. Suicide also is strongly associated with mental illness and substance use disorders.

Individuals who die from suicide, however, represent a fraction of those who consider or attempt suicide. In 2003, there were 348,830 nonfatal emergency department (ED) visits by adults aged 18 or older who had harmed themselves. Research suggests that there may be between eight and twenty-five attempted suicides for every suicide death. As with suicide completions, risk factors for attempted suicide in adults include depression and substance use.

The mission of the Office of Applied Studies (OAS) in the Substance Abuse and Mental Health Services Administration (SAMHSA) is to collect, analyze, and disseminate critical public health data. OAS manages two national surveys that offer insight into suicidal ideation and attempts and, in particular, drug-related suicide attempts: the National Survey on Drug Use and Health (NSDUH) and the Drug Abuse Warning Network (DAWN).

NSDUH is the nation's primary source of information on the prevalence of illicit drug use among the civilian, noninstitutionalized population aged 12 or older and also provides estimates of alcohol and tobacco use and mental health problems in that population. NSDUH data provide information about the relationships between suicidal thoughts, suicide attempts, and substance use among adults aged 18 or older who have had at least one major depressive episode (MDE) during the past year.

DAWN is a public health surveillance system that measures some of the health consequences of drug use by monitoring drug-related visits to hospital emergency departments (EDs) in the United States. Data from DAWN provide information about the patients, types of drugs, and other characteristics of suicide-related DAWN ED visits.

NSDUH Methods and Findings

NSDUH asks adults aged 18 or older questions to assess lifetime and past year major depressive episodes (MDEs). MDE is defined using diagnostic criteria from the fourth edition of the *Diagnostic and Statistical Manual of Mental Disorders* (*DSM-IV*), which specifies a period of two weeks or longer during which there is either depressed mood or loss of interest or pleasure and at least four other symptoms that reflect a change in functioning, such as problems with sleep, eating, energy, concentration, and self-image. Suicide-related questions are administered to respondents who report having had a period of two weeks or longer during which they experienced either depressed mood or loss of interest or pleasure. These questions ask if (during their worst or most recent episode of depression) respondents thought it would be better if they were dead, thought about committing suicide, and, if they had thought about committing suicide, whether they made a suicide plan and whether they made a suicide attempt.

NSDUH also asks all respondents about their use of alcohol and illicit drugs during the 12 months prior to the interview. Binge alcohol use is defined as drinking five or more drinks on the same occasion (at the same time or within a couple of hours of each other) on at least one day in the past 30 days. Any illicit drug refers to marijuana/ hashish, cocaine (including crack), inhalants, hallucinogens, heroin, or prescription-type drugs used nonmedically.

This section examines the prevalence of suicidal thoughts among adults who experienced at least one MDE during the past year. Because mental illness and substance use commonly co-occur, the prevalence of past year MDE, suicidal thoughts, and suicide attempts is also examined by substance use status.

Prevalence of MDE: In 2004–2005, 14.5% of persons aged 18 or older (31.2 million adults) experienced at least one MDE in their lifetime, and 7.6% (16.4 million adults) experienced an MDE in the past year. Females were almost twice as likely as males to have experienced a past year MDE (9.8% versus 5.4%). Rates of past year MDE varied by age group, with adults aged 55 or older being less likely to have had a past year MDE than adults in all other age groups.

Suicidal thoughts among adults with MDE: Among adults aged 18 or older who experienced a past year MDE, 56.3% thought, during their worst or most recent MDE, that it would be better if they were dead, and 40.3% thought about committing suicide. There were some differences in suicidal thoughts by gender and age. Although males and females with past year MDE did not differ significantly in the percentage who thought that it would be better if they were dead, males were more likely than females to have thought about committing suicide (45.5% versus 37.6%). Among adults with a past year MDE, those aged 55 or older were less likely than individuals in all other age groups to have thought that it would be better if they were dead and to have thought about committing suicide. There were no significant differences in the prevalence of suicidal thoughts by region or urbanicity.

Past Month Substance Use, MDE, and Suicidal Thoughts and Behaviors

Adults aged 18 or older who reported binge alcohol use were more likely to report past year MDE than their counterparts who had not engaged in binge drinking (8.7% versus 7.3%). In addition, adults with past year MDE and past month binge alcohol use were more likely to report past year suicidal thoughts and past year suicide attempts than those with MDE who did not binge drink.

Table 42.1. Percentages Reporting Suicidal Thoughts and Suicide Attempts among Adults Aged 18 or Older with a Past Year Major Depressive Episode, by Past Month Binge Alcohol Use: 2004 and 2005 NSDUHs

	Past Month Binge Alcohol Use	No Past Month Binge Alcohol Use
Past Year Suicidal Thoughts	61.8	57.1
Past Year Suicide Attempt	13.7	9.1

Source: SAMHSA, 2004 and 2005 NSDUHs.

Similarly, adults aged 18 or older who reported having used illicit drugs during the past month were more likely to report past year MDE than adults who had not used illicit drugs during the past month (14.2% versus 7.1%). Rates of past year suicidal thoughts and suicide attempts were also higher among adults with past year MDE who had used illicit drugs during the past month than adults with past year MDE who had not used illicit drugs.

Table 42.2. Percentages Reporting Suicidal Thoughts and Suicide Attempts among Adults Aged 18 or Older with a Past Year Major Depressive Episode, by Past Month Illicit Drug Use: 2004 and 2005 NSDUHs

	Past Month Illicit Drug Use	No Past Month Illicit Drug Use
Past Year Suicidal Thoughts	67.0	56.9
Past Year Suicide Attempt	19.0	8.9

Source: SAMHSA, 2004 and 2005 NSDUHs.

DAWN Methods and Findings

DAWN is a public health surveillance system that monitors drug-related ED visits in the United States. Data are collected from a nationally representative sample of short-stay, general, non-federal hospitals that operate 24-hour emergency departments (ED). In DAWN, a drug-related ED visit is defined as any ED visit related to drug use. The drug must be implicated in the ED visit, either as the direct cause or as a contributing factor. For each drug-related ED visit, information is gathered from medical records about the number and types of drugs involved. These include illegal or illicit drugs, such as cocaine, heroin, and marijuana; prescription drugs; over-the-counter medications; dietary supplements; inhalants; and alcohol. DAWN differs from NSDUH in that it captures medical as well as nonmedical use of pharmaceuticals and includes pharmaceuticals sold over the counter as well as by prescription. DAWN also collects demographic information about the patients, their diagnoses, and their disposition (outcome) at the time of their discharge from the ED.

In this report, ED visits associated with drug-related suicide attempts among persons aged 18 or older are examined. Although DAWN includes only those suicide attempts that involve drugs, these attempts are not limited to overdoses. Also included are suicide attempts made by other means (by firearm) when drugs are involved. National estimates of the number of ED visits involving drug-related suicide attempts in 2004 are presented, along with percentages of visits and visit rates per 100,000 population. The patients, types of drugs, and other characteristics of drug-related suicide attempts treated in EDs are described.

Substances involved in drug-related suicide attempts treated in EDs: In 2004, an average of 2.3 drugs were implicated in suicide attempts by adults aged 18 or older that were treated in the ED. Over 33% (35,560 visits) involved only one drug, 51.3% involved two or three drugs, and 15.2% involved four or more drugs.

Table 42.3. Selected Drugs Involved in Emergency Department (ED) Visits for Drug-Related Suicide Attempts among Persons Aged 18 or Older: National Estimates, 2004 DAWN

Selected Drug Category/Drug	Estimated ED Visits	Percentage of ED Visits
Alcohol	35,242	33.2
Illicit Drugs	30,109	28.4
Cocaine	13,620	12.8
Marijuana	8,490	8.0
Psychotherapeutic Medications	62,502	58.9
Antidepressants	23,359	22.0
Anxiolytics/sedatives/hypnotics	41,188	38.8
Antipsychotics	11,968	11.3
Pain Medications	38,238	36.0
Opioids	15,706	14.8
Nonsteroidal anti-inflammatory agents (NSAIDs)	8,167	7.7
Acetaminophen/combinations	14,410	13.6
Anticonvulsants	7,961	7.5
Cardiovascular Medications	5,859	5.5

Source: SAMHSA, 2004 DAWN (September 2005 update).

About one-third of the drug-related suicide attempts treated in the ED involved alcohol. Alcohol is always reported to DAWN if the patient was younger than age 21. If the patient was aged 21 or older, alcohol is reported only if it was used with another drug. Although it is an illegal substance for persons under age 21, alcohol was involved in approximately 25% (2,504 visits) of the suicide-related DAWN ED visits by patients aged 18 to 20 and frequently was combined with another drug (2,504 visits). The suicide-related DAWN ED visits involving patients aged 55 or older had the lowest rate of alcohol involvement, although it should be noted that DAWN only captured these visits for adults if alcohol was used with another drug.

Outcomes from drug-related suicide attempts: The disposition of an ED visit provides information about the patient's outcome, as well as clues to the suicide attempt's severity. Of the estimated 106,079 drug-related suicide attempts treated in EDs, less than 1% ended in death in the ED. However, this estimate is based solely on ED records, which do not include patients who died before coming to the ED or after leaving the ED (after admission to the hospital). Patients in about 81% (85,789) of the visits received further treatment, either as inpatients at the same hospital (60,020) or by transfer to another health care facility (25,769). In an estimated 16% (16,811) of visits, the patients were released after treatment in the ED.

Section 42.2

Alcohol and Suicide among Racial/Ethnic Populations

Excerpted from "Alcohol and Suicide among Racial/Ethnic Populations—17 States, 2005–2006," *MMWR Weekly* 58(23); 637–641, Centers for Disease Control and Prevention (CDC), June 19, 2009. The complete document with references is available at http://www.cdc.gov/mmwr/preview/mmwrhtml/mm5823a1.htm.

During 2001–2005, an estimated annual 79,646 alcohol-attributable deaths (AAD) and 2.3 million years of potential life lost (YPLL) were attributed to the harmful effects of excessive alcohol use. An estimated 5,800 AAD and 189,667 YPLL were associated annually with suicide. The burden of suicide varies widely among racial and ethnic populations in the United States, and limited data are available to describe the role of alcohol in suicides in these populations. To examine the relationship between alcohol and suicide among racial/ethnic populations, Centers for Disease Control and Prevention (CDC) analyzed data from the National Violent Death Reporting System (NVDRS) for the two-year period 2005–2006 (the most recent data available). This report summarizes the results of that analysis, which indicated that the overall prevalence of alcohol intoxication (blood alcohol concentration [BAC] at or above the legal limit of 0.08 g/dL) was nearly 24% among suicide decedents tested for alcohol, with the highest percentage occurring among American Indian/Alaska Natives (AI/ANs) (37%), followed by Hispanics (29%) and persons aged 20–49 years (28%).

NVDRS is an active, state-based surveillance system that collects information on homicides, suicides, deaths of undetermined intent, deaths from legal intervention (involving a person killed by an on-duty police officer), and unintentional firearm deaths. CDC used five racial/ethnic categories: Hispanic, non-Hispanic White, non-Hispanic Black, non-Hispanic AI/AN, and non-Hispanic Asian/Pacific Islander (A/PI). Analysis was limited to persons aged ten years and older. Data from two years, 2005 and 2006, were aggregated to produce more stable estimates than could be obtained from an analysis of data from a single year.

A total of 19,255 suicides occurred in the 17 states contributing data to NVDRS during 2005–2006 (Alaska, California [covering four major metropolitan counties], Colorado, Georgia, Kentucky, Massachusetts, Maryland, North Carolina, New Jersey, New Mexico, Oklahoma, Oregon, Rhode Island, South Carolina, Utah, Virginia, and Wisconsin). This analysis excluded 21 decedents because they were aged less than ten years or of unknown age and 240 decedents who were classified as "other" race or unknown race and/or ethnicity, resulting in a final sample of 18,994.

Alcohol-related information was assessed by NVDRS through questions asked of next of kin, judgment by medical or law enforcement officials, or laboratory data. Information collected related to 1) the decedent's alcohol dependence or problem (whether the victim was perceived by self or others to have a problem with, or to be addicted to, alcohol); 2) suspected alcohol use (whether alcohol use by the decedent in the hours preceding the incident was suspected, based on witness or investigator reports or circumstantial evidence, such as empty alcohol containers around the decedent); 3) testing for alcohol (whether the decedents blood was tested for the presence of alcohol); 4) alcohol test results (recorded as positive, negative, not applicable [not tested], or unknown); and 5) the decedent's blood alcohol content (BAC) measured in g/dL. A BAC of 0.08 g/dL or greater was used to define intoxication consistent with the standard set by the U.S. Department of Transportation. Coroner and medical examiner records indicated that nearly 70% of the decedents were tested for BAC. The analysis of BAC excluded persons not tested for alcohol and persons who were tested for alcohol but for whom no quantitative values were recorded.

The highest percentage of suicide decedents characterized as dependent on alcohol was observed among non-Hispanic AI/ANs (21%); the lowest percentage was observed among non-Hispanic Blacks (7%). Recent alcohol use was suspected in approximately 46% of non-Hispanic AI/ANs, nearly 30% of Hispanics, and 26% of non-Hispanic Whites.

The highest percentage of suicide decedents tested for alcohol was among non-Hispanic Blacks (76%). Alcohol was detected in the blood of 33.2% of decedents tested, with the highest percentages occurring among non-Hispanic AI/AN (45.5%) and Hispanic (39.0%) subjects tested.

For all age groups, the highest percentage of decedents with BACs of 0.08 g/dL or greater was among AI/ANs aged 30–39 years (54.3%), followed by AI/AN and Hispanic decedents aged 20–29 years (50.0% and 37.3%, respectively). Among decedents tested who were aged 10–19 years (all of whom were under the legal drinking age in the United States), 12% had BACs of 0.08 g/dL or greater; the levels ranged from 1.3% in non-Hispanic Blacks to 28.6% in non-Hispanic A/PIs. Among male decedents tested, 25% tested above legal intoxication; among females tested, 18% tested above legal intoxication. Males had a significantly higher percentage with BACs greater than 0.08 g/dL than females in all racial/ethnic populations except non-Hispanic AI/ANs, for whom the percentages for each sex were equal (37%).

Discussion

Researchers have proposed various mechanisms regarding the role of acute or chronic alcohol use in suicidal behavior. These include alcohol's effect on promoting depression and hopelessness, promoting disinhibition of negative behavior and impulsivity, impairing problem solving, and contributing to disruption in interpersonal relationships. Although numerous studies show that alcohol use often plays a role in suicide, the association can vary from population to population. The results of this analysis indicate that alcohol intoxication likely was present in nearly one quarter of the tested suicide deaths recorded by NVDRS in 17 states during 2005–2006; especially among non-Hispanic AI/ANs and Hispanics. Racial/ethnic differences in the prevalence of problem drinking cannot explain the pattern in alcohol-associated suicides. Data from the Behavioral Risk Factor Surveillance System that examined binge drinking among different racial/ethnic populations showed that the highest percentage occurred among Hispanics.

The analysis by sex reveals that the percentage(s) of tested subjects with BACs at or over the legal limit for intoxication was higher for males than females in all racial/ethnic populations except non-Hispanic AI/ANs, for whom the percentage(s) for each sex were equal. Among suicide decedents, other studies also show higher levels of intoxication among males compared with females.

Effective, comprehensive suicide-prevention programs have been developed. These programs focus on an array of risk or protective factors, including alcohol consumption, substance misuse, and social support; however, few have been developed specifically for minority populations. Some international studies suggest that measures to restrict alcohol use can reduce suicides. The measures include raising the minimum legal drinking age; increasing taxes on alcohol sales; limiting the sale of alcohol products by age of purchaser, time of day available, or business type; and mandating that workplaces be alcohol-free. An example of a successful comprehensive prevention program that included a component addressing alcohol misuse and was implemented in an AI/AN community is the Natural Helpers program. This multi-component program involved personnel who were trained to respond to young persons in crisis, notify mental health professionals in the event of a crisis, and provide health education in the schools and community. Other program components included outreach to families after a suicide or traumatic death, immediate response and follow-up for reported at-risk youth, alcohol and substance-abuse programs, community education about suicide prevention, and suicide-risk screening in mental health and social service programs.

In Figure 42.1, among male decedents tested, 25% tested above legal intoxication; among females tested, 18% tested above legal intoxication. Males had a significantly higher percentage with BACs greater than 0.08 g/dL than females in all racial/ethnic populations except non-Hispanic American Indians/Alaska Natives, for whom the percentages for each sex were equal (37%)

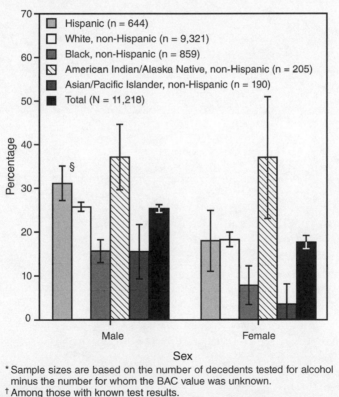

* Sample sizes are based on the number of decedents tested for alcohol minus the number for whom the BAC value was unknown.
† Among those with known test results.
§ 95% confidence interval.

Figure 42.1. *Percentage of suicide decedents with blood alcohol concentrations (BACs) 0.08 g/dL or greater,* by race/ethnicity and sex†—National Violent Death Reporting System, 17 states, 2005–2006*

Part Six

Alcohol's Impact on Family, Work, and the Community

Chapter 43

Children Living with Alcohol-Abusing Parents

Chapter Contents

Section 43.1

The Number of Children Living with Substance-Abusing Parents

Excerpted from "Children Living with Substance-Dependent or Substance-Abusing Parents," Substance Abuse and Mental Health Services Administration (SAMHSA), April 16, 2009. The complete document with references is available at http://www.oas.samhsa.gov/2k9/SAparents/SAparents.htm.

Parental substance dependence and abuse can have profound effects on children, including child abuse and neglect, injuries and deaths related to motor vehicle accidents, and increased odds that the children will become substance dependent or abusers themselves. Up-to-date estimates of the number of children living with substance-dependent or substance-abusing parents are needed for planning both adult treatment and prevention efforts and programs that support and protect affected children.

The National Survey on Drug Use and Health (NSDUH) can be used to address this data need. NSDUH annually collects data on alcohol or illicit drug dependence or abuse. It defines dependence or abuse using criteria specified in the *Diagnostic and Statistical Manual of Mental Disorders* (*DSM-IV*), which includes such symptoms as withdrawal, tolerance, use in dangerous situations, trouble with the law, and interference in major obligations at work, school, or home during the past year. The NSDUH sample includes representative subsamples of mothers and fathers, as well as mother-father pairs who live in the same household. The survey obtains information about children living in the household, including age and relationship to the adult respondent.

This section examines the number of children living with substance-dependent or substance-abusing parents. It focuses on biological, step-, adoptive, and foster children under 18 years of age who were living with one or both parents at the time of the survey interview. All findings are based on annual averages from the combined 2002 to 2007 NSDUH data.

Children Living with Substance-Dependent or Substance-Abusing Parents

Over 8.3 million children under 18 years of age (11.9%) lived with at least one parent who was dependent on or abused alcohol or an illicit drug during the past year. Of these, almost 7.3 million (10.3%) lived with a parent who was dependent on or abused alcohol, and about 2.1 million (3.0%) lived with a parent who was dependent on or abused an illicit drug. Past year substance dependence or abuse by parents involved almost 14.0% of children aged five or younger compared with 12.0% of children aged 6–11 and 9.9% of youths aged 12–17.

Table 43.1. Estimated Numbers of Children* under 18 Years of Age Living with One or More Parents with Past Year Substance Dependence or Abuse: 2002 to 2007

Substance Dependence or Abuse	Number in Millions
Illicit Drugs	2.1
Alcohol	7.3
Alcohol or Illicit Drugs	8.3

* Includes biological, step-, adoptive, or foster children. Children under 18 years of age who were not living with one or more parents were excluded from this analysis. Approximately 4.0% of children under age 18 were not living with one or more parents.

Source: 2002 to 2007 SAMHSA National Surveys on Drug Use and Health (NSDUHs).

Table 43.2. Percentages of Children* under 18 Years of Age Living with One or More Parents with Past Year Substance Dependence or Abuse, by Child's Age: 2002 to 2007

Age	Percent
Younger than three	13.9%
3–5	13.6%
6–11	12.0%
12–17	9.9%

* Includes biological, step-, adoptive, or foster children. Children under 18 years of age who were not living with one or more parents were excluded from this analysis. Approximately 4.0% of children under age 18 were not living with one or more parents.

Source: 2002 to 2007 SAMHSA National Surveys on Drug Use and Health (NSDUHs).

Parental Gender and Household Structure

About 5.4 million children under 18 years of age lived with a father who met the criteria for past year substance dependence or abuse, and 3.4 million lived with a mother who met the criteria. These population estimates are equivalent to 10.2% of all children in this age range who lived with their father and 5.1% of those who lived with their mother. One in eight (12.8%) children under age 18 in two-parent households had one or more parents who were dependent on or abused alcohol or illicit drugs in the past year. Among children residing in single-parent households, living with a substance dependent or abusing parent was more likely in father-only households (16.1%) than in mother-only households (8.4%).

Discussion: Substance use disorders can have a profound influence on the lives of individuals and their families, particularly their children. The data in this report indicate that more than one in ten children in the United States under the age of 18 were living in homes with a substance-dependent or substance-abusing parent. These data highlight the potential breadth of needs for the whole family—from substance abuse treatment for the affected adults to prevention and supportive services for the children.

Section 43.2

Coping with an Alcoholic Parent

Anthony is in bed when he hears the front door slam. He covers his head with his pillow so he doesn't have to listen to the sound of his parents arguing. Anthony knows that his mother has been drinking again. He starts worrying about getting to school on time and realizes he will probably have to help get his younger sister ready too.

Why do people drink too much?

Lots of people live with a parent or caregiver who is an alcoholic or who drinks too much. Alcoholism has been around for centuries, yet no one has discovered an easy way to prevent it. Alcohol can affect people's health and also how they act. People who are drunk might be more aggressive or have mood swings. They may act in a way that is embarrassing to them or other people.

Alcoholism is a disease: Like any disease, it needs to be treated. Without professional help, a person with alcoholism will probably continue to drink and may even become worse over time. Diseases like alcoholism are no one's fault. Some people are more susceptible to wanting to drink too much. Scientists think it has to do with genetics, as well as things like family history, and life events.

Sometimes what starts as a bad habit can become a very big problem. For example, people may drink to cope with problems like boredom, stress, or money troubles. Maybe there's an illness in the family, or parents are having marriage problems. No matter what anyone says, people don't drink because of someone else's behavior. So if you live with someone who has a drinking problem, don't blame yourself.

How does alcoholism affect families?

If you live with a parent who drinks, you may feel embarrassed, angry, sad, hurt, or any number of emotions. You may feel helpless: When parents promise to stop drinking, for example, it can end in frustration when they don't keep their promises.

Problem drinking can change how families function. A parent may have trouble keeping a job and problems paying the bills. Older kids may have to take care of younger siblings.

Some parents with alcohol problems might mistreat or abuse their children emotionally or physically. Others may neglect their kids by not providing sufficient care and guidance. Parents with alcohol problems might also use other drugs.

Despite what happens, most children of alcoholics love their parents and worry about something bad happening to them. Kids who live with problem drinkers often try all kinds of ways to prevent them from drinking. But, just as family members don't cause the addiction, they can't stop it either. The person with the drinking problem has to take charge. Someone who has a bad habit or an addiction to alcohol needs to get help from a treatment center. Alcoholism affects family members just as much as it affects the person drinking. Because of this, there are lots of support groups to help children of alcoholics cope with the problem.

What if a parent doesn't see a problem?

Drinking too much can be a problem that nobody likes to talk about. In fact, lots of parents may become enraged at the slightest suggestion that they are drinking too much. Sometimes, parents deny that they have a problem. A person in denial refuses to believe the truth about a situation. So problem drinkers may try to blame someone else because it is easier than taking responsibility for their own drinking.

Some parents make their families feel bad by saying stuff like, "You're driving me crazy!" or "I can't take this anymore." That can be harmful, especially to kids: Most young children don't know that the problem has nothing to do with their actions and that it's all in the drinker's mind. Some parents do acknowledge their drinking, but deny that it's a problem. They may say stuff like, "I can stop anytime I want to," "Everyone drinks to unwind sometimes," or "My drinking is not a problem."

Lots of people fall into the trap of thinking that a parent's drinking is only temporary. They tell themselves that, when a particular problem is over, like having a rough time at work, the drinking will stop. But even if a parent who drinks too much has other problems, drinking is a separate problem. And that problem won't go away unless the drinker gets help.

Why do I feel so bad?

If you're like most teens, your life is probably filled with emotional ups and downs, regardless of what's happening at home. Add a parent with a drinking problem to the mix, and it can all seem like too much. There are many reasons why a parent's drinking can contribute to feelings of anger, frustration, disappointment, sadness, embarrassment, worry, loneliness, and helplessness. For example:

- You might be subjected to a parent's changing moods. People who drink can behave unpredictably. Kids who grow up around them may spend a lot of energy trying to figure out a parent's mood or guess what that parent wants. One day you might walk on eggshells to avoid an outburst because the dishes aren't done or the lawn isn't mowed. The next day, you may find yourself comforting a parent who promises that things will be better.

- It may be hard to do things with friends or other people. For some people, it feels like too much trouble to have a friend over or do the things that everyone else does. You just never know how your parent will act. Will your mom or dad show up drunk for school events or drive you (and your friends) home drunk?

- You might be stressed or worried. It can be scary to listen to adults in the house yell, fight, or break things by accident. Worrying about a parent just adds to all the other emotions you may be feeling. Are you lying awake waiting for mom or dad to get home safely? Do you feel it's not fair that you have to be the grown up and take care of things around the house? These are all normal reactions.

Although each family is different, people who grow up with alcoholic parents often feel alone, unloved, depressed, or burdened by the secret life they lead at home. You know it's not possible to cause or stop the behavior of an alcoholic. So what can you do to feel better (or help a friend feel better)?

What can I do?

Acknowledge the problem: Many kids of parents who drink too much try to protect their parents or hide the problem. Admitting that your parent has a problem—even if he or she won't—is the first step in taking control. Start by talking to a friend, teacher, counselor, or coach. If you can't face telling someone you know, call an organization like Al-Anon/Alateen (they have a 24-hour hotline at 800-344-2666) or go online for help.

Be informed: Being aware of how your parent's drinking affects you can help put things in perspective. For example, some teens who live with alcoholic adults become afraid to speak out or show any normal anger or emotion because they worry it may trigger a parent's drinking. Remind yourself that you are not responsible for your parent drinking too much, and that you cannot cause it or stop it.

Be aware of your emotions: When you feel things like anger or resentment, try to identify those feelings. Talk to a close friend or write down how you are feeling. Recognizing how a parent's problem drinking makes you feel can help you from burying your feelings and pretending that everything's okay.

Learn healthy coping strategies: When we grow up around people who turn to alcohol or other unhealthy ways of dealing with problems, they become our example. Watching new role models can help people learn healthy coping mechanisms and ways of making good decisions.

Coaches, aunts, uncles, parents of friends, or teachers all have to deal with things like frustration or disappointment. Watch how they do it. School counselors can be a great resource here. Next time you have a problem, ask someone you trust for help.

Find support: It's good to share your feelings with a friend, but it's equally important to talk to an adult you trust. A school counselor, favorite teacher, or coach may be able to help. Some teens turn to their school D.A.R.E. (Drug and Alcohol Resistance Education) officer. Others prefer to talk to a family member or parents of a close friend.

Because alcoholism is such a widespread problem, several organizations offer confidential support groups and meetings for people living with alcoholics. Alateen is a group specifically geared to young people living with adults who have drinking problems. Alateen can also help teens whose parents may already be in treatment or recovery. The group Alcoholics Anonymous (AA) also offers resources for people living with alcoholics.

Find a safe environment: Do you find yourself avoiding your house as much as possible? Are you thinking about running away? If you feel that the situation at home is becoming dangerous, you can call the National Domestic Violence Hotline at 800-799-SAFE (7233). And don't hesitate to dial 911 if you think you or another family member is in immediate danger.

Stop the cycle: Teenage children of alcoholics are at higher risk of becoming alcoholics themselves. Scientists think this is because of genetics and the environment that kids grow up in. For example, people might learn to drink as a way to avoid fear, boredom, anxiety, sadness, or other unpleasant feelings. Understanding that there could be a problem and finding adults and peers to help you can be the most important thing you do to reduce the risk of problem drinking.

Alcoholism is a disease. You can show your love and support, but you won't be able to stop someone from drinking. Talking about the problem, finding support, and choosing healthy ways to cope are choices you can make to feel more in control of the situation. Above all, don't give up.

Chapter 44

Interpersonal Violence and Alcohol

Interpersonal violence and harmful and hazardous alcohol use are major challenges to global public health. Harmful use of alcohol is defined as a pattern of alcohol use that causes damage to health. Hazardous alcohol use is defined as a pattern of alcohol use that increases the risk of harmful consequences for the user (World Health Organization, http://www.who.int/substance_abuse/terminology/who_lexicon/en/). Both place large burdens on the health of populations, the cohesion of communities and the provision of public services including health care and criminal justice. Globally, alcohol is responsible for 4% of all years of health lost through premature death or disability (DALYs, disability-adjusted life years), ranging from 1.3% in countries in the Middle East and Indian subcontinent to 12.1% in Eastern Europe and Central Asia. Through homicide, interpersonal violence results in around 520,000 deaths per year (a rate of 8.8 per 100,000 population, ranging from 3.4 in the World Health Organization (WHO) Western Pacific Region to 27.5 in the WHO Region of the Americas). For every death resulting from interpersonal violence, scores of further victims require hospital treatment and many more remain untreated and unrecorded by either health or criminal justice agencies. Although levels of alcohol consumption, patterns of drinking and rates of interpersonal violence vary widely between countries, across all cultures there are strong links between the two. Each exacerbates the effects of the other with a strong association between alcohol consumption and an individual's risk of being either a perpetrator or a victim of violence.

Interpersonal Violence

Interpersonal violence is the intentional use of physical force or power, threatened or actual, against another person, that either results in or has a high likelihood of resulting in injury, death, psychological harm, maldevelopment or deprivation. Interpersonal violence can be categorized into these groups:

- **Youth violence:** Violence committed by young people.

- **Child maltreatment:** Violence and neglect towards children by parents and caregivers.

- **Intimate partner violence:** Violence occurring within an intimate relationship.

- **Elder abuse:** Violence and neglect towards older people by family, caregivers, or others where there is an expectation of trust.

- **Sexual violence:** Sexual assault, unwanted sexual attention, sexual coercion, and sexual trafficking.

The links between alcohol use and interpersonal violence: The mechanisms linking alcohol and interpersonal violence are manifold:

- Harmful alcohol use directly affects physical and cognitive function. Reduced self-control and ability to process incoming information makes drinkers more likely to resort to violence in confrontations, while reduced ability to recognize warning signs in potentially violent situations makes them appear easy targets for perpetrators.

- Individual and societal beliefs that alcohol causes aggressive behavior can lead to the use of alcohol as preparation for involvement in violence, or as a way of excusing violent acts.

- Dependence on alcohol can mean individuals fail to fulfill care responsibilities or coerce relatives into giving them money to purchase alcohol or cover associated costs.

- Experiencing or witnessing violence can lead to the harmful use of alcohol as a way of coping or self-medicating.

- Uncomfortable, crowded, and poorly managed drinking settings contribute to increased violence among drinkers.

- Alcohol and violence may be related through a common risk factor (antisocial personality disorder) that contributes to the risk of both heavy drinking and violent behavior.

- Prenatal alcohol exposure resulting in fetal alcohol syndrome or fetal alcohol effects are associated in infants with increased risk of their maltreatment, and with delinquent and sometimes violent behavior in later life, including delinquent behavior, sexual violence, and suicide.

Magnitude of alcohol-related interpersonal violence: Levels and patterns of alcohol consumption vary widely between countries (Table 44.1). Similarly, levels of violence differ between countries. Rates of mortality for intentional injury range from around four per 100,000 population in Georgia, Kuwait, and Greece to over 50 per 100,000 in the Russian Federation, El Salvador, and Colombia.

Few countries routinely measure the involvement of alcohol in violence. Further, most recording systems and research examining alcohol use by victims and perpetrators of violence derive from high-income countries. Even where estimates of alcohol's role in violence are available, methodological differences between studies complicate direct comparisons between countries. However, across countries, harmful alcohol use is estimated to be responsible for 26% of male and 16% of female DALYs lost through homicide. Furthermore, the role of harmful alcohol consumption as a risk factor for violent victimization and perpetration, and the impact of violent experiences on future drinking behaviors, are increasingly being identified throughout the world. Findings from a review of global scientific literature include the following:

Harmful alcohol consumption by perpetrators of violence:

- In the USA, among victims that were able to report whether their attacker had been using alcohol, 35% believed the offender had been drinking.

- In England and Wales, 50% of victims of interpersonal violence reported the perpetrator to be under the influence of alcohol at the time of assault.

- In Russia, around three-quarters of individuals arrested for homicide had consumed alcohol shortly before the incident.

- In South Africa, 44% of victims of interpersonal violence believed their attacker to have been under the influence of alcohol.

- In Tianjin, China, a study of inmates found that 50% of assault offenders had been drinking alcohol prior to the incident.

403

Table 44.1. Levels and patterns of alcohol consumption by WHO Region

WHO Regions[a]	Total consumption (all people)[b]	Proportion of drinkers	Consumption per drinker[c]	Pattern[d]
Low to Middle Income Countries				
Very high or high mortality: lowest consumption	Islamic middle east and Indian subcontinent (EMR-D, SEAR-D)	1.88	15.0%	12.27	2.9
Very high or high mortality: low consumption	Poorest countries in Africa and America (AFR-D, AFR-E, AMR-D)	5.93	42.8%	14.21	2.8
Low mortality emerging economies	Better-off developing countries in America, Asia, Pacific (AMR-B, EMR-B, SEAR-B, WPR-B)	5.23	51.0%	10.53	2.4
High Income Countries				
Very low mortality	North America, Western Europe, Japan, Australasia. (AMR-A, EUR-A, WPR-A)	10.90	77.8%	14.00	1.5
Former socialist: low mortality	Eastern Europe and Central Asia (EUR-B, EUR-C)	11.42	74.5%	15.09	3.3
World		6.03	48.6%	12.26	2.5

Source: Room et al 2005

[a] Regional sub groupings defined by WHO on the basis of mortality levels (see World Health Report 2002, available from: http://www.who.int/whr/2002/en/index.html).

[b] Litres of pure alcohol per resident aged 15 and over per year (recorded and unrecorded consumption).

[c] Liters of pure alcohol per resident drinker aged 15 and over per year (recorded and unrecorded consumption).

[d] Indicator of hazard per liter of alcohol consumed, composed of several indicators of heavy drinking occasions, frequency of drinking in public places plus frequency of drinking with meals (reverse scored). Range, 1=least detrimental, 4=most detrimental.

Harmful alcohol consumption by victims of violence:

- In Australia, 26% of male and 17% of female homicide victims (2002–2003) had been drinking just prior to death.

- Between 1970 and 1998, 36% of victims of violence presenting to a trauma department in the Netherlands had consumed alcohol.

- Among victims of violent injuries presenting to emergency rooms in six countries (Argentina, Australia, Canada, Mexico, Spain, and the USA), the percentage testing positive for alcohol, for countries where 95% or more patients were tested, ranged from 24% in Argentina to 43% in Australia.

- Between 1999 and 2001, between 43% and 90% of victims presenting to hospital trauma units in three South African cities tested positive for alcohol.

- In São Paulo, Brazil, 42% of homicide victims were shown to have used alcohol prior to death (2001); and 46% of assault victims presenting to a trauma center tested positive for alcohol (1998–1999).

Harmful alcohol use is a risk factor across all types of interpersonal violence. Victims are less likely than perpetrators to be under the influence of alcohol during an incident, and for many victims harmful levels of alcohol use can occur later as a consequence of violent experiences (Table 44.2).

Risk Factors for Alcohol-Related Interpersonal Violence

A wide range of factors can increase individuals' risks of being either a perpetrator or victim of alcohol-related violence. To help understand these factors and how they interact, an ecological model is used to divide risk factors into those associated with the individual, relationships between individuals, communities and society. Risk factors for each are summarized here.

Individual Factors

Victims:

- *Age:* Alcohol-related assaults are experienced more frequently among young adults. For instance in England and Wales and Australia, 16–29 year olds, and 15–34 year olds respectively are at increased risk.

- *Gender:* In general, males are at higher risk of alcohol-related interpersonal violence requiring hospital treatment. In studies

Table 44.2. Alcohol Misuse as a Risk Factor for and a Consequence of Violence

	Alcohol misuse as a risk factor for violence	Alcohol misuse as a consequence of violence
Child maltreatment	In Germany, 32% of offenders of fatal child abuse (1985–90) were thought to have consumed alcohol prior to the offence. Parental alcohol or drug use was reported in 34% of child welfare investigations in Canada.	Globally, a history of child sexual abuse is estimated to cause 4–5% of alcohol misuse in men and 7–8% in women.
Youth violence	In Israel, 11–16 year olds who reported both drinking five or more drinks per occasion and having ever been drunk were twice as likely to be a perpetrator of bullying, five times as likely to be injured in a fight, and six times as likely to carry a weapon.	In the USA, victims of violence during adolescence report higher levels of alcohol consumption in later life.
Intimate partner violence	In Russia, 60–75% of male perpetrators of intimate partner homicides had been drinking. In Iceland, 71% of female victims of intimate partner violence stated partner alcohol use as the main cause of their assault.	In Iceland, 22% of female intimate partner violence victims reported using alcohol following the event as a mechanism for coping.
Elder abuse	In the USA, 44% of male and 14% of female abusers of elderly parents (age 60 years and over) were dependent on alcohol or drugs, along with 7% of victims.	In Canada, an outreach program for seniors with alcohol or other substance misuse problems reported 15–20% of clients experiencing some form of elder abuse. For some, alcohol use was a way of coping with violent experiences.
Sexual violence	In the United Kingdom, 58% of men imprisoned for rape reported having consumed alcohol in the six hours preceding the offence, and 37% were considered to be alcohol dependent.	In the USA, victims of sexual assault report higher levels of psychological distress and the consumption of alcohol, in part, to self-medicate.

of hospital admissions, males accounted for the majority of all alcohol-related assault victims (for example, Australia 74%, England 80%) and in one Kenyan study of emergency department presentations for injury, were approximately twice as likely as females to have been drinking alcohol prior to assault.

- *Drinking patterns:* High levels of alcohol consumption have been associated with increased risk of experiencing violence, with those who report more frequent intoxication most likely to be involved in an alcohol-related assault. Further, early initiation into alcohol use has been associated with increased risk of sexual victimization in adolescence.

- *Experience of violence:* Individuals who experience violence in childhood and adulthood can be at greater risk of alcohol dependence later in life. Further, adults who have suffered more than one type of violence (for example, by an intimate partner and a stranger) have higher rates of alcohol problems than those who have experienced only one type.

Perpetrators:

- *Age:* Risk of perpetration varies with age. In the USA, 38% of offenders of alcohol-related violent crime are aged 30–39, and a further 29% aged 21–29. In the United Kingdom, alcohol-related violence towards strangers is more likely to be committed by 16–24 year olds and that towards acquaintances by those aged 25 years and older.

- *Gender:* Perpetrators of alcohol-related violence are more likely to be male (Norway; England and Wales).

- *Drinking patterns:* Heavier and more frequent drinkers are more at risk of perpetrating violence (Norway, Latin America, and Spain), as are those that start drinking alcohol at an earlier age.

- *Personality:* The relationship between alcohol and violence is mediated by certain characteristics such as an antisocial personality, which increases the risk of a person becoming aggressive after drinking.

Relationship factors:

- *Drinking patterns:* Discrepant drinking patterns (for example, only one partner is a heavy drinker) have been found to increase the risk of intimate partner violence.

- *Exposure to violence:* Experience of parental violence in childhood is associated with the development of alcohol-related problems later in life.

- *Parental use of alcohol:* A young person's risk of violent offending is increased if their parent (particularly their mother) engages in harmful use of alcohol.

- *Acquaintances:* A higher risk of alcohol-related criminal and disorderly offending is found among those who associate with delinquent acquaintances.

Community factors:

- *Time of day and day of week:* Alcohol-related assaults occur most frequently at night and particularly at weekend nights (England and Wales, Kenya).

- *Drinking venues:* Greater concentrations of drinking venues within an area have been found to increase the risk of interpersonal violence in that area.

- *Characteristics of licensed premises:* Premises that are uncomfortable (such as crowded, lacking seating and ventilation, hot and noisy); unattractive and poorly maintained; offer discounted alcoholic drinks; employ aggressive door supervisors; have a high proportion of intoxicated patrons, or have a permissive attitude towards anti-social behavior (serving underage or drunk customers and allowing swearing and overt sexual activity) are more associated with violent behavior.

Societal factors:

- *Risky drinking culture:* Across studies in seven countries (Argentina, Australia, Canada, Mexico, Poland, Spain, and the USA), the percentage of violence-related injuries associated with harmful alcohol use was higher in societies that had greater alcohol consumption per capita. Societies characterized by heavy episodic drinking suffer higher levels of alcohol-related violence than societies where alcohol use is high but more integrated into daily routines (for example, mealtimes).

- *Societal beliefs and attitudes:* Beliefs that alcohol has disinhibiting effects encourage the harmful use of alcohol as an excuse for violent behavior (such as youth violence; Sweden) or to fuel the audacity necessary to commit crimes (including violent crimes; South Africa). Also in South Africa, rape can result from men who buy drinks for women and subsequently think they are owed sexual favors in return.

Impact

Across all countries, alcohol-related violence has far-reaching consequences, affecting the health and well-being of victims, relationships with family and friends, levels of fear within communities, and pressures on health and other public services. For victims, health impacts include physical injuries and emotional harm such as depression, anxiety, and sleep problems. In England and Wales, around three-quarters of victims of assault experience some form of subsequent emotional harm. Harmful alcohol use is often cited as a method of coping with violent experiences and victims are more likely to develop problematic drinking habits later in life. Other longer-term health effects can include suicide and post-traumatic stress disorder.

Research in high-income countries has found that alcohol consumption by both victims and perpetrators of violence can increase the severity of injuries. Furthermore, in serious assaults alcohol may play a role in determining victims' survival, for example by reducing their ability to seek urgent medical assistance or reducing perceptions of the seriousness of injury.

Social problems resulting from the experience of violence often affect victims' relationships with family, friends, and future intimate partners, as well as their ability to work or attend school. Children who witness violence or threats of violence between their parents are more likely to develop emotional and behavioral problems during childhood and heavy drinking patterns or alcohol dependency later in life, increasing their risk of becoming perpetrators of violence. A high prevalence of alcohol-related violence within a community can also affect quality of life, reducing community cohesion, increasing fear of crime, and preventing people from visiting places associated with disorder such as city centers at night, or using public transport.

Economic Costs of Alcohol-Related Violence

The economic costs of alcohol-related violence include direct costs such as those to health care and judicial services, and indirect costs such as work and school absenteeism. Estimates of the economic costs of violence and the proportion of violence related to alcohol include:

- **USA:** US$ 46.8 billion to US$ 425 billion per year, depending on the type of costs included. An estimated 35% of violence is related to alcohol.

- **England and Wales:** £24.4 billion per year (approximately US$ 42.7 billion) (excluding violence towards children aged less than 16 years and elders over 65 year of age), around 2% of gross domestic product (GDP). An estimated 50% of violence is related to alcohol.

- **Latin America:** Estimated percentages of GDP lost due to violent crime (1997) including collective violence range from 1.3% in Mexico to 24.9% in El Salvador, although the proportion related to alcohol is not known.

The burden of alcohol-related violence on public service provision and the economy can be immense. For health and criminal justice agencies, apprehending and treating offenders and victims of alcohol-related violence is financially costly and diverts resources from other health and crime issues. Furthermore, health and judicial staff can frequently be victims of alcohol-related violence themselves while at work, and this may encourage both employees and prospective employees to consider alternative careers.

Alcohol and Suicide

Suicide can be a consequence of interpersonal violence. There is also a strong relationship between alcohol consumption and suicide or attempted suicide, especially among those who drink heavily. In this group the risk of suicidal behavior increases if other mental health problems such as depression are present. Approximately 7% of people with alcohol dependence die through suicide. Suicide rates rise with increased per capita consumption, and tend to be higher in drinking cultures characterized by irregular heavy drinking, in common with interpersonal violence. Effective interventions that reduce heavy drinking may reduce both assaults and suicide.

Prevention

Although alcohol consumption is a normal and acceptable part of society throughout much of the world, violence associated in particular with hazardous and harmful consumption poses an important but preventable problem. Central to prevention is creating societies and environments that discourage risky drinking behaviors and do not allow alcohol to be used as an excuse for violence. The evidence base for the effective prevention of alcohol-related violence is mainly from high-income countries. Much less is known about the effectiveness of interventions elsewhere with differences in drinking cultures, societal attitudes towards violence, and laws surrounding the sale and consumption of alcohol being important considerations.

For interpersonal violence in general, early interventions such as pre- and postnatal services can be effective prevention measures and these strategies have been thoroughly reviewed elsewhere. Specifically for alcohol-related violence, interventions to reduce population alcohol consumption (for example, regulating alcohol sales) have proven effective in reducing levels of violence both in low-to middle-income and high-income countries. However, interventions to modify drinking settings (such as improving licensed premise management), screen for harmful drinking and conduct brief interventions, treat alcohol dependence, and improve drinking environments have been found to be effective in high-income countries, but are largely untested elsewhere.

Several important factors impinge on the applicability of prevention strategies in low- to middle-income countries. In many low- to middle-income societies, a large proportion of alcohol consumed is produced at home. Thus, strategies to reduce alcohol consumption through increased price (higher taxation) may be less effective and may switch drinkers to cheaper, home-produced alcohol. In some low- and middle-income countries, the enactment and enforcement of legislation on the legal minimum age for purchase of alcohol, and efforts to strengthen and expand the licensing of liquor outlets could be of great value in reducing alcohol-related violence. For example, there is no legal minimum age of sale for alcohol in the Gambia, and in South Africa it is estimated that 80–90% of liquor outlets are unlicensed. In contrast, in high-income countries the majority of alcohol outlets are licensed, most alcohol is produced by industry, and laws to restrict access to alcohol by minors are enforced. More research is needed in low- to middle-income countries to identify successful interventions for preventing alcohol-related violence and to examine opportunities to regulate production and sale.

Chapter 45

Alcohol-Impaired Vehicle Operation

Chapter Contents

Section 45.1

How Alcohol Affects Drivers

Text in this section is from "Impaired Driving: Myths and Facts about Alcohol" and "Impaired Driving: How Alcohol and Drugs Affect Driving," undated fact sheets produced by the U.S. Department of Labor (www.dol.gov).

Myths and Facts about Alcohol and Driving

Myths and misconceptions about alcohol and its effects on safe driving are widespread. Knowing the truth could mean the difference between life and death.

Myth: Alcohol is a stimulant.

Fact: Alcohol is a depressant. It acts on the central nervous system like an anesthetic to lower or depress the activity of the brain.

Myth: "Drinking coffee sobers me up."

Fact: Coffee cannot rid your system of alcohol. It just makes you a nervous, wide-awake drunk. Only time reverses the impairment.

Myth: "I always stay away from the hard stuff."

Fact: Alcohol is alcohol. One 12-ounce glass of beer has as much alcohol as a 1.5-ounce shot of whiskey or a 5-ounce glass of wine.

Myth: "I am bigger so I can handle my liquor better than other people."

Fact: Size is only one factor in how much you can drink. Metabolism, amount of rest and food intake all play a part in how you handle liquor. Impairment in motor reflexes and judgment can begin with the first drink.

Myth: "Once I roll down my car window, I am okay to drive."

Fact: No amount of fresh, chilly air can reverse impairment. You gain nothing by rolling down a window or turning on the air conditioner.

Myth: "I just drive slower after drinking."

Fact: Many people believe that by driving more slowly, they can compensate for being impaired. The truth is, drunk drivers are dangerous at any speed.

Myth: "All I have to do is splash my face with cold water."

Fact: Cold water or even a cold shower will not sober you up or make you a safer driver.

How Alcohol and Drugs Affect Driving

Alcohol (beer, wine, whiskey, gin, rum, vodka, tequila, and so forth):

- Dulls judgment and concentration
- Slows releases and reaction time
- Leads to multiple, blurred, and restricted side and night vision
- Hinders muscle control and coordination
- Exaggerates emotions
- Increases drowsiness

Alcohol plus marijuana (any alcoholic beverage and pot, hash or tetrahydrocannabinol [THC]) adds the following to the effects of alcohol:

- Dulls concentration and reasoning abilities
- Slows reaction time
- Leads to multiple vision and slowed glare recovery time
- Hinders muscle control coordination, maneuvering ability, and ability to recognize traffic signals
- Affects short term memory and tracking ability
- Increases distraction and drowsiness

Alcohol plus antihistamines (any alcoholic beverage and cold remedies such as Sudafed, Coricidin) adds the following to the effects of alcohol:

- Dulls judgment and concentration
- Slows reaction time
- Leads to reduced vision
- Hinders coordination
- Increases drowsiness, confusion, and anxiety

Alcohol plus tranquilizers (any alcoholic beverage and sleep medication such as Valium, Librium, Seconal, and so forth) adds the following to the effects of alcohol:

- Dulls judgment and concentration
- Slows reflexes and reaction time
- Leads to multiple, blurred, and restricted side and night vision
- Hinders coordination and motor skills
- Increases drowsiness

Section 45.2

Crashes and Fatalities Involving Alcohol-Impaired Drivers

Excerpted from "Alcohol-Impaired Driving 2008 Data," National Highway Traffic Safety Administration (NHTSA), 2009.

Drivers are considered to be alcohol-impaired when their blood alcohol concentration (BAC) is .08 grams per deciliter (g/dL) or higher. Thus, any fatality occurring in a crash involving a driver with a BAC of .08 or higher is considered to be an alcohol-impaired-driving fatality. The term driver refers to the operator of any motor vehicle, including a motorcycle. In 2008, 11,773 people were killed in alcohol-impaired-driving crashes. These alcohol-impaired-driving fatalities accounted for 32% of the total motor vehicle traffic fatalities in the United States. Traffic fatalities in alcohol-impaired-driving crashes decreased nearly 10% from 13,041 in 2007 to 11,773 in 2008. The alcohol-impaired-driving fatality rate per 100 million vehicle miles traveled (VMT) decreased to 0.40 in 2008 from 0.43 in 2007. Estimates of alcohol-impaired driving are generated using BAC values reported to the Fatality Analysis Reporting System (FARS) and imputed BAC values when they are not reported. The term alcohol-impaired does not indicate that a crash or a fatality was caused by alcohol impairment. The 11,773 fatalities in alcohol-impaired-driving crashes during 2008 represent an average of one alcohol-impaired-driving fatality every 45 minutes. In 2008, all 50 states, the District of Columbia, and Puerto Rico had by law created a threshold making it illegal per se to drive with a BAC of .08 or higher. Of the 11,773 people who died in alcohol-impaired-driving crashes in 2008, 8,027 (68%) were drivers with a BAC of .08 or higher. The remaining fatalities consisted of 3,054 (26%) motor vehicle occupants and 692 (6%) nonoccupants.

Table 45.1. Fatalities, by Role, in Crashes Involving at Least One Driver with a BAC of .08 or Higher, 2008

Role	Number	Percent of Total
Driver with BAC=.08+	8,027	68%
Passenger Riding w/Driver with BAC=.08+	1,875	16%
Subtotal	9,902	84%
Occupants of Other Vehicles	1,179	10%
Nonoccupants	692	6%
Total Fatalities	11,773	100%

Children: In 2008, a total of 1,347 children age 14 and younger were killed in motor vehicle traffic crashes. Of those 1,347 fatalities, 216 (16%) occurred in alcohol-impaired-driving crashes. Out of those 216 deaths, 99 (46%) were occupants of a vehicle with a driver who had a BAC level of .08 or higher. Another 34 children age 14 and younger who were killed in traffic crashes in 2008 were pedestrians or pedalcyclists who were struck by drivers with a BAC of .08 or higher.

Time of day and day of week: The rate of alcohol impairment among drivers involved in fatal crashes was four times higher at night than during the day (36% versus 9%). In 2008, 15% of all drivers involved in fatal crashes during the week were alcohol-impaired, compared to 32% on weekends.

Drivers: In fatal crashes in 2008 the highest percentage of drivers with a BAC level of .08 or higher was for drivers ages 21 to 24 (34%), followed by ages 25 to 34 (31%) and 35 to 44 (25%). The percentages of drivers involved in fatal crashes with a BAC level of .08 or higher in 2008 were 29% for motorcycle riders and 23% for both passenger cars and light trucks. The percentage of drivers with BAC levels of .08 or higher in fatal crashes was the lowest for large trucks (2%). In 2008, 6,316 passenger vehicle drivers killed had a BAC of .08 or higher. Out of those 6,316 driver fatalities, for which restraint use was known, 73% were unrestrained. Drivers with a BAC of .08 or higher involved in fatal crashes were eight times more likely to have a prior conviction for driving while impaired (DWI) than were drivers with no alcohol (8% and 1%, respectively).

In 2008, 84% (10,946) of the 13,029 drivers with a BAC of .01 or higher who were involved in fatal crashes had BAC levels at or above .08, and 57% (7,378) had BAC levels at or above .15 or greater. The most frequently recorded BAC level among drinking drivers in fatal crashes was .16.

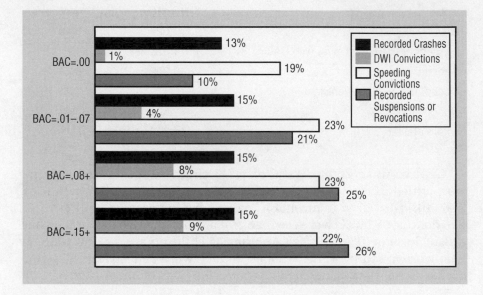

Figure 45.1. Previous Driving Records of Drivers involved in Fatal Crashes, by BAC, 2008.

Section 45.3

Driving after Binge Drinking

Nearly one in eight binge drinkers say they get behind the wheel and drive within two hours of drinking, United States (U.S.) government researchers report. The new research adds a timeline and other new information to what's known about drinking and driving, said study author Dr. Timothy Naimi, a physician with the alcohol team at the U.S. Centers for Disease Control and Prevention (CDC). The report was published in the October 2009 issue of the *American Journal of Preventive Medicine*.

"A lot of studies, including ours, have established a strong connection between binge drinking and impaired driving, which is sort of obvious on some level," he said. "What hasn't been looked at is how many people actually do get behind the wheel after a binge drinking episode."

So Naimi and his colleagues evaluated data from more than 14,000 adults in 13 states in 2003 and 14 states in 2004, who reported binge drinking and then answered additional questions. They were part of the Behavior Risk Factor Surveillance System survey.

Binge drinking was defined as having five or more drinks during an occasion, such as an evening out or at a party. Overall, 11.9% of the binge drinkers drove within two hours of their binge drinking, Naimi found. "It's a pretty awesome number when you link it up with the number of binge drinking episodes in the U.S.," he said. According to the CDC, about 1.5 billion binge drinking episodes occur in the United States each year. "If you were to spread that out [equally among the population], that would be over seven binge drinking episodes per adult per year," Naimi said.

Two other statistics shed more light on the binge drinking and driving issue, he said. For starters, 50% of the binge drinkers were aged 25 to 44. And the binge drinkers were often coming from bars, clubs and restaurants—54.3% of them, in fact. Just 23% had been drinking at someone else's home.

Laws make it illegal for bars, clubs, and restaurants to sell alcohol to intoxicated people, Naimi pointed out. But those laws are not well-enforced. "The key thing about this study is, it's really illustrating the shared responsibility between individual drinkers and the places that are selling them alcohol."

Another expert, Nick Ellinger, a spokesman for Mothers Against Drunk Driving (MADD), said one unique aspect of the study is that "they looked at the incidence of binge drinking as it related to drunk driving by location." If you look only at bars and clubs, he said, one of five binge drinkers who drink at those locations drive afterwards. The message? Not binge drinking is best, of course. But if you think you may over-indulge, make plans in advance for safe transport home, Ellinger said. "A lot of people drive to bars and restaurants to drink. It's wise ahead of time to make your plans for how you are going to get home safely because after you have begun drinking that decision-making process breaks down."

"The research shows that driving after binge drinking is a preventable problem," said David Jernigan, an associate professor at the Bloomberg School of Public Health at Johns Hopkins University, in Baltimore. "There are things to do" to remedy the problem, he said, including training servers to stop serving people who are intoxicated and strengthening the liability of club and restaurant owners.

For consumers, planning transportation home ahead of time is crucial, he said. But designated drivers have not been shown to work, he added. "It creates a carload of designated drunks," he said, some of whom may insist on driving. Public transportation is another, and sometimes safer, option.

Section 45.4

Boating Under the Influence of Alcohol

Excerpted from "Boating Under the Influence Initiatives," U.S. Coast Guard, April 2009.

Boating under the influence (BUI) is just as deadly as drinking and driving. Did you know?

- A boat operator is likely to become impaired more quickly than a driver, drink for drink.

- The penalties for BUI can include large fines, revocation of operator privileges, and serious jail terms.

- The use of alcohol is involved in about a third of all recreational boating fatalities.

Every boater needs to understand the risks of boating under the influence of alcohol or drugs (BUI). It is illegal to operate a boat while under the influence of alcohol or drugs in every state. The Coast Guard also enforces a federal law that prohibits BUI. This law pertains to all boats (from canoes and rowboats to the largest ships)—and includes foreign vessels that operate in U.S. waters, as well as U.S. vessels on the high seas.

Dangers of BUI

Alcohol affects judgment, vision, balance, and coordination. These impairments increase the likelihood of accidents afloat—for both passengers and boat operators. U.S. Coast Guard data shows that in boating deaths involving alcohol use, over half the victims capsized their boats and/or fell overboard.

Alcohol is even more hazardous on the water than on land. The marine environment—motion, vibration, engine noise, sun, wind, and spray—accelerates a drinker's impairment. These stressors cause fatigue that makes a boat operator's coordination, judgment, and reaction time decline even faster when using alcohol.

421

Alcohol can also be more dangerous to boaters because boat operators are often less experienced and less confident on the water than on the highway. Recreational boaters don't have the benefit of experiencing daily boat operation. In fact, boaters average only 110 hours on the water per year.

Alcohol effects: Alcohol has many physical effects that directly threaten safety and well-being on the water. When a boater or passenger drinks, the following occur:

- Cognitive abilities and judgment deteriorate, making it harder to process information, assess situations, and make good choices.

- Physical performance is impaired as evidenced by balance problems, lack of coordination, and increased reaction time.

- Vision is affected, including decreased peripheral vision, reduced depth perception, decreased night vision, poor focus, and difficulty in distinguishing colors (particularly red and green).

- Inner ear disturbances can make it impossible for a person who falls into the water to distinguish up from down.

- Alcohol creates a physical sensation of warmth which may prevent a person in cold water from getting out before hypothermia sets in.

As a result of these factors, a boat operator with a blood alcohol concentration above .10 BAC is estimated to be more than ten times as likely to die in a boating accident than an operator with zero blood alcohol concentration. Passengers are also at greatly increased risk for injury and death, especially if they are also using alcohol.

Many factors, including prescription medications and fatigue, can affect an individual's response to alcohol, and impairment can occur much more quickly as a result. There is no safe threshold for drinking and operating a boat, so do not assume you are safe just because you fall into the rarely or possibly influenced categories.

Enforcement and Penalties

The Coast Guard and every state have stringent penalties for violating BUI laws. Penalties can include large fines, suspension or revocation of boat operator privileges, and jail terms. The Coast Guard and the states cooperate fully in enforcement in order to remove impaired boat operators from the waters.

In waters that are overseen solely by the states, the states have the authority to enforce their own BUI statutes. In state waters that are also subject to U.S. jurisdiction, there is concurrent jurisdiction. That means if a boater is apprehended under federal law in these waters, the Coast Guard will (unless precluded by state law) request that state law enforcement officers take the intoxicated boater into custody.

When the Coast Guard determines that an operator is impaired, the voyage may be terminated. The vessel will be brought to mooring by the Coast Guard or a competent and un-intoxicated person on board the recreational vessel. Depending on the circumstances, the Coast Guard may arrest the operator, detain the operator until sober, or turn the operator over to state or local authorities.

Tips for avoiding BUI: Boating, fishing, and other water sports are fun in their own right. Alcohol can turn a great day on the water into the tragedy of a lifetime.

Consider these alternatives to using alcohol while afloat:

- Take along a variety of cool drinks, such as sodas, water, iced tea, lemonade, or non-alcoholic beer.

- Bring plenty of food and snacks.

- Wear clothes that will help keep you and your passengers cool.

- Plan to limit your trip to a reasonable time to avoid fatigue. Remember that it's common to become tired more quickly on the water.

- If you want to make alcohol part of your day's entertainment, plan to have a party ashore at the dock, in a picnic area, at a boating club, or in your backyard. Choose a location where you'll have time between the fun and getting back into your car or boat.

- If you dock somewhere for lunch or dinner and drink alcohol with your meal, wait a reasonable time (estimated at a minimum of an hour per drink) before operating your boat.

- Having no alcohol while aboard is the safest way to enjoy the water—intoxicated passengers are also at risk of injury and falls overboard.

- Spread the word on the dangers of BUI. Many recreational boaters forget that a boat is a vehicle, and that safe operation is a legal and personal responsibility.

Chapter 46

Preventing Alcohol-Impaired Driving

Chapter Contents

Section 46.1

Impaired Driving Research

Excerpted from "Impaired Driving," Centers for Disease Control and
Prevention (CDC), January 26, 2009.

Every day 32 people in the United States die in motor vehicle crashes
that involve an alcohol-impaired driver. This amounts to one death
every 45 minutes. The annual cost of alcohol-related crashes totals
more than $51 billion. But, there are effective measures that can help
prevent injuries and deaths from alcohol-impaired driving.

How can deaths and injuries from impaired driving be prevented?
Effective measures include:

- Aggressively enforcing existing 0.08% blood alcohol content
  (BAC) laws, minimum legal drinking age laws, and zero tolerance laws for drivers younger than 21 years old in all states.

- Promptly revoking the driver's licenses of people who drive while
  intoxicated.

- Using sobriety checkpoints.

- Implementing health promotion efforts that use an ecological
  framework to influence economic, organizational, policy, and
  school/community action.

- Using multi-faceted community-based approaches to alcohol control and driving while intoxicated (DWI) prevention.

- Requiring mandatory substance abuse assessment and treatment for DWI offenders.

Other suggested measures include:

- Reducing the legal BAC limit to 0.05%.

- Raising state and federal alcohol excise taxes.

- Implementing compulsory blood alcohol testing when traffic
  crashes result in injury.

Centers for Disease Control and Prevention (CDC) Research and Program Activities

A systematic review conducted by CDC researchers on behalf of the Task Force on Community Preventive Services concluded that well-executed multi-component interventions with community mobilization are effective in reducing alcohol-related crashes. The interventions included most or all of following: responsible beverage service training, other efforts to limit alcohol access, sobriety checkpoints, and a strong local media component.

Ignition interlock programs recommended: Ignition interlocks are installed in vehicles to prevent operation by anyone with a blood alcohol concentration (BAC) above a specified safe level (usually 0.02%–0.04%). CDC reviewed the effectiveness of ignition interlocks programs to reduce alcohol-impaired driving recidivism and alcohol-related crashes. The review, conducted on behalf of the Task Force on Community Preventive Services, drew on findings from a 2004 review conducted by Willis, Lybrand and Bellamy (Willis 2004). It concluded that ignition interlocks are associated with a median 73% reduction in re-arrest rates for alcohol-impaired driving. Based on strong evidence of the effectiveness of interlocks in reducing re-arrest rates, the Task Force recommended that ignition interlock programs be implemented.

Systematic reviews support maintaining and enforcing current minimum legal drinking age (MLDA) laws: Some college administrators have suggested that minimum legal drinking age (MLDA) laws contribute to the problem of underage alcohol use and that lowering MLDA could reduce binge drinking among underage students. Two systematic reviews conducted on behalf of the Task Force on Community Preventive Services provide evidence to support maintaining and enforcing the existing MLDA of 21 years.

Last Call intervention aims to reduce alcohol-related crashes: CDC funded researchers at the Harborview Injury Prevention and Research Center to design and evaluate a multifaceted social marketing campaign, Last Call. The program goal was to increase the use of designated drivers and safe rides home among 21–34 year olds who drink in bars and restaurants. The researchers established permanent taxi stands in five of Seattle Washington's primary entertainment districts and mounted a mass media campaign promoting designated drivers and safe-ride home options. The program appeared to increase use of taxis and reduce use of privately-own cars after drivers spent evenings out drinking with friends. There was also an increase in the use of designated drivers. Among the heaviest drinkers, the program significantly increased the use of designated drivers and increased the use of taxis by 63%.

Section 46.2

Mass Media Campaigns to Prevent Alcohol-Impaired Driving

Excerpted from "Mass Media Campaigns Are Effective in Preventing Alcohol-Impaired Driving," Centers for Disease Control and Prevention (CDC), January 19, 2009.

A Centers for Disease Control and Prevention (CDC)-led systematic review of the research literature revealed that, under certain conditions, mass media campaigns are effective in preventing alcohol-impaired driving. Based on these findings, the Task Force on Community Preventive Services, a 15-member, nonfederal group with expertise in public health policy, behavioral and social sciences, issued a recommendation for mass media campaigns that are carefully planned, well executed, attain adequate audience exposure, and are implemented in conjunction with other ongoing alcohol-impaired driving prevention activities.

Evidence of effectiveness: Findings from the systematic review are based on eight studies that evaluated the effectiveness of mass media campaigns on fatal crashes, fatal and nonfatal injury crashes combined, crashes that damage property, and drivers' blood alcohol levels. The campaigns reviewed had several components in common: pretesting of messages; high levels of audience exposure, generally achieved through paid advertising; and corresponding prevention efforts at the local level (such as high-visibility enforcement of impaired driving laws).

Of the campaigns evaluated, three focused on increasing public awareness of local law enforcement activities and the legal consequences of drinking and driving, the remaining five studies evaluated campaigns that emphasized the social and health consequences of alcohol-impaired driving. Overall, the evaluated studies showed median decreases of 13% for total alcohol-related crashes and 10% for injury crashes. No clear differences were noted in the effectiveness of campaign messages that emphasized legal consequences versus social and health consequences, though certain messages and delivery channels may be more effective with particular audiences.

Cost-benefit analyses were available for two of the reviewed campaigns. The estimated societal benefits exceeded the costs of developing and airing the campaign messages by factors of eight and twenty-one, respectively.

Section 46.3

Sobriety Checkpoints

Text in this section is from "Research Update: Sobriety Checkpoints Are Effective in Reducing Alcohol-Related Crashes," Centers for Disease Control and Prevention (CDC), January 19, 2009.

Fewer alcohol-related crashes occur when sobriety checkpoints are implemented, according to a report published in *Traffic Injury Prevention*. This conclusion is based on a systematic review of research on sobriety checkpoints. The review was conducted by a team of experts led by Centers for Disease Control and Prevention (CDC) scientists, under the oversight of the Task Force on Community Preventive Services. The review combined the results of 23 scientifically sound studies from around the world. Results indicated that sobriety checkpoints consistently reduced alcohol-related crashes, typically by about 20%. The results were similar regardless of how the checkpoints were conducted, and results were similar for short-term blitzes or when checkpoints were used continuously for several years. This suggests that the effectiveness of checkpoints does not diminish over time.

What are sobriety checkpoints?

Sobriety checkpoints are traffic stops where law enforcement officers systematically select drivers to assess their level of alcohol impairment. The goal of these interventions is to deter alcohol-impaired driving by increasing drivers' perceived risk of arrest. Two types of sobriety checkpoints exist. Selective breath testing (SBT) checkpoints are the only type used in the United States. At these checkpoints, police must have a reason to suspect that drivers have been drinking before testing their blood alcohol levels. At random breath testing (RBT) checkpoints, all drivers who are stopped have their blood alcohol levels tested. These checkpoints are used in Australia and several European countries.

Issues for Implementation

Legal issues: Although the U.S. Supreme Court ruled in 1990 that sobriety checkpoints are constitutional, some states prohibit them based on statutes or from interpretation of state constitutions.

Financial issues: Sobriety checkpoints result in substantial savings to society as a whole. Nonetheless, for the agencies that implement them, it can be costly to initiate and maintain checkpoint programs. For this reason, it is important that sobriety checkpoint programs are adequately funded.

Community involvement and support: Most Americans support sobriety checkpoints, and levels of public support often increase after checkpoints are implemented. Building on this support can lead to partnerships between the general public, advocacy groups, federal, state, and local government, and law enforcement agencies. Broad-based community support can help law enforcement agencies develop and maintain strong checkpoint programs.

Support among law enforcement: Support among the police officers conducting checkpoints is important. Because checkpoints tend to result in few arrests for alcohol-impaired driving, it is important for officers to understand that the primary goal is to prevent such occurrences. Checkpoints can also lead to the arrest of drivers for other offenses, such as weapons possession.

Section 46.4

Designated Driver Promotion Programs

Text in this section is from "Research Update: Effectiveness of Designated Driver Promotion Programs to Reduce Alcohol-Impaired Driving Is Unknown," Centers for Disease Control and Prevention (CDC), January 19, 2009.

What are designated drivers?

The varying definition of a designated driver is among the challenges facing researchers who study the effectiveness of designated driver programs. The most common definition requires that the designated driver abstain from alcohol, be assigned before anyone in the group starts drinking, and drive group members to their homes at the end of the event or gathering. Another definition is based on the concept of risk- or harm-reduction. Under this definition, the designated driver needs only to maintain a blood alcohol content (BAC) limit that is under the legal limit. In practice, many people may apply the designated driver concept in ways that are unsafe (for example, by choosing the person in the group who is least drunk to be the designated driver).

Systematic Review of the Research

Despite the popularity of designated driver promotion programs, few studies have evaluated their effectiveness in reducing alcohol-impaired driving, according to a report published in the *American Journal of Preventive Medicine*. A team of experts led by CDC scientists, under the oversight of the Task Force on Community Preventive Services conducted a systematic review of research on population-based campaigns and incentive programs designed to increase the use of designated drivers. The review combines the results of nine peer-reviewed papers and technical reports.

Designated Driver Promotion Programs

Population-based campaigns promote the concept of designated drivers through mass media outlets. Only one study from Australia

431

met the criteria for the review. Results showed a 13% increase among survey respondents who always select a designated driver, but no significant change in self-reported alcohol-impaired driving or riding with an alcohol-impaired driver.

Incentive programs increase the use of designated drivers via drinking establishments offering free incentives such as soft drinks, exotic non-alcohol drinks, food, or free admission. The seven studies that measured the number of patrons who identified themselves as designated drivers reported that incentive programs had a median increase of 0.9 designated drivers per drinking establishment per night. The public health impact of the small increase in self-identified designated drivers at each drinking venue is unknown.

Review Results

The review found insufficient evidence of effectiveness to recommend either type of designated driver promotion program (population-based campaigns or incentive programs) due to the limited number of studies, the small effect sizes observed, and limitations of the outcome measures. It is important to note that researchers focused exclusively on programs to promote the use of designated drivers; they did not address the question of whether the use of designated drivers reduces alcohol-impaired driving.

Chapter 47

Alcohol Impacts the Workplace

Substance use in the workplace negatively affects U.S. industry through lost productivity, workplace accidents and injuries, employee absenteeism, low morale, and increased illness. The loss to U.S. companies due to employees' alcohol and drug use and related problems is estimated at billions of dollars a year. Research shows that the rate of substance use varies by occupation and industry. Studies also have indicated that employers vary in their treatment of substance use issues and that workplace-based employee assistance programs (EAP) can be a valuable resource for obtaining help for substance-using workers.

Worker Substance Use

Reflecting the fact that almost two-thirds of the adult population (64.3%) were employed full time, a majority of past month illicit drug and heavy alcohol users also were employed full time. From 2002 to 2004, over half of all past month illicit drug users (57.5%) and past month heavy alcohol users (67.3%) aged 18 to 64 were employed full time.

Among full-time workers aged 18 to 64, the highest rates of past month heavy alcohol use were found in construction (15.9%); arts, entertainment, and recreation (13.6%); and mining (13.3%) (Table

---

This chapter includes excerpts from "Worker Substance Use, by Industry Category," Substance Abuse and Mental Health Services Administration (SAMHSA), August 23, 2007; excerpts from "Workplace Substance Use: Quick Facts to Inform Managers," SAMHSA, 2008; and "Impaired Driving: A Safe and Sober Message about Workplace Parties and Drinking," U.S. Department of Labor.

47.2). The industry categories with the lowest rates of heavy alcohol use were educational services (4.0%) and health care and social assistance (4.3%).

Table 47.1. Past Month Illicit Drug Use and Heavy Alcohol Use among Persons Aged 18 to 64, by Employment Status: 2002–2004 Combined

	Illicit Drug Use		Heavy Alcohol Use	
Employment Status	Percent	Number in Thousands	Percent	Number in Thousands
Total	9.2	16,363	8.4	15,017
Full-Time	8.2	9,413	8.8	10,113
Part-Time	11.9	2,903	8.6	2,094
Unemployed	18.6	1,405	13.6	1,028
Other*	8.3	2,642	5.6	1,783

*Retired persons, disabled persons, homemakers, students, or other persons not in the labor force are included in the other employment category.
Source: SAMHSA, 2002, 2003, and 2004 NSDUHs.

Among full-time workers who used alcohol heavily in the past month, 37.2% worked for an employer who provided educational information about drug and alcohol use, 73.7% were aware of written policies about drug and alcohol use, and 51.1% had access to an EAP at their workplace.

Substance Use: Facts to Inform Managers

Effect of Substance Abuse on Businesses

Regardless of where illicit drug use or heavy alcohol use takes place, workers reporting substance use and abuse have higher rates of turnover and absenteeism.

• Workers reporting heavy alcohol use or illicit drug use, as well as workers reporting dependence on or abuse of alcohol or illicit drugs, are more likely to have worked for more than three employers in the past year.

• Likewise, those workers are more likely to have skipped work more than two days in the past month.

- Workers reporting past-month illicit drug use or dependence on or abuse of alcohol or illicit drugs were also more likely to have missed more than two days of work due to illness or injury in the past month.

Furthermore, the impact of employee substance use and abuse is a problem that extends beyond the substance-using employee.

- There is evidence that co-worker job performance and attitudes are negatively affected.

- Workers have reported being put in danger, having been injured, or having had to work harder, to redo work, or to cover for a co-worker as a result of a fellow employee's drinking.

Table 47.2. Past Month Heavy Alcohol Use among Full-Time Workers Aged 18 to 64, by Industry Categories: 2002–2004 Combined

Industry Categories	Percent
Construction	15.9
Arts, entertainment, recreation	13.6
Mining	13.1
Accommodations and food services	12.0
Wholesale trade	11.5
Management of companies and enterprises, administrative, support, waste management, and remediation services	10.4
Information	10.4
Utilities	10.1
Other services (except public administration)	9.9
Real estate, rental, and leasing	9.8
Agriculture, forestry, fishing, and hunting	9.7
Manufacturing	9.5
Retail trade	8.8
Transportation and warehousing	8.6
Professional, scientific, and technical services	7.1
Finance and insurance	6.9
Public administration	5.9
Health care and social assistance	4.3
Educational services	4.0

Source: SAMHSA, 2002, 2003, and 2004 National Survey on Drug Use and Health (NSDUH).

Fast Facts: Prevention in the Workplace

Workplace prevention programs—minimizing risk, mitigating workplace injuries: Workplace prevention programs, like Peer-Care, attempt to reduce substance abuse on the job and, in turn, reduce workplace injuries. The program, which trained employees in PeerCare from 1968–1999 saw annual workplace injury costs fall from almost $90 million in 1986 to about $40 million in 1999 at an annual cost to the company of just 1.8 million. The National Registry of Evidence-Based Programs and Practices provides information on programs available for workplaces which have been tested for efficacy.

Employer costs—short-term and long-term: Data suggest that substance abuse prevention may result in higher healthcare costs and utilization in the short term, but a reduction in health risk behaviors such as heavy drinking may result in lower health care costs and utilization in the long run. Employees accessing the company employee assistance program (EAP) had a higher number of outpatient visits for a substance abuse and/or mental health problem compared to those not accessing the EAP. However, employed drug abusers cost their employers about twice as much in medical and worker compensation claims as their drug-free coworkers.

A Safe and Sober Message about Workplace Parties and Drinking

The workplace is frequently a place where employees and employers get together to celebrate special events. Workplace parties typically mean lots of music, food, and drinks. If the drinks include alcohol the potential for unfortunate consequences greatly increases. Opinions vary regarding the appropriateness of making alcoholic beverages available at workplace parties or other company-sponsored events. Ignoring the possibility that some employees or guests may drive home under the influence invites trouble.

Improper use of alcohol may expose employers to liability under tort, workers' compensation or other laws. For example, an employer may be held liable if a person consumes alcoholic beverages at a company-sponsored party and subsequently causes a crash. Some employers have been held liable because negligent acts by employees under the influence of alcohol consumed at employer-sponsored events were found to be within the scope of their employment. In other cases, individuals have been held liable merely because they provided alcohol to social guests.

Each time an employee is involved in an impaired driving crash, businesses pay in the form of increased absenteeism and use of health care benefits. According to the National Highway Traffic Safety Administration's (NHTSA), the annual employer cost of motor vehicle crashes in which at least one driver was alcohol-impaired is more than $9 billion, including wage-risk premiums. Furthermore, if the employee caused the crash or is arrested for impaired driving even if a crash did not occur, administrative and legal procedures such as court time and traffic school may require further time away from work. And certainly no employer can deny the emotional difficulty and decreased morale employees experience when a colleague suffers from a severe injury or dies—two unfortunate, but not uncommon, outcomes of mixing alcohol and driving.

Depending on the nature of their business, some employers may have additional incentives to ensure their employees are educated about the potential legal vulnerabilities associated with impaired driving. Employers whose businesses serve or sell alcohol may be held liable if an individual consumes alcohol at their establishment and subsequently causes a crash. Employers with employees who drive as part of their job—such as couriers, delivery persons, and sales representatives—may also be subject to legal action if the impaired employee causes a crash while conducting business. These employers must consider the costs of insuring and maintaining company vehicles, in addition to the time managers spend taking care of these procedures. The return on investment for employer-sponsored impaired driving prevention is considerable when compared to the financial burden caused by just one crash, especially for small businesses.

All employers run a risk if they serve alcoholic beverages at workplace celebrations and other company-sponsored events because they may be held liable if a person causes a crash subsequent to consuming alcoholic beverages at such an event. However, if an employer does decide to provide or allow alcoholic beverages at an office event, state laws regarding their use and resulting employer legal responsibilities should be consulted and addressed. Also, there are several measures employers can take in attempt to minimize any negative consequences of alcohol consumption.

The good news is that employers have enormous power to protect their businesses from the negative impact of impaired driving by educating employees about its harmful effects and supporting efforts to prevent it in their communities. By doing so, employers do more than just safeguard their business assets-they contribute to the nationwide campaign to eliminate a devastating and preventable crime and play a part in making their communities safer for their friends and families and those of their employees.

Chapter 48

Alcohol-Related Fire Fatalities

Alcohol intoxication may increase the risk of starting a fire by impairing one's judgment and coordination. A smoker under the influence of alcohol is more susceptible to falling asleep and dropping a lit cigarette on upholstery or clothing. The effect of alcohol may cause a failure to notice the smell of smoke or hear a smoke alarm, and escaping from a fire can be hampered by the loss of motor coordination and mental clarity even when warning signs are heeded.

Case Study Findings: Contribution of Alcohol to Fire Fatalities in Ontario

- Over a seven-year period (1995–2001), 19% of fire fatalities were alcohol impaired.

- Fatalities increase from noon to midnight and then decline. Alcohol-related deaths begin climbing at 4:00 p.m. and peak at 5:00 a.m.

- Alcohol-related fatalities are relatively constant throughout the year.

- Nearly 70% of all alcohol-related fire fatalities were between the ages of 25 and 54.

Text in this chapter is from "Focus on Fire Safety: Alcohol and Fire," U.S. Fire Administration, March 20, 2009.

Case Study Findings: Contribution of Alcohol to Fire Fatalities in Minnesota

- From 1996 to 2002, 36% of Minnesota's fire fatalities had alcohol levels of 0.1 or higher.

- 13% of children under age 15 died in fires during the 1995–2002 time period. None were alcohol impaired, but alcohol may have contributed to a number of these deaths by virtue of an alcohol- or drug-impaired caregiver.

- 69% of the alcohol-impaired fire victims in Minnesota were aged 35–54.

- Although the elderly (75+) are at high risk from fire, only 8% of the elderly victims in Minnesota were alcohol impaired.

- The cause of 26% of fire deaths was smoking. Of these deaths, 62% were alcohol impaired. There is a strong connection between smokers, drinkers, and fire deaths.

Understanding the Risk

According to the Centers for Disease Control and Prevention (CDC), alcohol use and the resulting impairment may be the strongest independent factor for death from fire. One study found that intoxication contributed to an estimated 40% of deaths due to residential fires. By altering ones cognitive, physiological, and motor functions, alcohol increases the chance of starting a serious fire while at the same time reduces the chance of survival from a fire or burn injury.

Young children, older adults, and those who are dependent on a caregiver are most vulnerable to fire deaths and injuries due to their dependence on others. According to the American Medical Association (AMA), the presence of an adult with no physical or cognitive disability who was unimpaired by alcohol or other drugs reduced the risk of death in this group.

Men have been found to consistently outnumber women among fire casualties and do so with even greater disparity for fire victims under the influence of alcohol. In addition, the younger adult population (ages 15–24) seems to incur the greatest number of alcohol-impaired fire casualties. Drinking behaviors that are characteristic of each gender and various age groups may explain these findings.

Researchers have suggested that alcohol-related unintentional injuries have more to do with alcohol drinking patterns than the total amount of alcohol consumed per capita. Who drinks, where they drink, what they drink, and under what social, cultural and religious circumstances they drink are perhaps more significant factors than the amount of alcohol consumed. A lone drinker at home is probably at greater risk of a fire emergency than a group of people drinking in a bar or restaurant. Moreover, the number of drinks consumed in a single sitting seems to matter a great deal.

Alcohol and College Students

In cases where fire fatalities have occurred on college campuses, alcohol was a factor. There is a strong link between alcohol and fire deaths. In more than 40% of adult fire fatalities, victims were under the influence at the time of the fire. Alcohol abuse often impairs judgment and hampers evacuation efforts.

Tragic scenarios, too often repeated:

- Chapel Hill, North Carolina: In the 1996 fraternity fire that killed five students, four of them had blood alcohol levels of over 0.14. This fire broke out following a party the evening before, as had the fire in Bloomsburg, Pennsylvania where three males were killed.

- Amherst, Massachusetts: A fire the day following a party destroyed the fraternity. There were large numbers of empty beer cans. The smoke alarms had all been covered with bags so they would not activate during the party.

Minimize Your Risk

It is possible to minimize fire risk by increasing the awareness of those who drink and those who are surrounded by regular drinkers. Understand the dangers and don't become a fire statistic.

Chapter 49

Raising Alcohol Taxes Reduces Harm

Increasing taxes and prices on alcoholic beverages is an effective public health strategy for reducing alcohol consumption and alcohol-related harm.[1]

- Higher prices result in lower consumption, which reduces alcohol harm overall.[2]

- Increasing alcohol taxes is a highly effective tool in reducing a wide range of harm and consequences among all age groups.[2]

- Types of alcohol-related harm that are reduced with higher taxes include: alcohol dependence,[3] liver cirrhosis,[4] risky sexual behaviors leading to STDs,[5] and traffic fatalities.[2]

- Significant reductions in the numbers of deaths (ranging from 11%–29%) were attributed to alcohol tax increases in 1983 and in 2002 in the state of Alaska.[6]

Alcohol-Related Car Crashes

- Adjusting the federal beer tax for the inflation rate since 1951 would have reduced auto fatalities among youth between the ages of 18 and 20 by 15%.[7]

- A 10% increase in price would reduce traffic crashes by 5%–10%, with even larger reductions (7%–17%) for youth.[2]

This chapter includes "Raising Alcohol Taxes Reduces Harm," and "Alcohol Tax FAQ," © 2009 The Marin Institute (www.marininstutute.org). Reprinted with permission.

- A 10% increase in price would reduce drinking and driving by 7.4% among males and by 8.1% among females, with even larger reductions (12.6% and 21.1%) among those 21 years or younger.[8]

Alcohol-Related Illness

- A 10% increase in price would reduce cirrhosis mortality from 8.3%–12.8% after the levels of heavy drinking adjusted to the price change in future years.[9]

- A $1 increase in state alcohol taxes would reduce gonorrhea rates by 2.1%, while a 20-cent increase in the tax on a six-pack of beer would reduce gonorrhea rates by 8.9%, with similar effects on syphilis rates.[10]

- A 10% increase in the average state excise tax on beer reduced AIDS rates by a range of 5.1%–8.5% in males between the ages of 12 and 21.[11]

Alcohol-Related Violence

- Higher alcohol prices can reduce rates of homicide and suicide.[12]

- A 10% increase in beer tax would reduce the probability of any child abuse by 1.2%, and reduce the probability of severe child abuse by 2.1%.[13]

- Increased prices on alcohol would reduce the rate of domestic violence.[14]

- A 10% increase in beer tax would reduce the overall number of college students involved in some sort of violent behavior by 200,000 or about 4%.[15]

Academic Achievement

- Increased prices on alcohol would improve study habits among college students.[16]

- A 10-cent per case of beer price increase would improve a student's probability of attending and graduating from a four-year college or university by 6.3%.[17]

- A 10% increase in beer tax would raise the probability of high school graduation by approximately 3%.[18]

Bottom line: Raising alcohol taxes and prices is one of the most effective public health policies available to reduce alcohol-related harm. Even heavy drinkers will consume less when prices go up.

Alcohol Tax FAQ

Won't alcohol taxes have the biggest impact on "Joe Six-Pack," the average moderate drinker who just wants to blow off steam at the end of the day? Contrary to popular belief, studies have shown that increasing alcohol taxes will have a negligible effect on moderate drinkers. The tax will most dramatically impact heavy drinkers, who account for 15% of the population. This is the segment responsible for the vast majority of the costs related to alcohol abuse.

Could fair alcohol taxes reduce underage drinking? We believe it would. Extremely low taxes allow products such as beer and alcopops to be sold remarkably cheap. This low price gives underage drinkers easy access to the products. In fact, a report issued by the Institute of Medicine specifically recommended raising taxes on alcohol as the most comprehensive and effective method of reducing underage drinking.

Would alcohol higher taxes mean fewer jobs? It is unlikely that big alcohol companies would produce less if taxes went up. After the tax increase in 1991, the Bureau of Labor Statistics of the U.S. Department of Labor reported that beer-industry wholesale trade employment actually rose by 8,000 jobs.

Why would the average American support increasing alcohol taxes? Actually, a majority of Americans support an increased tax on alcohol, particularly when they learn that alcohol-related harms are estimated at a cost of $184 billion nationwide.

Are there any other benefits that may come out of appropriately taxing alcohol? Increasing alcohol taxes has proven to reduce the rates of sexually-transmitted diseases. For example, the Centers for Disease Control and Prevention found that a beer-tax increase of 20 cents per six-pack would reduce gonorrhea rates by 8.9% and syphilis rates by 32.7%. Increases in the state excise tax on beer decreases the probability of overall violence toward children. Higher beer taxes are also associated with lower rates of traffic fatalities. Specifically, every 1% increase in the price of beer results in the decline of traffic fatality rates by 0.9%.

References

1. Cook PJ, *Paying the Tab: The Costs and Benefits of Alcohol Control*. Princeton: Princeton University Press, 2007.

2. Chaloupka FJ, The effects of price on alcohol use, abuse, and their consequences. In Bonnie RJ, O'Connell ME. *Reducing Underage Drinking: A Collective Responsibility*. The National Academies Press, Washington, DC. 2004:541–564.

3. Farrell S, Manning WG, Finch MD. Alcohol dependence and the price of alcoholic beverages. *J Health Econ*. 2003;22:117–147.

4. Cook PJ, Tauchen G. The effect of liquor taxes on heavy drinking. *Bell J Econ*. 1982;13:379–390.

5. Markowitz S, Kaestner R, Grossman M. An investigation of the effects of alcohol consumption and alcohol policies on youth risky sexual behaviors. *Am Econ Rev*. 2005;95:263-266.

6. Wagenaar AC, Maldonado-Molina MM, Wagenaar BH. Effects of Alcohol Tax Increases on Alcohol-Related Disease Mortality in Alaska: Time-Series Analyses from 1976 to 2004. *Am J Public Health*. 2009;99(1):1–8.

7. Saffer H, Grossman M. Beer taxes, the legal drinking age, and youth motor vehicle fatalities. *J Legal Stud*. 1987a;16:351–374.

8. Kenkel DS. Drinking, driving and deterrence: The effectiveness and social costs of alternative policies. *J Law Econ*. 1993;36: 877–914.

9. Grossman M. The economic analysis of addictive behavior. In Hilton ME, Bloss G. Economics and the prevention of alcohol-related problems. *National Institute on Alcohol Abuse and Alcoholism Research Monograph No. 25*, NIH Publication No. 93–513. Rockville, MD: National Institute on Alcohol Abuse and Alcoholism.1993:91–123.

10. Chesson H, Harrison P, Kassler WJ. Sex under the influence: The effect of alcohol policy on sexually transmitted disease rates in the United States. *J Law Econ*. 2000;43:215–238.

11. Grossman M, Kaestner R, Markowitz S. An investigation of the effects of alcohol policies on youth STD's. *Am Econ Rev*. 2004;95:263–266.

12. Sloan FA, Reilly BA, Schenzler C. Effects of prices, civil and criminal sanctions, and law enforcement on alcohol-related mortality. *J Stud Alcohol*. 1994;55:454–465.

13. Markowitz S, Grossman M. Alcohol regulation and domestic violence towards children. *Contemp Econ Pol*. 1998;16:309–320.

14. Markowitz S. The price of alcohol, wife abuse and husband abuse. *South Econ J*. 2000;67:279–303.

15. Grossman M, Markowitz S. Alcohol regulation and violence on college campuses. In M. Grossman and C.R. Hsieh (Eds.),

Economic analysis of substance use and abuse: The experience of developed countries and lessons. 2001.

16. Powell LM, Williams J, Wechsler H. Study habits and the level of alcohol use among college students. *Impact Teen Research Paper Series #19.* Chicago: University of Illinois. 2002. Available at: http://www.alcoholpolicymd.com/pdf/studyhabits_powellfinal.pdf. Accessed August 18, 2009.

17. Cook PJ, Moore MJ. Drinking and schooling. *J Health Econ.* 1993;12:411–429.

18. Yamada T, Kendix M, Yamada T. The impact of alcohol consumption and marijuana use on high school graduation. *Health Econ.* 1996;5:77–92.

Part Seven

Treatment and Recovery

Chapter 50

Helping Someone Who Has a Problem with Alcohol

The person who has someone close who drinks too much or who uses other drugs has plenty of company. People experiencing alcohol and other drug problems often feel they hurt only themselves. That isn't true. They also hurt their families, friends, coworkers, employers, and others.

There are millions of people with alcohol and other drug problems in this country. A recent study reported that 28 million people age 12 and older used illicit drugs during the past year. By current estimates, more than 76 million people have been exposed to alcoholism in the family. Experience shows that for every person with an alcohol or other drug problem, at least four others are affected by their behavior. However, looking at it another way—as we should—millions of Americans have a personal stake in helping "someone close" find the way to overcome alcohol and other drug problems.

The person who sets out to help someone with an alcohol or other drug problem may at first feel quite alone, possibly embarrassed, not knowing where to turn for help. We have preserved so many wrong ideas and attitudes about problem drinking and other drug abuse, too often thinking of them as moral weakness or lack of willpower.

You may have learned to better understand alcohol and other drug problems and already made contact with nearby sources of services. This does not mean that "someone close" will cooperate at once by going for treatment. Those with alcohol and other drug problems may deny they have a problem. They may find it difficult to ask for or accept help.

"If Someone Close Has a Problem with Alcohol or Other Drugs," Substance Abuse and Mental Health Services Administration (SAMHSA).

If there is one thing true about alcohol and other drug abusers, it is that, as with all people, each one is different—different in human needs and responses, as well as in their reasons for drinking and taking other drugs, their reactions to these drugs, and their readiness for treatment.

You are in a good position to help your relative or friend, because you know a good deal about their unique qualities and their way of life. And having made the effort to gain some understanding of the signs and effects of problem drinking or other drug abuse, you should be in a better position to consider a strategy for helping.

Be active, get involved. Don't be afraid to talk about the problem honestly and openly. It is easy to be too polite, or to duck the issue by saying, "After all, it's their private affair." But it isn't polite or considerate to let someone destroy their family and life. You may need to be persistent to break through any denial they have. You also may need to let them know how much courage it takes to ask for help, or to accept it. You will find that most people with drinking- or other drug-related troubles really want to talk it out if they find out you are concerned about them.

To begin, you may need to reject certain myths that in the past have done great harm to alcoholics and other drug abusers and hampered those who would help them. These untruths come from ingrained public attitudes that see alcoholism and other drug problems as personal misconduct, moral weakness, or even sin. They are expressed in such declarations as, "Nothing can be done unless the alcohol or drug abuser wants to stop," or "They must hit bottom," that is, lose health, job, home, family, "before they will want to get well." These stubborn myths are not true, and have been destructive. One may as well say that you cannot treat cancer or tuberculosis until the gross signs of disease are visible to all. The truth is that with alcohol and other drug problems, as with other kinds of acute and chronic illness, early recognition and treatment intervention are essential—and rewarding.

Be compassionate, be patient—but be willing to act. Experience proves that preaching does not work. A nudge or a push at the right time can help. It also shows that you care. Push may even come to shove when the person with alcohol or other drug troubles must choose between losing family or job, or going to treatment. Thousands of alcohol and other drug abusers have been helped when a spouse, employer, or court official made treatment a condition of continuing family relationships, job, or probation. You cannot cure the illness, but when the crucial moment comes you can guide the person to competent help.

Treatment attempts to discover the relationship between a person's problematic drinking and other drug use to their real needs—an understanding of what they would really strive for it they were not disabled by their problems. One goal is building up their capacity for control which becomes possible in periods of sobriety.

Persons with drinking and other drug problems have the same needs as all other people—food, clothing, shelter, health care, job, social contact and acceptance and, particularly, the need for self-confidence and feelings of competence, self-worth, and dignity. This is where support comes in. What may be needed most is warm, human concern. The kinds of support given depend, of course, on finding out from the person what they feel they need. Strained family and friend relationships, money troubles, worry about the job or business, sometimes matters that may seem trivial to us, all confuse their situation and may contribute to their drinking and other drug problems. Moral support in starting and staying with treatment, reassurances from employer or business associates, willing participation by spouse or children in group therapy sessions are examples of realistic support. The long range goal is healthy living for the person and their family—physical health, social health, emotional health—an objective we all share.

Three out of four alcohol and drug abusing men and women are married; living at home; holding onto a job, business, or profession; and are reasonably well accepted members of their communities. For those in this group who seek treatment, the outlook is good. Regardless of life situation, the earlier treatment starts after troubles are recognized, the better the chances for success.

Many therapists now use rehabilitation as a measure of outcome—success is considered achieved when the patient maintains or reestablishes a good family life and work record, and a respectable position in the community. Relapse may occur but does not mean that the person or the treatment effort has failed. A successful outcome, on this basis, can be expected for 50%–70% depending upon the personal characteristics of the patient; early treatment intervention; competence of the therapists; availability of hospital and outpatient facilities; and the strong support of family, friends, employer, and community.

"It is doubtful that any specific percentage figure has much meaning by itself," says one authority. "What does have a great deal of meaning is the fact that tens of thousands of such cases have shown striking improvement over many years."

The Center for Substance Abuse Prevention offers information on all aspects of the prevention of alcohol and other drug problems. It also maintains a state-by-state listing of most public and private alcohol and other drug information, counseling, and treatment facilities. Call or write:

The National Clearinghouse for Alcohol and Drug Information
P.O. Box 2345
Rockville, MD 20847-2345
Toll-Free: 800-729-6686

What Not to Do

- Don't attempt to punish, threaten, bribe, or preach.

- Don't try to be a martyr. Avoid emotional appeals that may only increase feelings of guilt and the compulsion to drink or use other drugs.

- Don't allow yourself to cover up or make excuses for the alcoholic or drug addict or shield them from the realistic consequences of their behavior.

- Don't take over their responsibilities, leaving them with no sense of importance or dignity.

- Don't hide or dump bottles, throw out drugs, or shelter them from situations where alcohol is present.

- Don't argue with the person when they are impaired or high.

- Don't try to drink along with the problem drinker or take drugs with the drug abuser.

- Above all, don't feel guilty or responsible for another's behavior.

What to Do

- Try to remain calm, unemotional, and factually honest in speaking about their behavior and its day-to-day consequences.

- Let the person with the problem know that you are reading and learning about alcohol and other drug abuse, attending Al-Anon, Nar-Anon, Alateen, and other support groups.

- Discuss the situation with someone you trust—someone from the clergy, a social worker, a counselor, a friend, or some individual who has experienced alcohol or other drug abuse personally or as a family member.

- Establish and maintain a healthy atmosphere in the home, and try to include the alcohol/drug abuser in family life.

- Explain the nature of alcoholism and other drug addiction as an illness to the children in the family.

- Encourage new interests and participate in leisure time activities that the person enjoys. Encourage them to see old friends.

- Be patient and live one day at a time. Alcoholism and other drug addiction generally take a long time to develop, and recovery does not occur overnight. Try to accept setbacks and relapses with calmness and understanding.

- Refuse to ride with anyone who's been drinking heavily or using other drugs.

Chapter 51

Screening for Alcohol Use and Alcohol-Related Problems

Doctors routinely screen patients for an increasing number of conditions. The term screening refers to the testing of members of a certain population (such as all the patients in a physician's practice) to estimate the likelihood that they have a specific disorder, such as alcohol abuse or dependence.

Screening is not the same as diagnostic testing, which establishes a definite diagnosis of a disorder. Instead, screening is used to identify people who are likely to have a disorder, as determined by their responses to certain key questions. People with positive screening results may be advised to undergo more detailed diagnostic testing to definitively confirm or rule out the disorder. A clinician might initiate further assessment, provide a brief intervention, and/or arrange for clinical followup when a screening test indicates that a patient may have a problem with alcohol. There is good evidence that even patients who do not meet the criteria for alcohol dependence or abuse, but who are drinking at levels that place them at risk for can be helped through screening and brief intervention.

Excerpted from "Screening for Alcohol Use and Alcohol-Related Problems," National Institute on Alcohol Abuse and Alcoholism (NIAAA), April 2005. The complete document with references is available at http://pubs.niaaa.nih.gov/publications/aa65/AA65.pdf. Reviewed in May 2010, by Dr. David A. Cooke, MD, FACP, Diplomate, American Board of Internal Medicine.

Screening in Different Settings

In primary care: Screening for alcohol disorders in primary care can vary from one simple question to an extensive assessment using a standardized questionnaire. The level of screening used by a clinician typically depends on the patient's characteristics, whether he or she has other medical or psychiatric problems, the physician's skills and interest, and the amount of time available.

Clinicians under strict time constraints may have time to ask a patient only one screening question about his or her alcohol consumption. One study has shown that a positive response to the question "On any single occasion during the past three months, have you had more than five drinks containing alcohol?" accurately identifies patients who meet either National Institute on Alcohol Abuse and Alcoholism (NIAAA) criteria for at-risk drinking or the criteria for alcohol abuse or dependence specified in the *Diagnostic and Statistical Manual of Mental Disorders, Fourth Edition (DSM–IV)*.

Whenever possible, questions about alcohol use should be asked of all patients on an annual basis or in response to problems that may be alcohol related. The questions can be included in a pre-exam interview and conducted as part of the patient's check-in process. If the patient appears to be at risk for alcohol-related medical problems, or if the clinician suspects that the patient is minimizing his or her alcohol use, more qualitative questions should be asked to better determine the nature and extent of the problem.

The CAGE questionnaire is popular for screening in the primary care setting because it is short, simple, easy to remember, and because it has been proven effective for detecting a range of alcohol problems.

CAGE

C Have you ever felt you should cut down on your drinking?

A Have people annoyed you by criticizing your drinking?

G Have you ever felt bad or guilty about your drinking?

E Eye opener: Have you ever had a drink first thing in the morning to steady your nerves or to get rid of a hangover?

Longer tests, such as the 25-question Michigan Alcoholism Screening Test (MAST) or the 10-question Alcohol Use Disorders Identification Test (AUDIT), may be used to obtain more qualitative information about a patient's alcohol consumption. The MAST includes questions about drinking behavior and alcohol-related problems; it is particularly useful for identifying alcohol dependence. The AUDIT includes questions about the quantity and frequency of alcohol use, as well as binge drinking, dependence symptoms, and alcohol-related problems. Its strength lies in its ability to identify people who have problems with alcohol but who may not be dependent. Research shows that the AUDIT may be especially useful when screening women and minorities. This screening tool also has shown promising results when tested in adolescents and young adults; it is less accurate in older patients, though further research is needed with these populations. Computerized versions of the AUDIT and other screening instruments now are available and can be used in conjunction with other health assessment questionnaires.

Screening in the emergency department: Many of the estimated 110 million emergency department (ED) visits in the United States each year are related to alcohol use. Up to 31% of patients treated in ED and 50% of severely injured trauma patients (those requiring hospital admission, usually to an intensive care unit) screen positive for alcohol problems. Patients treated in ED also are 1.5–3 times more likely than those treated in primary care clinics to report heavy drinking, to experience the adverse effects of drinking (for example, alcohol-related injuries, illnesses, and legal or social problems), and to have been treated previously for an alcohol problem.

Screening is feasible in the ED setting; however, barriers to screening in an ED setting are clear. This environment typically is chaotic and time is precious. Emergency practitioners and trauma physicians may believe that interventions for alcoholism are ineffective, or they may lack confidence in their ability or the ability of their staffs to screen patients effectively. And resources may not be available for conducting screening and brief interventions in the ED. Ethical and insurance issues also present obstacles to screening. For example, because of existing laws, third-party payers (insurers) may deny reimbursement for medical services if a patient has a positive blood alcohol level at the time of the ED visit. This can place a large financial burden on the patient or on the treating hospital (if it does not receive payment from the patient or the insurance company). Another legal issue related to screening for alcohol use in the ED is the possible denial of benefits because the patient was injured while committing a crime. In many states, driving while impaired (DWI) is a felony, especially if a crash is severe enough to result in the need for medical attention. Many insurance policies will not pay benefits for injuries sustained during the commission of a felony (but will provide for injuries sustained in the commission of a lesser crime). Other policies, however, exclude benefits for injuries sustained in the commission of any criminal act; in these cases, lesser offenses such as public intoxication or illegal consumption of an alcoholic beverage could be used as justification to deny benefits.

T-ACE

T Tolerance: How many drinks does it take to make you feel high?

A Have people annoyed you by criticizing your drinking?

C Have you ever felt you ought to cut down on your drinking?

E Eye opener: Have you ever had a drink first thing in the morning to steady your nerves or get rid of a hangover?

The T-ACE, which is based on the CAGE, is valuable for identifying a range of use, including lifetime use and prenatal use, based on the *DSM–III–R* criteria. A score of two or more is considered positive. Affirmative answers to questions A, C, or E = 1 point each. Reporting tolerance to more than two drinks (the T question) = two points.

Screening in prenatal care settings: Women who drink during pregnancy come from all walks of life. Anywhere from 14%–22.5% of women report drinking some alcohol while pregnant. The U.S. Surgeon General issued an advisory warning pregnant women and women who might become pregnant to abstain from any alcohol use to eliminate the chance of giving birth to a baby with fetal alcohol spectrum disorders (FASD)—a range of preventable birth defects caused by prenatal alcohol exposure.

Identifying women who are drinking during pregnancy clearly is important. Yet determining a woman's prenatal alcohol consumption can be difficult. Many women alter their drinking once they learn they are pregnant. But a woman may have been drinking harmful levels of alcohol prior to learning about her pregnancy, and some injury already could have been done to the fetus. The standard questions about a woman's current quantity and frequency of alcohol use may not show her true risk for problems. Asking her about her drinking patterns before she became pregnant would solicit more accurate measures of her first-trimester consumption.

A woman also may not report her alcohol consumption accurately because she is embarrassed or afraid to admit to drinking while pregnant. And popular screening instruments, such as the CAGE, although effective in other populations, may not identify harmful drinking by pregnant women.

The T-ACE, a four-item questionnaire based on the CAGE, is a simple screening instrument that can identify women's prenatal consumption. T-ACE has been tested in a wide variety of obstetric practices and has proven to be a valuable and efficient tool for identifying a range of alcohol use, including any current prenatal alcohol consumption, prepregnancy risk drinking (defined as more than two drinks per drinking day), and lifetime alcohol diagnoses.

Women who screen positive using the T-ACE or another screening questionnaire, such as the AUDIT, should receive further assessment and brief intervention to help reduce the risk to the developing fetus and to maximize pregnancy outcome.

Screening in the criminal justice system: Most states mandate screening and assessment of driving while impaired (DWI) offenders to evaluate the extent of their problem with alcohol and their need for treatment. Current sentencing guidelines also recommend that all DWI offenders be screened for alcohol use problems and recidivism risk, but the existing screening programs for DWI offenders differ in how they evaluate clients. Some programs conduct a simple screening—typically, a brief questionnaire—to determine whether the client should be transferred either to an education program or to treatment.

Screening for alcohol disorders in the criminal justice setting poses specific challenges. One factor that may limit the effectiveness of current screening procedures is that most instruments were developed in populations other than DWI offenders or other criminal justice populations and were not designed specifically for use in court-mandated screening. These instruments rely on the offenders' reports of their own alcohol use (that is, self-reports), without considering other information (such as court records for previous alcohol-related offenses, statements from the offender's family or others, or data obtained from biochemical tests to detect alcohol consumption), making it more difficult to truly gauge alcohol consumption.

Offenders also may feel coerced into screening and treatment, fearing that they may be penalized if they admit to alcohol use, perhaps losing custody of their children or receiving unfavorable probation conditions. Issues of confidentiality also may come into play. These factors can make it difficult to assess the true nature and severity of an offender's alcohol problems and underscore the need for adequately trained personnel to conduct screening in criminal justice populations so that any under-reporting of problems can be avoided. Many programs, however, cannot afford specially trained staff to conduct these evaluations.

Financial constraints are an issue in community and state criminal justice systems. Yet the costs to society of failing to properly identify and treat alcohol abusers in the criminal justice system also are substantial. Appropriately delivered treatment can be effective in changing behavior and reducing re-arrests—the result is a cost that's much less than incarceration.

Screening in college populations: Identifying those students at greatest risk for alcohol problems is the first step in prevention. Screening instruments must be selected that will accurately detect the problem within the population of interest, and be feasible to implement.

Screening may occur in the campus health center, counseling center, or local hospital emergency department (for example, students may answer questions as part of normal intake procedures). Incorporating screening into campus judicial systems has several advantages. Many campuses already have policies in place that mandate students cited for alcohol policy violations to complete assessment and interventions, and trained staff typically are available to respond to these policy violators.

Summary

Screening tests are a first-line defense in the prevention of disease. Screening for alcohol problems can take place in a wide variety of populations and settings. Research shows that a number of good screening instruments are available that can be tailored to specific audiences and needs. Detecting alcohol abuse and dependence early in the course of disease enables clinicians to get people the help they need, either by initiating a brief intervention or by referring the patient to treatment. Even patients who do not have an alcohol disorder, but who are drinking in ways that are harmful, can benefit from screening and brief intervention.

Chapter 52

Changing Alcohol Drinking Habits

Chapter Contents

Section 52.1

Strategies for Reducing Alcohol Consumption or Quitting

This section includes text excerpted from "Rethinking Drinking: Alcohol and Your Health," National Institute on Alcohol Abuse and Alcoholism (NIAAA), February 2009.

Thinking about a Change? It's Up to You

It's up to you as to whether and when to change your drinking; other people may be able to help, but in the end it's your decision. Weighing your pros and cons can help.

Pros: What are some reasons why you might want to make a change?

- Improve health
- Improve relationships
- Avoid hangovers
- Do better at work or school
- Lose weight or get fit
- Save money
- Avoid more serious problems
- Meet personal standards

Cons: List possible reasons why you might not want to change.

Compare your pros and cons: Put extra check marks by the most important one(s). Is there a difference between where you are and where you want to be?

Ready, or not? Are you ready to change your drinking? If so, continue reading for support. But don't be surprised if you continue to have mixed feelings. You may need to re-make your decision several times before becoming comfortable with it. If you're not ready to change yet, consider these suggestions in the meantime:

- Keep track of how often and how much you're drinking.

- Notice how drinking affects you.

- Make or re-make a list of pros and cons about changing.

- Deal with other priorities that may be in the way of changing.

- Ask for support from your doctor, a friend, or someone else you trust.

Don't wait for a crisis or to hit bottom: When someone is drinking too much, making a change earlier is likely to be more successful and less destructive to individuals and their families.

Cut down or quit? If you're considering changing your drinking, you'll need to decide whether to cut down or to quit. It's a good idea to discuss different options with a doctor, a friend, or someone else you trust. Quitting is strongly advised if you:

- try cutting down but cannot stay within the limits you set;

- have had an alcohol use disorder or now have symptoms;

- have a physical or mental condition that is caused or worsened by drinking;

- are taking a medication that interacts with alcohol; or

- are or may become pregnant.

If you do not have any of these conditions, talk with your doctor to determine whether you should cut down or quit based on factors such as family history of alcohol problems, your age, whether you've had drinking-related injuries, and symptoms such as sleep disorders and sexual dysfunction.

Planning for Change

Even when you have committed to change, you still may have mixed feelings at times. Making a written change plan will help you to solidify your goals, why you want to reach them, and how you plan to do it. Reinforce your decision with reminders.

Enlist technology to help: Change can be hard, so it helps to have concrete reminders of why and how you've decided to do it. Some standard options include carrying a change plan in your wallet or posting sticky notes at home. If you have a computer or mobile phone, consider these high-tech ideas:

- Fill out a change plan online at the Rethinking Drinking website (http://RethinkingDrinking.niaaa.nih.gov), email it to your personal (non-work) account, and review it weekly.

- Store your goals, reasons, or strategies in your mobile phone in short text messages or notepad entries that you can retrieve easily when an urge hits.

- Set up automated mobile phone or email calendar alerts that deliver reminders when you choose, such as a few hours before you usually go out.

- Create passwords that are motivating phrases in code, which you'll type each time you log in, such as 1Day@aTime, 1stThings1st, or 0Pain=0Gain.

Strategies for Cutting Down

Small changes can make a big difference in reducing your chances of having alcohol-related problems. Here are some strategies to try. Check off perhaps two or three to try in the next week or two, then add some others as needed. If you haven't made progress after 2–3 months, consider quitting drinking altogether, seeking professional help, or both.

Keep track of how much you drink: Find a way that works for you, such as a card in your wallet, check marks on a kitchen calendar, or notes in a mobile phone notepad or personal digital assistant. Making note of each drink before you drink it may help you slow down when needed.

Count and measure: Know the standard drink sizes so you can count your drinks accurately. Measure drinks at home. Away from home, it can be hard to keep track, especially with mixed drinks. At times you may be getting more alcohol than you think. With wine, you may need to ask the host or server not to top off a partially filled glass.

Set goals: Decide how many days a week you want to drink and how many drinks you'll have on those days. It's a good idea to have some days when you don't drink. Drinkers with the lowest rates of alcohol use disorders stay within these limits: For men, no more than four drinks on any day and 14 per week; and for women, no more than three drinks on any day and seven per week. Both men and women over age 65 generally are advised to have no more than three drinks on any day and seven per week. Depending on your health status, your doctor may advise you to drink less or not at all.

Pace and space: When you do drink, pace yourself. Sip slowly. Have no more than one standard drink with alcohol per hour. Have drink spacers—make every other drink a nonalcoholic one, such as water, soda, or juice.

Include food: Don't drink on an empty stomach. Have some food so the alcohol will be absorbed into your system more slowly.

Find alternatives: If drinking has occupied a lot of your time, then fill free time by developing new, healthy activities, hobbies, and relationships or renewing ones you've missed. If you have counted on alcohol to be more comfortable in social situations, manage moods, or cope with problems, then seek other, healthy ways to deal with those areas of your life.

Avoid triggers: What triggers your urge to drink? If certain people or places make you drink even when you don't want to, try to avoid them. If certain activities, times of day, or feelings trigger the urge, plan something else to do instead of drinking. If drinking at home is a problem, keep little or no alcohol there.

Plan to handle urges: When you cannot avoid a trigger and an urge hits, consider these options: Remind yourself of your reasons for changing (it can help to carry them in writing or store them in an electronic message you can access easily); or talk things through with someone you trust; or get involved with a healthy, distracting activity, such as physical exercise or a hobby that doesn't involve drinking; or, instead of fighting the feeling, accept it and ride it out without giving in, knowing that it will soon crest like a wave and pass.

Know your no: You're likely to be offered a drink at times when you don't want one. Have a polite, convincing "no, thanks" ready. The faster you can say no to these offers, the less likely you are to give in. If you hesitate, it allows you time to think of excuses to go along.

Support for Quitting

The suggestions in this section will be most useful for people who have become dependent on alcohol, and thus may find it difficult to quit without some help. Several proven treatment approaches are available. One size doesn't fit all, however. It's a good idea to do some homework on the Internet or at the library to find social and professional support options that appeal to you, as you are more likely to stick with them. Chances are excellent that you'll pull together an approach that works for you.

These strategies are especially helpful. But if you think you may be dependent on alcohol and decide to stop drinking completely, don't go it alone. Sudden withdrawal from heavy drinking can be life threatening. Seek medical help to plan a safe recovery.

Social Support

One potential challenge when people stop drinking is rebuilding a life without alcohol. It may be important to:

- educate family and friends,
- develop new interests and social groups,
- find rewarding ways to spend your time that don't involve alcohol, and
- ask for help from others.

When asking for support from friends or significant others, be specific. This could include:

- not offering you alcohol,
- not using alcohol around you,
- giving words of support and withholding criticism,
- not asking you to take on new demands right now, and
- going to a group like Al-Anon.

Consider joining Alcoholics Anonymous or another mutual support group. Recovering people who attend groups regularly do better than those who do not. Groups can vary widely, so shop around for one that's comfortable. You'll get more out of it if you become actively involved by having a sponsor and reaching out to other members for assistance.

Feeling depressed or anxious? It's common for people with alcohol problems to feel depressed or anxious. Mild symptoms may go away if you cut down or stop drinking. See a doctor or mental health professional if symptoms persist or get worse. If you're having suicidal thoughts, call your health care provider or go to the nearest emergency room right away. Effective treatment is available to help you through this difficult time.

Professional Support

Advances in the treatment of alcoholism mean that patients now have more choices and health professionals have more tools to help.

Medications to treat alcoholism: Newer medications can make it easier to quit drinking by offsetting changes in the brain caused by alcoholism. These options (naltrexone, topiramate, and acamprosate) don't make you sick if you drink, as does an older medication (disulfiram). None of these medications are addictive, so it's fine to combine them with support groups or alcohol counseling. A major clinical trial recently showed that patients can now receive effective alcohol treatment from their primary care doctors or mental health practitioners by combining the newer medications with a series of brief office visits for support.

Alcohol counseling: Talk therapy also works well. There are several counseling approaches that are about equally effective—12-step, cognitive-behavioral, motivational enhancement, or a combination. Getting help in itself appears to be more important than the particular approach used, as long as it offers empathy, avoids heavy confrontation, strengthens motivation, and provides concrete ways to change drinking behavior.

Specialized, intensive treatment programs: Some people will need more intensive programs. If you need a referral to a program, ask your doctor. Don't give up.

Ready to begin? If so, start by filling out a change plan (see a sample online at the Rethinking Drinking website, where you can print it out or email it to yourself). If you are cutting down as opposed to quitting, one tool you can use is a drinking tracker card or calendar where you mark down each drink before you have it.

Section 52.2

Technology That Helps Consumers Reduce Alcohol Use

This section includes excerpts from "Impact of Consumer Health Informatics Applications," Agency for Healthcare Research and Quality (AHRQ), October 2009.

Many people are excited about the potential to improve the health of the public by using health information technology (health IT) and e-Health solutions that are tailored to consumers. Despite growing interest in this field referred to as consumer health informatics (CHI), the value of CHI applications has not been rigorously reviewed. For the purposes of this review, CHI is defined as any electronic tool, technology, or electronic application that is designed to interact directly with consumers, with or without the presence of a health care professional that provides or uses individualized (personal) information and provides the consumer with individualized assistance, to help the patient better manage their health or health care.

Evidence of Impact of CHI Applications on Health Outcomes

Evaluated intermediate outcomes related to alcohol abuse included self-management, knowledge attainment, and change in health behaviors. All studies found significant positive effect on at least one intermediate outcome related to alcohol abuse. No study found any evidence of harm.

Alcohol Abuse and Smoking Cessation

Summary of the findings: Twenty-six studies evaluated the impact of CHI applications on a variety of intermediate health outcomes related to the use of alcohol and tobacco. Outcomes of interest include self-management, knowledge attainment (program adherence), and change in health behaviors. The quality of these 26 trials was good. All were randomized controlled trials (RCT) with sample sizes ranging from 83 to 288 respondents for the alcohol abuse studies and ranging from 139 to 3,971 respondents for the tobacco use studies. Post-intervention evaluation ranged from as little as 30 days to as long as 24 months. Upon review, the body of scientific evidence from these studies indicates that most CHI applications evaluated to date had statistically significant effects on intermediate health outcomes.

Outcomes of alcohol abuse reviews: Riper et al. investigated the effects of a web-based, multi-component, interactive, self-help intervention for problem drinkers without therapist guidance compared to a control intervention consisting of receiving access to an online psycho-educational alcohol use. Based on complete case analysis, the intervention group decreased their mean weekly alcohol consumption significantly more than the control group. In a subsequent secondary analysis of data from this study the authors demonstrated that at six and twelve month follow-up women and those with higher levels of education were more likely to have lower alcohol consumption levels, based on self report, as compared to controls.

Lieberman investigated program adherence to an online alcohol-use evaluation among study participants. After completing four standard questionnaires to evaluate problem drinking, an intervention consisting of a multimedia condition involving a personified guide was compared with a control treatment of feedback from the questionnaire results in text form. Increased levels of program adherence, as assessed by completion of greater numbers of modules of the online alcohol-use evaluation, were more strongly associated with the multimedia feedback via the personified guide.

Cunningham et al. investigated the effects of an internet-based personalized feedback intervention compared to the same intervention with the addition of a self-help book based on three outcomes: mean typical number of drinks per week, mean Alcohol Use Disorders Identification Test (AUDIT) scores, and mean number of alcohol consequences experienced. Study participants who received the additional self-help book reported decreased consumption of alcoholic drinks per week, a lower AUDIT score, and fewer alcohol-related consequences compared to participants who received the internet-based intervention alone

Hester et al. investigated the effect a computer-based brief motivational intervention, the Drinker's Checkup (DCU). The intervention was randomly assigned to participants in either an immediate treatment group or to a 4-week delayed treatment group and participants were followed over a 12-month period. Significant effects were reported for the immediate group when comparing baseline measurement to

471

measurement at 12 months for the outcomes of average drinks per day and average peak blood alcohol content (BAC). For the delayed group, significant effects were also reported when comparing baseline measurement to measurement at 12 months for the outcomes of average drinks per day and average peak BAC.

Kypri et al. investigated the effects 10–15 minutes of web-based assessment and personalized feedback for hazardous drinking as compared with a control treatment of an informational leaflet only. Six outcomes were measured at six weeks and six months: frequency of drinking; typical occasion quantity; total consumption; frequency of very episodic heavy drinking; personal, social, sexual, and legal consequences of episodic heavy drinking; and consequences related to academic performance. Significant effects of the intervention were seen on outcomes of total consumption at six weeks; frequency of very episodic heavy drinking at six weeks; and personal, social, sexual, and legal consequences of episodic heavy drinking at both six weeks and six months.

Neighbors et al. investigated the effects of a computer-delivered personalized normative feedback intervention in decreasing alcohol consumption among heavy-drinking college students. Outcomes assessed were effect size in perceived norms and the effect size in reduction in alcohol consumption. The effect size for the intervention effect on drinking was reported to be significant at three and six months. Significance of the effect size for the intervention effect on perceived norms was not reported.

Chapter 53

The Differences Between Brief Intervention and Treatment for Alcoholism

Chapter Contents

Section 53.1

Brief Interventions to Moderate Alcohol Consumption

Excerpted from "Brief Interventions," *Alcohol Alert: Number 66*, July 2005, National Institute on Alcohol Abuse and Alcoholism (NIAAA). Reviewed in May 2010, by Dr. David A. Cooke, MD, FACP, Diplomate, American Board of Internal Medicine.

Unlike traditional alcoholism treatment, which focuses on helping people who are dependent on alcohol, brief interventions—or short, one-on-one counseling sessions—are ideally suited for people who drink in ways that are harmful or abusive. Unlike traditional alcoholism treatment, which lasts many weeks or months, brief interventions can be given in a matter of minutes, and they require minimal follow-up.

The goals of brief interventions differ from formal alcoholism treatment. Brief interventions generally aim to moderate a person's alcohol consumption to sensible levels and to eliminate harmful drinking practices (such as binge drinking), rather than to insist on complete abstinence from drinking—although abstinence may be encouraged, if appropriate. (A binge is a pattern of drinking alcohol that brings blood alcohol concentration [BAC] to 0.08 gram percent or above. For a typical adult this pattern corresponds with consuming five or more drinks [male], or four or more drinks [female] in about two hours.)

Exactly what constitutes a brief intervention remains a source of debate. Brief interventions typically consist of one to four short counseling sessions with a trained interventionist (physician, psychologist, social worker). Studies have shown that people who received brief interventions when they were being treated for other conditions consistently showed greater reductions in alcohol use than comparable groups who did not receive an intervention. People seeking treatment specifically for alcohol abuse appeared to reduce their alcohol use about the same amount, whether they received brief interventions or extended treatments (five or more sessions). These findings show that brief interventions can be an effective way to reduce drinking, especially among people who do not have severe drinking problems requiring more intensive treatment.

The appropriate intervention depends on the patient—that is, on the severity of his or her problems with alcohol and whether he or she uses tobacco or other drugs, or has a co-occurring medical or psychiatric problem. The choice of intervention also is based on the clinical setting, the clinician's skills and interest, and time constraints. A brief intervention usually includes personalized feedback and counseling based on the patient's risk for harmful drinking. Often, simply providing this feedback is enough to encourage those at risk to reduce their alcohol intake

Brief interventions may include approaches—such as motivational interviewing—that are designed to persuade people who are resistant to moderating their alcohol intake or who do not believe they are drinking in a harmful or hazardous way. Motivational interviewing encourages patients to decide to change for themselves by using empathy and warmth rather than confrontation. Clinicians also can assist patients by helping them establish specific goals and build skills for modifying their drinking behavior.

Screening: People who would benefit from brief interventions may be identified through routine medical screenings, such as during a visit to a primary care physician. Standardized screening instruments exist that are specifically designed to identify alcohol use disorders.

Administering the intervention: Seeking treatment for problems with alcohol can be potentially embarrassing, stigmatizing, and inconvenient, taking time away from work or family responsibilities. Brief interventions give patients a simple way to receive care in a comfortable and familiar setting. Because they are brief, they can be easily incorporated into a variety of medical practices. Moreover, these approaches offer a lower cost alternative to more formal, specialist-led, alcoholism treatment.

Typically a nonspecialist authority figure who the patient may already trust or feel comfortable being treated by—such as a physician, a nurse, or physician's assistant in a primary care setting, or nurse or physician's assistant on a medical unit—delivers the brief intervention.

Supplemental handouts may be provided to patients during the intervention, including pamphlets, manuals, or workbooks to reinforce the strategies offered during the session. Clinicians also can follow up at a later date, either in person or through the mail, to provide additional assessment and further motivate the patient to achieve the goals set during the initial meeting. If the brief intervention does not motivate the patient to reduce alcohol consumption, clinicians can recommend more intensive treatment.

Many of the challenges involved in administering brief interventions—such as finding the time to administer them in busy doctors' offices, obtaining the extra training that helps staff become comfortable providing interventions, and managing the cost of using interventions—may be overcome through the use of technology. Patients may be encouraged to use computer programs in the doctor's waiting room or at home, or to access the intervention through the internet, which offers privacy and the ability to complete the program at any time of day.

Another potential tool for administering interventions is video doctor technology, in which an actor-doctor asks health questions in an interactive computer program.

Putting Research into Practice

Research shows that brief interventions can decrease alcohol consumption, and they work in a variety of populations—younger and older adults, men and women. Interventions that involve repeated contact generally are more effective than single-contact interventions. A review of studies reported that intervention participants reduced their alcohol consumption an average of 13%–34% compared with a control group. In addition, a recent analysis concluded that brief interventions may reduce mortality rates among problem drinkers by an estimated 23%–26%.

Primary care settings: Brief intervention in primary care can be simple and short—ranging from only a few questions (with appropriate responses)—or more extensive, including referral to a substance abuse specialist. Clinicians with limited time may want to use a basic intervention for all patients who use alcohol above the recommended limits; patients who do not respond to the basic intervention can be referred to an alcohol treatment specialist at the follow-up visit.

The most basic level of brief intervention consists of a simple statement or two. The clinician states that he or she is concerned about the patient's drinking, that it exceeds recommended limits and could lead to alcohol-related problems, and the clinician advises the patient to cut down or stop drinking.

Patients who have clear symptoms of alcohol abuse or dependence also may benefit from brief interventions in the primary care setting. Referral to a specialist for alcoholism treatment is a key component of this type of intervention. These interventions typically are more intense; the goal is abstinence from alcohol, not merely cutting down on drinking.

Despite evidence that brief interventions are useful in primary care settings, these short counseling sessions are not routine practice. One survey of primary care physicians found that although most (88%) reported asking their patients about alcohol use, only 13% used standard screening instruments. A survey of primary care patients revealed that more than 50% said their primary care physician did nothing about their substance abuse; 43% said their physician never diagnosed their condition.

The emergency department (ED): Up to 31% of all patients who are treated in an ED and as many as 50% of severely injured trauma patients (patients who require hospital admission, usually to an intensive care unit) test positive when screened for alcohol problems.

ED practitioners have reported that they considered performing a brief intervention for harmful and hazardous drinkers feasible and acceptable in their everyday practice. Other investigators have demonstrated that ED residents who receive training in screening and brief intervention in a skills-based workshop increase their knowledge and practice of these procedures. Fifty-eight percent of medical records of patients treated by trained residents contained evidence of screening and intervention, compared with 17% of records of patients treated by a control group of similar residents who did not receive training.

Many clinicians consider situations in which a patient receives acute medical care for an alcohol-related injury to be teachable moments—situations in which the patient may be particularly open to an alcohol intervention. Brief interventions delivered while patients are receiving trauma care may reduce those patients' alcohol consumption and risk of subsequent alcohol-related injuries.

Innovative methods for screening and intervention are being developed for use in the ED, including the use of computer-based approaches. These interventions are intended to help physicians use the patients' waiting time for health promotion and to target patients at risk for various health problems.

Prenatal care settings: Approximately 14%–22.5% of women report drinking some alcohol during pregnancy, and an estimated 1% of all newborns experience some prenatal alcohol-related damage. Routine screening in obstetrical offices may prove to be vital in preventing drinking during pregnancy—the leading cause of preventable birth defects.

Brief interventions have been recommended as the first step in approaching people with mild-to-moderate alcohol problems. Because pregnant women generally are motivated to change their behaviors and only infrequently have severe alcohol problems, they may be especially receptive to brief interventions. In addition, studies show that the people who change their drinking behavior do so within six months of receiving the brief intervention. Because most pregnant women seek prenatal care during their first trimester, this is an opportune time to help them to make the changes necessary for a healthy pregnancy.

Research also shows that these interventions are effective. In a recent study, 304 pregnant women were assigned to receive an intervention or to be in a control group. Some of these women tested positive for prenatal alcohol use, whereas others were selected randomly to participate in the study. A unique twist to this investigation was that women received the intervention along with their partners (usually their husbands or the fathers of their unborn children). Results indicated that the women with the highest levels of drinking had the greatest reductions in drinking when they received the brief intervention. The effects of the brief intervention were much greater when a partner participated.

An innovative approach in the prenatal setting, the Protecting the Next Pregnancy Project involves intervening with women who have been identified as drinking during their last pregnancy. The goal of this approach is to reduce alcohol use during the women's future pregnancies. Following the intervention, these women not only drank significantly less than those in a control group during their later pregnancies, they also had fewer low-birthweight babies and fewer premature deliveries. Moreover, children born to women in the brief intervention group had better neurobehavioral performance at 13 months when compared with control group children.

The criminal justice system: Alcohol use is closely linked to crime. Few studies have evaluated the impact of brief interventions in criminal justice populations. Davis and colleagues examined whether brief motivational feedback helped to increase offenders' participation in treatment after they completed their jail sentences. They found that offenders receiving feedback were more likely to schedule and keep appointments for follow-up treatment than were offenders in a control group. However, a study of driving while intoxicated (DWI) offenders found that brief individual interventions reduced recidivism only among offenders who showed evidence of depression, but not among offenders who were not depressed. This study suggests that brief interventions may be particularly useful in certain subgroups of DWI offenders.

College settings: Strong evidence has been found to support the use of brief motivational interventions. These interventions are especially useful in college settings because they often focus on moderating a person's alcohol consumption to sensible levels and eliminating harmful drinking practices (such as binge drinking). Brief interventions may be used in campus health centers, counseling centers, or local hospital emergency rooms. Incorporating these interventions into campus judicial systems has several advantages: Many campuses already have policies in place that require students cited for alcohol policy violations to complete an assessment and intervention, and trained staff usually is available to respond to policy violators.

Peer counseling has a long history on college campuses and generally has been found to be effective for solving both academic and health problems. Although few studies have looked at the effectiveness of brief interventions for alcohol problems, research indicates that trained peer counselors (college undergraduates) are as effective as professionals in encouraging drinking changes among college students. A disadvantage is that peer providers require considerable training and supervision; most research protocols recommend weekly individual or group supervision by a trained therapist.

Studies have found that students who most need alcohol-related interventions may be least likely to participate in these sessions. So motivating students to receive brief interventions, especially interventions delivered outside the health center and mandated contexts is key to reducing alcohol consumption on campus. Calling students when they miss appointments and using other program reminders may increase participation by heavier drinkers. Support also is emerging for the use of mailed or computerized feedback in place of personalized, individual feedback. Such approaches have been successful in producing at least short-term reductions in students' alcohol consumption. Another approach to implementing brief interventions is to use different levels or steps of care, perhaps starting with assessing and providing feedback through the Internet, then moving to in-person interventions for those students who have more severe alcohol-related problems or those who do not respond to the initial intervention.

Conclusion: Brief interventions can be useful in a variety of settings and are potentially cost-effective in reducing hazardous or harmful alcohol consumption. Medical settings such as emergency departments or trauma centers also may provide opportunities, or teachable moments, when people may be open to making changes in their alcohol consumption. New technology, such as computerized interventions, may offer an effective means for implementing brief interventions, especially in settings in which time constraints or lack of resources or training in intervention techniques are issues.

Section 53.2

Examples of Early and Brief Interventions

Excerpted from *Examples of Early and Brief Interventions* (Washington, DC: U.S. Department of Education, Office of Safe and Drug-Free Schools, Higher Education Center for Alcohol and Other Drug Abuse and Violence Prevention, 2008). For more information, please contact the Center at 800-676-1730 or visit the Center's website at www.highered center.org.

This list of early and brief interventions is not meant to be exhaustive but rather to provide a few examples of the application of effective strategies.

The Alcohol Skills Training Program (ASTP) was developed by the Addictive Behaviors Research Center at the University of Washington. The three key underlying elements of the ASTP approach are the application of cognitive-behavioral self-management strategies, the use of motivational enhancement techniques, and the use of harm reduction principles. The primarily cognitive behavioral alcohol prevention program provides information about alcohol use and addiction, and teaches skills for avoiding, resisting, and setting limits on alcohol use. The program consists of eight ninety-minute sessions with facilitated group discussions. Research indicates that the program effectively decreases participants' peak blood alcohol level, and the amount of alcohol consumed per week, per month, and in heavy drinking situations.

BASICS (Brief Alcohol Screening and Intervention for College Students) is another program, derived from ASTP, that uses a combination of strategies to reduce individual drinking. The program consists of two short individualized sessions with a counselor. The first session is used to assess the student's drinking patterns, attitudes, and expectancies of alcohol. Then during the second session the student is provided with non-confrontational, non-judgmental feedback regarding his/her habits. Studies indicate that students receiving BASICS report less drinking and fewer negative consequences of drinking than those that do not receive BASICS. In addition, research indicates that these decreases in consumption are still significant months and years after BASICS participation.

CHUG (Check-Up to Go) is a brief assessment that assesses drinking behavior. Encouraging findings suggest that mailed personalized feedback based on the CHUG assessment may reduce heavy drinking among college students. CHUG is available in a paper-pencil format and an electronic assessment-plus-feedback version called e-CHUG. Using normative feedback and motivational interviewing approaches, feedback is delivered online and is designed to motivate students to reduce their consumption using personalized information about their own drinking and risk factors.

MyStudentBody (http://www.mystudentbody.com) provides information about alcohol and other drugs and the consequences of substance abuse. One component is a risk assessment which is based on BASICS. Research indicates MyStudentBody participants report significant decreases in rate and frequency of drinking and fewer negative consequences in follow-up.

Additional Applications of the Research

AlcoholEdu (http://www.outsidetheclassroom.com) is an interactive assessment and personalized feedback tool for college students. Evaluations have shown AlcoholEdu to reduce consumption levels and negative behaviors associated with alcohol use.

CHOICES (http://www.thechangecompanies.com) is a brief alcohol prevention and harm reduction program that uses interactive journaling to provide students with non-judgmental normative, psychological, and biological education about alcohol consumption. In addition, the intervention provides strategies for harm reduction. The program is administered to a group in one or two sessions lasting a total of three hours or less.

Section 53.3

Brief Intervention Helps Emergency Patients Reduce Drinking

Text in this section is from "Brief Intervention Helps Emergency Patients Reduce Drinking," National Institute on Alcohol Abuse and Alcoholism (NIAAA), December 26, 2007.

Asking emergency department patients about their alcohol use and talking with them about how to reduce harmful drinking patterns is an effective way to lower rates of risky drinking in these patients, according to a nationwide collaborative study supported by the National Institute on Alcohol Abuse and Alcoholism (NIAAA) and the Substance Abuse and Mental Health Services Administration (SAMHSA). Emergency department patients who underwent a regimen of alcohol screening and brief intervention reported lower rates of risky drinking at three-month follow-up than did those who received only written information about reducing their drinking.

"This encouraging finding raises the prospect of reaching many individuals whose alcohol misuse might otherwise go untreated," says NIAAA Director Ting-Kai Li, MD. Previous studies of screening, brief intervention, and referral conducted in primary care and in-patient trauma centers have shown positive outcomes in decreasing or eliminating alcohol use, reducing injury rates, and reducing costs to society.

In the current study, investigators at 14 university-based emergency centers throughout the United States used a brief questionnaire to assess the alcohol use patterns of 7,751 emergency patients, regardless of whether they had signs of alcohol use on admission. They found that more than one-fourth of the patients exceeded the limits for low-risk drinking—defined by NIAAA as no more than: four drinks per day for men and three drinks per day for women; and not more than 14 drinks per week for men, and seven drinks per week for women. More than 1,100 patients who exceeded these limits agreed to continue to participate in the study and were divided into intervention and control groups. The study enrolled patients with all levels of risky drinking and visit type.

The primary intervention consisted of a brief negotiated interview (BNI) that emergency practitioners performed with each member of the intervention group. Patients in the intervention group also received a written handout explaining low-risk drinking and a referral list of alcohol treatment providers. Patients in the control group received only the low-risk drinking handout and referral list.

"The BNI, a conversation between emergency care providers and patients that involves listening rather than telling, and guiding rather than directing, is designed to review the patient's current drinking patterns, assess their readiness to change, offer advice about the low-risk guidelines and the next steps to pursue, and negotiate a written prescription for change or a drinking agreement with the patient," explains co-author Edward Bernstein, MD, professor and vice chair for academic affairs in the department of emergency medicine at Boston University School of Medicine. Dr. Bernstein, who coordinated the training of emergency department personnel in the study, notes that the interview typically takes less than ten minutes to complete.

Researchers contacted members of each group three months later to assess any changes in drinking habits. The intervention group reported drinking three fewer drinks per week than the controls, and more than one-third of individuals in the intervention group reported drinking at low-risk levels, compared with about one-fifth of those in the control group.

"This study demonstrates that a broad group of emergency practitioners can learn how to perform the intervention and that it is effective across multiple practice sites," says co-author Gail D'Onofrio, MD, professor and chief of emergency medicine at Yale University. "The emergency department visit is often the only access to care for many patients and thus is an ideal opportunity to begin the conversation regarding unhealthy alcohol use."

The researchers conclude that widespread use of these techniques by emergency personnel could significantly reduce unhealthy alcohol use. "Our results should provide the impetus for broader implementation of screening, brief intervention, and referral for treatment in the emergency department setting," notes co-author Robert Aseltine, PhD, associate professor in the division of behavioral science and community health and director of the Institute for Public Health Research at the University of Connecticut Health Center.

Chapter 54

Alcohol Treatment: Need, Utilization, and Barriers

Alcohol abuse affects the physical, mental, and fiscal health of millions of people every year. A number of programs can effectively treat alcohol dependence or abuse; however, many people who need treatment may not use these services or even recognize the need for them. Increasing the public's awareness of the signs of alcohol problems, expanding screening for alcohol problems in primary care and in emergency departments, and ensuring that individuals are matched to appropriate intervention and/or treatment services may help to save or improve the lives of alcohol abusers, their families, and other citizens in our communities.

The National Survey on Drug Use and Health (NSDUH) gathers information that can help to provide a better understanding of alcohol treatment needs, service utilization, and barriers. NSDUH classifies persons as needing treatment for an alcohol problem if they met the criteria for alcohol dependence or abuse or if they received specialty alcohol use treatment in the past year. Respondents were asked if there was any time in the past year when they felt they needed treatment for their alcohol use but did not receive it. Persons who felt the need for treatment but did not receive it were asked about their reasons for not receiving treatment.

Excerpted from "Alcohol Treatment: Need, Utilization, and Barriers," Substance Abuse and Mental Health Services Administration (SAMHSA), April 9, 2009. The complete document with references is available at http://www.oas.samhsa.gov/2k9/AlcTX/AlcTX.htm.

Need for alcohol treatment: In 2007, 7.8% of persons aged 12 or older (an estimated 19.3 million persons) needed treatment for an alcohol problem in the past year. The rate of treatment need for an alcohol problem was twice as high for males as for females (10.9 versus 4.8%), and the rate of treatment need for young adults aged 18 to 25 was 2–3 times higher than that of other age groups (17.2% for persons aged 18–25 versus 5.5% for those aged 12–17 and 6.5% for those aged 26 or older).

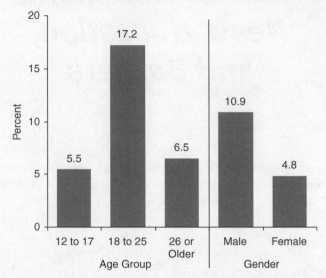

Figure 54.1. *Needed Treatment for an Alcohol Problem in the Past Year among Persons Aged 12 or Older, by Demographic Characteristics: 2007 (Source: 2007 SAMHSA National Survey on Drug Use and Health [NSDUH]).*

Service utilization: Of the 19.3 million persons who needed alcohol treatment in the past year, 8.1% (1.6 million) received treatment at a specialty facility in the past year (Figure 54.2). Among persons who needed treatment for alcohol use, adults aged 26 or older were more likely than adolescents and young adults to have received treatment at a specialty facility (9.7% versus 5.9% and 5.1%, respectively). There was little difference by gender.

Nearly nine-tenths (87.4%) of individuals who needed treatment neither received it nor perceived the need for it (Figure 54.2). Only 4.5% perceived a need for treatment but did not receive it (had a perceived unmet need). About one-quarter (27.9%) of the 859,000 persons who had a perceived unmet need for alcohol treatment made an effort to get it in the past year.

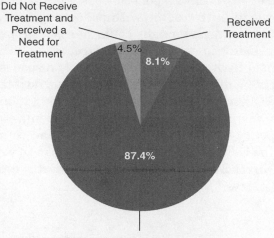

Did Not Receive
Treatment and
Perceived a
Need for
Treatment

Received
Treatment

4.5%

8.1%

87.4%

Did Not Receive Treatment and
Did Not Perceive a Need for Treatment

Figure 54.2. Receipt* of and Perceived Need for Alcohol Treatment in the
Past Year among Persons Aged 12 or Older Who Needed Treatment: 2007
(Source: 2007 SAMHSA National Survey on Drug Use and Health [NSDUH]).

Barriers to receiving alcohol treatment: Individuals who needed but did not receive alcohol treatment at a specialty facility and who
felt a need for alcohol treatment were asked to indicate the reasons for
not receiving it. Averages for 2004 to 2007 show that the most common
reasons given for not receiving treatment were not being ready to stop
using alcohol (42.0%) and cost or insurance barriers (34.5%) (Figure
54.3). Other reasons included social stigma associated with receiving
treatment (18.8%), access issues (11.7%), not feeling the need for treatment or thinking they could handle the problem without treatment
(11.6%), and not knowing where to go for treatment (11.1%).

Figure Notes

* Refers to receipt of treatment in a specialty facility.

** Respondents could indicate multiple reasons; thus, these response
categories are not mutually exclusive. "Cost/insurance barriers" include
"no health coverage and could not afford cost," "had health coverage but
it did not cover treatment or did not cover cost," and other-specify responses of "could not afford cost; health coverage not indicated." "Social
stigma" include "might cause neighbors/community to have negative
opinion," "might have negative effect on job," "did not want others to

find out," and other-specify responses of "ashamed/embarrassed/afraid" and "afraid would have trouble with police/social services." "Did not think needed treatment/thought could handle the problem without treatment" include "did not feel need for treatment," "could handle the problem without treatment," and other-specify responses of "could do it with support of family/friends/others" and "could do it through religion/spirituality." "Other barriers" include "no transportation/inconvenient," "no program having type of treatment," "no openings in a program," and other-specify responses of "no program had counselors/doctors with whom you were comfortable," "services desired were unavailable or you were currently ineligible," and "attempted to get treatment but encountered delays."

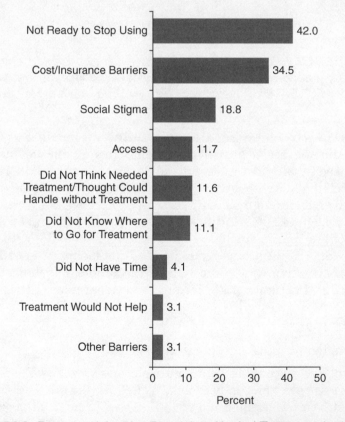

Figure 54.3. Reasons** for Not Receiving Alcohol Treatment in the Past Year among Persons Aged 12 or Older Who Needed Treatment and Who Perceived a Need for It: 2004 to 2007 (Source: 2007 SAMHSA National Survey on Drug Use and Health [NSDUH]).

Chapter 55

Detoxification: One Part of Substance Abuse Treatment

Detoxification is a set of interventions aimed at managing acute intoxication and withdrawal. It denotes a clearing of toxins from the body of the patient who is acutely intoxicated and/or dependent on substances of abuse. Detoxification seeks to minimize the physical harm caused by the abuse of substances. Detoxification alone is not sufficient in the treatment and rehabilitation of substance use disorders.

Evaluation entails testing for the presence of substances of abuse in the bloodstream, measuring their concentration, and screening for co-occurring mental and physical conditions. Evaluation also includes a comprehensive assessment of the patient's medical, psychological, and social situation.

Stabilization includes the medical and psychosocial process of assisting the patient through acute intoxication and withdrawal to the attainment of a medically stable, fully supported, substance-free state.

Fostering the patient's entry into treatment involves preparing a patient for entry into treatment by stressing the importance of following through with a complete continuum of care.

This chapter includes text excerpted from "Quick Guide for Clinicians: Detoxification and Substance Abuse Treatment (Based on TIP 45)," Substance Abuse and Mental Health Services Administration (SAMHSA), 2006.

Guiding Principles Recognized by the Treatment Improvement Protocol (TIP) 45 Consensus Panel

1. Detoxification alone is not sufficient treatment for substance dependence but it is one part of a continuum of care for substance-related disorders.

2. The detoxification process consists of evaluation, stabilization, and fostering patient readiness for and entry into treatment. A detoxification process that does not incorporate all three critical components is considered incomplete and inadequate by the consensus panel.

3. Detoxification can take place in a wide variety of settings and at a number of levels of intensity within these settings. Placement should be appropriate to the patient's needs.

4. Persons seeking detoxification should have access to the components of the detoxification process described, no matter what the setting or the level of treatment intensity.

5. All persons requiring treatment for substance use disorders should receive treatment of the same quality and appropriate thoroughness and should be put into contact with a substance abuse treatment program after detoxification.

6. Ultimately, insurance coverage for the full range of detoxification services is cost-effective. If reimbursement systems do not provide payment for the complete detoxification process, patients may be released prematurely, leading to medically or socially unattended withdrawal.

7. Patients seeking detoxification services have diverse cultural and ethnic backgrounds as well as unique health needs and life situations. Organizations that provide detoxification services need to ensure that they have standard practices in place to address cultural diversity.

8. A successful detoxification process can be measured, in part, by whether an individual who is substance dependent enters, remains in, and is compliant with the treatment protocol of a substance abuse treatment/rehabilitation program after detoxification.

Overarching principles for care during detoxification services:

- Detoxification services do not offer a cure for substance use disorders; they are often a first step toward recovery and a first door through which patients pass to treatment.

- Substance use disorders are treatable and there is hope for recovery.

- Substance use disorders are brain disorders and not evidence of moral weakness.

- Patients should be treated with respect and dignity at all times.

- Patients should be treated in a nonjudgmental and supportive manner.

- Services planning should be completed in partnership with the patient and his or her social support network, including family, significant others, or employers.

- All health professionals involved in the care of the patient will maximize opportunities to promote rehabilitation and maintenance activities and to link the patient to appropriate substance abuse treatment immediately after the detoxification phase.

- Active involvement of the family and other support systems, while respecting the patient's right to privacy and confidentiality, are to be encouraged.

- Patients should be treated with due consideration for individual background, culture, preferences, sexual orientation, disability, vulnerabilities, and strengths.

Levels of Care and Patient Placement

In addition to the general placement criteria for treatment for substance-related disorders, American Society of Addiction Medicine (ASAM) also has developed a second set of placement criteria—the five adult detoxification placement levels of care within Dimension 1 (ASAM 2001).

1. **Level I-D:** Ambulatory detoxification without extended onsite monitoring (physician's office, home health care agency). This level of care is an organized outpatient service monitored at predetermined intervals.

2. **Level II-D:** Ambulatory detoxification with extended onsite monitoring (day hospital service). This level of care is monitored by appropriately credentialed and licensed nurses.

3. **Level III.2-D:** Clinically managed residential detoxification (nonmedical or social detoxification setting). This level emphasizes peer and social support and is intended for patients whose intoxication and/or withdrawal is sufficient to warrant 24-hour support.

4. **Level III.7-D:** Medically monitored inpatient detoxification (freestanding detoxification center). Unlike Level III.2.D, this level provides 24-hour medically supervised detoxification services.

5. **Level IV-D:** Medically managed intensive inpatient detoxification (psychiatric hospital inpatient center). This level provides 24-hour care in an acute care inpatient setting.

It is important to note that ASAM PPC-2R criteria are only guidelines, and that there are no uniform protocols for determining which patients are placed in which level of care.

Biomedical and Psychosocial Issues

Detoxification presents an opportunity to intervene during a period of crisis and to encourage a client to make changes in the direction of health and recovery. Hence, a primary goal of the detoxification staff should be to build a therapeutic alliance and motivate patients to enter treatment. This process should begin as the patient is being medically stabilized.

Symptoms and signs of conditions that require immediate medical attention:

- Change in mental status

- Increasing anxiety

- Hallucinations

- Temperature greater than 100.4°F (these patients should be considered potentially infectious)

- Significant increases and/or decreases in blood pressure and heart rate

- Insomnia

- Abdominal pain

- Upper and lower gastrointestinal bleeding

- Changes in responsiveness of pupils

- Heightened deep tendon reflexes and ankle clonus, a reflex beating of the foot when pressed rostrally, indicating profound central nervous system irritability and the potential for seizures

Immediate mental health needs include suicidality or anger and aggression.

Strategies for Engagement and Recovery

It is essential that all clinicians offer hope and the expectation of recovery. Throughout detoxification, staff should be unified in their message that detoxification is only the beginning of the treatment process and that rehabilitation and maintenance activities are critical to sustained recovery.

Educate the patient on the withdrawal process:

- During intoxication and withdrawal, it is useful to provide information on the typical withdrawal process based on the particular drug of abuse.

- Providing information concerning withdrawal symptoms may reduce discomfort and the likelihood the individual will leave detoxification prematurely.

- Settings that routinely encounter individuals in withdrawal should have written materials available on drug effects and withdrawal from specific drugs. This material should also be available for non-English speaking patients.

- Interventions that assist the client in identifying and managing urges to use also may be helpful in retaining the client in detoxification and ensuring the initiation of rehabilitation.

Use support systems:

- The use of client advocates to intervene with clients wishing to leave early is often an effective strategy for promoting retention.

- Visitors should be instructed about the importance of supporting the individual in both detoxification and substance abuse treatment.

- If available and if the patient is stable, he or she can attend onsite 12-step or other support group meetings while receiving detoxification services.

Maintain a drug-free environment:

- Maintaining a safe and drug-free environment is essential to retaining clients in detoxification.

- Providers should be alert to drug-seeking behaviors.

- Visiting areas should be easy for staff to monitor.

- Explain to patients and visitors why substances are not allowed in the facility.

Foster a therapeutic alliance:

- A relationship between the clinician and patient that is supportive, empathic, and nonjudgmental is the hallmark of a strong therapeutic alliance.

- Efforts to establish a therapeutic alliance should begin upon admission.

Detoxification programs should focus their evaluation on areas that are essential to make an appropriate linkage to substance abuse treatment. The following are recommended:

- Medical conditions and complications
- Motivation/readiness to change
- Physical, sensory, or mobility limitations
- Relapse history and potential
- Substance abuse/dependence
- Development and cognitive issues
- Family and social support
- Co-occurring psychiatric disorders
- Dependent children
- Trauma and violence
- Treatment history
- Cultural background
- Strengths and resources
- Language

Providing Linkages to Treatment and Maintenance Activities

Research indicates that patients are more likely to initiate and remain in treatment if they believe the services will help them with specific life problems. The following are strategies that detoxification personnel can use with their patients to promote the initiation of treatment:

- Perform an assessment of urgency for treatment.

- Reduce time between initial call and appointment.

- Call to reschedule missed appointments.

- Provide information about what to expect at the first session.

- Provide information about confidentiality.

- Offer tangible incentives such as the prospect of improved relations with family and friends and improved self-image.

- Engage the support of family members.

- Introduce the client to the counselor who will deliver rehabilitation services.

- Offer services that address basic needs, such as housing, employment, and child care.

Chapter 56

Withdrawal from Alcohol

Chapter Contents

497

Section 56.1

Acute and Post-Acute Withdrawal

Information in this section is reprinted with permission from "Withdrawal" and "Post-Acute Withdrawal" by Dr. Steven M. Melemis, © 2009. For additional information, visit www.AddictionsAndRecovery.org.

Withdrawal

Withdrawal occurs because your brain works like a spring when it comes to addiction. Drugs and alcohol are brain depressants that push down the spring. They suppress your brain's production of neurotransmitters like noradrenaline. When you stop using drugs or alcohol it is like taking the weight off the spring, and your brain rebounds by producing a surge of adrenaline that causes withdrawal symptoms.

Every drug is different: Some drugs produce significant physical withdrawal (alcohol, opiates, and tranquilizers). Some drugs produce little physical withdrawal, but more emotional withdrawal (cocaine, marijuana, and ecstasy). Every person's physical withdrawal pattern is also different. You may experience little physical withdrawal. That does not mean that you are not addicted. You may experience more emotional withdrawal.

Following are two lists of withdrawal symptoms. The first list is the emotional withdrawal symptoms produced by all drugs. You can experience them whether you have physical withdrawal symptoms or not. The second list is the physical withdrawal symptoms that usually occur with alcohol, opiates, and tranquilizers.

Emotional Withdrawal Symptoms

- Anxiety
- Restlessness
- Irritability
- Insomnia
- Headaches
- Poor concentration
- Depression
- Social isolation

Physical Withdrawal Symptoms

- Sweating
- Racing heart
- Palpitations
- Muscle tension
- Tightness in the chest
- Difficulty breathing
- Tremor
- Nausea, vomiting, or diarrhea

Dangerous Withdrawal Symptoms

Alcohol and tranquilizers produce the most dangerous physical withdrawal: Suddenly stopping alcohol or tranquilizers can lead to seizures, strokes, or heart attacks in high risk patients. A medically supervised detox can minimize your withdrawal symptoms and reduce the risk of dangerous complications. Some of the dangerous symptoms of alcohol and tranquilizer withdrawal are:

- grand mal seizures,
- heart attacks,
- strokes,
- hallucinations, and
- delirium tremens (DTs).

Withdrawal from opiates like heroin and OxyContin® is extremely uncomfortable, but not dangerous unless they are mixed with other drugs. Heroin withdrawal on its own does not produce seizures, heart attacks, strokes, or delirium tremens. (Reference: www.AddictionsAnd Recovery.org)

Post-Acute Withdrawal (PAWS)

There are two stages of withdrawal. The first stage is the acute stage, which usually lasts at most a few weeks. During this stage, you may experience physical withdrawal symptoms. But every drug is different, and every person is different.

The second stage of withdrawal is called the post-acute withdrawal syndrome (PAWS). During this stage you will have fewer physical symptoms, but more emotional and psychological withdrawal symptoms.

Post-acute withdrawal occurs because your brain chemistry is gradually returning to normal. As your brain improves, the levels of your brain chemicals fluctuate as they approach the new equilibrium causing post-acute withdrawal symptoms.

Most people experience some post-acute withdrawal symptoms: Whereas in the acute stage of withdrawal every person is different, in post-acute withdrawal most people have the same symptoms.

The Symptoms of Post-Acute Withdrawal

The most common post-acute withdrawal symptoms are:

- mood swings,
- anxiety,
- irritability,
- tiredness,
- variable energy,
- low enthusiasm,
- variable concentration, and
- disturbed sleep.

Post-acute withdrawal feels like a roller coaster of symptoms: In the beginning, your symptoms will change minute to minute and hour to hour. Later, as you recover further, they will disappear for a few weeks or months only to return again. As you continue to recover, the good stretches will get longer and longer. But, the bad periods of post-acute withdrawal can be just as intense and last just as long.

Each post-acute withdrawal episode usually lasts for a few days: Once you have been in recovery for a while, you will find that each post-acute withdrawal episode usually lasts for a few days. There is no obvious trigger for most episodes. You will wake up one day feeling irritable and have low energy. If you hang on for just a few days, it will lift just as quickly as it started. After a while, you will develop confidence that you can get through post-acute withdrawal because you will know that each episode is time limited.

Post-acute withdrawal usually lasts for two years: This is one of the most important things you need to remember. If you are up for the challenge, you can get through this. But if you think that post-acute withdrawal will only last for a few months, then you will get caught off guard, and when you are disappointed you are more likely to relapse. (Reference: www.AddictionsAndRecovery.org)

How to Survive Post-Acute Withdrawal

Be patient: Two years can feel like a long time if you are in a rush to get through it. You cannot hurry recovery. But you can get through it one day at a time.

If you try to rush your recovery, or resent post-acute withdrawal, or try to bulldoze your way through, you will become exhausted. And when you are exhausted you will think of using to escape.

Post-acute withdrawal symptoms are a sign that your brain is recovering. They are the result of your brain chemistry gradually going back to normal. Therefore, don't resent them. But remember, even after one year, you are still only half way there.

Go with the flow: Withdrawal symptoms are uncomfortable. But the more you resent them the worse they will seem. You will have lots of good days over the next two years. Enjoy them. You will also have lots of bad days. On those days, don't try to do too much. Take care of yourself, focus on your recovery, and you will get through this.

Practice self-care: Give yourself lots of little breaks over the next two years. Tell yourself "what I am doing is enough." Be good to yourself. That is what most addicts cannot do, and that is what you must learn in recovery. Recovery is the opposite of addiction.

Sometimes you will have little energy or enthusiasm for anything. Understand this and don't overbook your life. Give yourself permission to focus on your recovery.

Post-acute withdrawal can be a trigger for relapse: You will go for weeks without any withdrawal symptoms, and then one day you will wake up and your withdrawal will hit you like a ton of bricks. You will have slept badly. You will be in a bad mood. Your energy will be low. And if you are not prepared for it, if you think that post-acute withdrawal only lasts for a few months, or if you think that you will be different and it will not be as bad for you, then you will get caught off guard. But if you know what to expect you can do this.

Being able to relax will help you through post-acute with-drawal: When you are tense, you tend to dwell on your symptoms and make them worse. When you are relaxed, it is easier to not get caught up in them. You are not as triggered by your symptoms which means you are less likely to relapse.

Remember: Every relapse, no matter how small, undoes the gains your brain has made during recovery. Without abstinence, everything will fall apart. With abstinence, everything is possible. (Reference: www.AddictionsAndRecovery.org)

Section 56.2

Delirium Tremens

"Delirium Tremens," © 2010 A.D.A.M., Inc. Reprinted with permission.

Delirium tremens is a severe form of alcohol withdrawal that involves sudden and severe mental or neurological changes.

Causes: Delirium tremens can occur after a period of heavy alcohol drinking, especially when the person does not eat enough food. It may also be triggered by head injury, infection, or illness in people with a history of heavy alcohol use. It is most common in people who have a history of alcohol withdrawal. It is especially common in those who drink the equivalent of 4–5 pints of wine or 7–8 pints of beer (or one pint of hard alcohol) every day for several months. Delirium tremens also commonly affects those who have had a history of habitual alcohol use or alcoholism for more than ten years.

Symptoms: These most commonly occur within 72 hours after the last drink, but may occur up to 7–10 days after the last drink. Symptoms may get worse rapidly, and can include the following:

- Body tremors
- Mental status changes such as:
  - agitation, irritability;
  - confusion, disorientation;

- decreased attention span;
- decreased mental status (such as deep sleep that persists for a day or longer; stupor, sleepiness, lethargy that usually occurs after acute symptoms);
- delirium (severe, acute loss of mental functions);
- excitement;
- fear;
- hallucinations (such as seeing or feeling things that are not present are most common);
- high sensitivity to light, sound, touch;
- increased activity;
- rapid mood changes;
- restlessness, excitement.

Seizures are:

- most common in first 24–48 hours after last drink;
- most common in people with previous complications from alcohol withdrawal;
- usually generalized tonic-clonic seizures.

Symptoms of alcohol withdrawal include the following:

- Anxiety
- Depression
- Difficulty thinking clearly
- Fatigue
- Feeling jumpy or nervous
- Feeling shaky
- Headache, general, pulsating
- Insomnia (difficulty falling and staying asleep)
- Irritability or easily excited
- Loss of appetite
- Nausea

- Pale skin
- Palpitations (sensation of feeling the heart beat)
- Rapid emotional changes
- Sweating, especially the palms of the hands or the face
- Vomiting

Additional symptoms that may occur include chest pain, fever, and stomach pain.

Exams and tests: Delirium tremens is a medical emergency. The health care provider will perform a physical exam. Signs may include:

- heavy sweating,
- increased startle reflex,
- irregular heartbeat,
- problems with eye muscle movement,
- rapid heart rate,
- rapid muscle tremors.

The following tests may be done:

- Chem-20
- electrocardiogram (ECG)
- electroencephalogram (EEG)
- toxicology screen

Treatment: The goals of treatment are to:

- save the person's life,
- relieve symptoms,
- prevent complications.

A hospital stay is required. The health care team will regularly check:

- blood chemistry results, such as electrolyte levels;
- body fluid levels;
- vital signs (temperature, pulse, rate of breathing, blood pressure).

Symptoms such as seizures and heart arrhythmias are treated with the following medications:

- Anticonvulsants such as phenytoin or phenobarbital
- Central nervous system depressants such as diazepam
- Clonidine to reduce cardiovascular symptoms and reduce anxiety
- Sedatives

The patient may need to be put into a sedated state for a week or more until withdrawal is complete. Benzodiazepine medications such as diazepam or lorazepam are often used. These drugs also help treat seizures, anxiety, and tremors.

Antipsychotic medications such as haloperidol may sometimes be necessary for persons with hallucinations.

Long-term preventive treatment should begin after the patient recovers from acute symptoms. This may involve a drying out period, in which no alcohol is allowed. Total and lifelong abstinence is recommended for most people who go through withdrawal. The person should receive treatment for alcohol use or alcoholism, including counseling and support groups such as Alcoholics Anonymous.

The patient should be tested, and if necessary, treated for other medical problems associated with alcohol use. Such problems may include:

- alcoholic cardiomyopathy,
- alcoholic liver disease,
- alcoholic neuropathy,
- blood clotting disorders,
- Wernicke-Korsakoff syndrome.

Outlook (prognosis): Delirium tremens is serious and may be life threatening. Symptoms such as sleeplessness, feeling tired, and emotional instability may persist for a year or more.

Possible complications:

- Heart arrhythmias, may be life threatening
- Injury from falls during seizures
- Injury to self or others caused by mental state (confusion/delirium)
- Seizures

When to contact a medical professional: Go to the emergency room or call the local emergency number (such as 911) if you have symptoms. Delirium tremens is an emergency condition.

Prevention: Avoid or reduce the use of alcohol. Get prompt medical treatment for symptoms of alcohol withdrawal.

Reference: O'Connor PG. Alcohol abuse and dependence. In: Goldman L, Ausiello D, eds. *Cecil Medicine. 23rd ed*. Philadelphia, Pa: Saunders Elsevier; 2007:chap 31.

Section 56.3

Repeated Alcohol Withdrawal: Sensitization and Implications for Relapse

Text in this section is excerpted from "Alcohol Dependence, Withdrawal, and Relapse," by Howard C. Becker, PhD, National Institute on Alcohol Abuse and Alcoholism (NIAAA), 2008.

Given that alcoholism is a chronic relapsing disease, many alcohol dependent people invariably experience multiple bouts of heavy drinking interspersed with periods of abstinence (withdrawal) of varying duration. A convergent body of preclinical and clinical evidence has demonstrated that a history of multiple detoxification/withdrawal experiences can result in increased sensitivity to the withdrawal syndrome—a process known as kindling. For example, clinical studies have indicated that a history of multiple detoxifications increases a person's susceptibility to more severe and medically complicated withdrawals in the future.

Effects of Repeated Withdrawals on Emotional State and Stress Response

Most studies demonstrating this sensitization or kindling of alcohol withdrawal primarily have focused on withdrawal-related excessive activity (hyperexcitability) of the central nervous system (CNS), as indicated by seizure activity, because this parameter is relatively easy to observe in experimental as well as clinical settings. More recently, however, researchers have been turning their attention to the evaluation of changes in withdrawal symptoms that extend beyond physical signs of withdrawal—that is, to those symptoms that fall within the domain of psychological distress and dysphoria. This new focus is clinically relevant because these symptoms (anxiety, negative affect, and altered reward set point) may serve as potent instigators driving motivation to drink. Sensitization resulting from repeated withdrawal cycles and leading to both more severe and more persistent symptoms therefore may constitute a significant motivational factor that underlies increased risk for relapse.

Furthermore, multiple withdrawal episodes provide repeated opportunities for alcohol dependent individuals to experience the negative reinforcing properties of alcohol—that is, to associate alcohol consumption with the amelioration of the negative consequences (withdrawal-related malaise) experienced during attempts at abstinence. This association not only may serve as a powerful motivational force that increases relapse vulnerability, but also favors escalation of alcohol drinking and sustained levels of potentially harmful drinking. Thus, for many dependent individuals, repeated withdrawal experiences may be especially relevant in shaping motivation to seek alcohol and engage in excessive drinking behavior.

Effects of Repeated Withdrawals on Tolerance to Subjective Alcohol Effects and Alcohol Self-Administration

Researchers also have explored the effects of repeated withdrawal episodes on the perceived subjective effects of alcohol. In animal studies using operant discrimination procedures, the animals' ability to detect (perceive) the subjective cues associated with alcohol intoxication was diminished during withdrawal from chronic alcohol exposure, and this tolerance effect was enhanced in mice that experienced multiple withdrawals during the course of the chronic alcohol treatment. Similarly, rats with a history of repeated cycles of chronic alcohol exposure and withdrawal exhibited long-lasting tolerance to the sedative/hypnotic effects of alcohol. Because changes in sensitivity as well as in the ability to detect (perceive) subjective effects associated with alcohol intoxication may influence decisions about drinking and, in particular, control over the amount consumed during a given drinking occasion, these observations may be relevant to the problem of relapse and excessive drinking. Indeed, clinical studies have indicated that heavy drinkers exhibit a reduced capacity to detect (discriminate) internal cues associated with alcohol intoxication. Future studies will need to further explore the potential relationship between increased tolerance to subjective effects of alcohol produced by repeated withdrawal experience and enhanced propensity to imbibe.

Effects of Repeated Withdrawals on Sensitivity to Treatment

Some studies using animal models involving repeated withdrawals have demonstrated altered sensitivity to treatment with medications designed to quell sensitized withdrawal symptoms. Moreover, after receiving some of these medications, animals exhibited lower relapse vulnerability and/or a reduced amount consumed once drinking was (re) initiate. These findings have clear clinical relevance from a treatment perspective. Indeed, clinical investigations similarly have reported that a history of multiple detoxifications can impact responsiveness to and efficacy of various pharmaco-therapeutics used to manage alcohol dependence. Future studies should focus on elucidating neural mechanisms underlying sensitization of symptoms that contribute to a negative emotional state resulting from repeated withdrawal experience. Such studies will undoubtedly reveal important insights that spark development of new and more effective treatment strategies for relapse prevention as well as aid people in controlling alcohol consumption that too often spirals out of control to excessive levels.

Chapter 57

Prescription Medicines Used for Alcohol Abuse Treatment

Three oral medications (naltrexone, acamprosate, and disulfiram) and one injectable medication (extended-release injectable naltrexone) are currently approved for treating alcohol dependence. Topiramate, an oral medication used to treat epilepsy and migraine, has recently been shown to be effective in treating alcohol dependence, although it is not approved by the Food and Drug Administration (FDA) for this indication. All of these medications have been shown to help patients reduce drinking, avoid relapse to heavy drinking, achieve and maintain abstinence, or gain a combination of these effects. As is true in treating any chronic illness, addressing patient adherence systematically will maximize the effectiveness of these medications.

When should medications be considered for treating an alcohol use disorder?

The drugs noted have been shown to be effective adjuncts to the treatment of alcohol dependence. Thus, consider adding a medication whenever you're treating someone with active alcohol dependence or someone who has stopped drinking in the past few months but is experiencing problems such as craving or slips. Patients who previously failed to respond to psychosocial approaches alone are particularly strong candidates for medication treatment.

Text in this chapter is excerpted from "Prescribing Medication for Alcohol Dependence," National Institute on Alcohol Abuse and Alcoholism (NIAAA), October 2008.

Must patients agree to abstain?

No matter which alcohol dependence medication is used, patients who have a goal of abstinence, or who can abstain even for a few days prior to starting the medication, are likely to have better outcomes. Still, it's best to determine individual goals with each patient. Some patients may not be willing to endorse abstinence as a goal, especially at first. If a patient with alcohol dependence agrees to reduce drinking substantially, it's best to engage him or her in that goal while continuing to note that abstinence remains the optimal outcome.

A patient's willingness to abstain has important implications for the choice of medication. Most studies on effectiveness have required patients to abstain before starting treatment. A notable exception is topiramate, which was prescribed to study volunteers who were still drinking. Both oral and extended-release injection naltrexone also may be helpful in reducing heavy drinking and encouraging abstinence in patients who are still drinking. However, its efficacy is much higher in patients who can abstain for 4–7 days before initiating treatment. Acamprosate, too, is only approved for use in patients who are abstinent at the start of treatment, and patients should be fully withdrawn before starting. Disulfiram is contraindicated in patients who wish to continue to drink, because a disulfiram-alcohol reaction occurs with any alcohol intake at all.

Which of the medications should be prescribed?

Which medication to use will depend on clinical judgment and patient preference. Each has a different mechanism of action. Some patients may respond better to one type of medication than another.

Naltrexone blocks opioid receptors that are involved in the rewarding effects of drinking alcohol and the craving for alcohol. It's available in two forms: oral (Depade®, ReVia®), with once-daily dosing, and extended-release injectable (Vivitrol®), given as once-monthly injections.

Oral naltrexone reduces relapse to heavy drinking, defined as four or more drinks per day for women and five or more for men. It cuts the relapse risk during the first three months by about 36% (about 28% of patients taking naltrexone relapse versus about 43% of those taking a placebo). Thus, it is especially helpful for curbing consumption in patients who have drinking slips. It is less effective in maintaining abstinence. In the single study available when this update was published, extended-release injectable naltrexone resulted in a 25% reduction in the proportion of heavy drinking days compared with a placebo, with a higher rate of response in males and those with lead-in abstinence.

Topiramate is thought to work by increasing inhibitory neurotransmission and reducing stimulatory neurotransmission. It is available in oral form and requires a slow upward titration of dose to minimize side effects.

Topiramate has been shown in two randomized controlled trials to significantly improve multiple drinking outcomes, compared with placebo. Over the course of a 14-week trial, topiramate significantly increased the proportion of volunteers with 28 consecutive days of abstinence or non-heavy drinking. In both studies, the differences between topiramate and placebo groups were still diverging at the end of the trial, suggesting that the maximum effect may not have been reached. The magnitude of topiramate's effect may be larger than that for naltrexone or acamprosate. Importantly, efficacy was established in volunteers who were drinking at the time of starting the medication.

Acamprosate (Campral®) acts on the neurotransmitter systems and is thought to reduce symptoms of protracted abstinence such as insomnia, anxiety, restlessness, and dysphoria. It's available in oral form (three times daily dosing).

Acamprosate increases the proportion of dependent drinkers who maintain abstinence for several weeks to months, a result demonstrated in multiple European studies and confirmed by a meta-analysis of 17 clinical trials. The meta-analysis reported that 36% of patients taking acamprosate were continuously abstinent at six months, compared with 23% of those taking a placebo.

More recently, two large United States (U.S.) trials failed to confirm the efficacy of acamprosate, although secondary analyses in one of the studies suggested possible efficacy in patients who had a baseline goal of abstinence. A reason for the discrepancy between European and U.S. findings may be that patients in European trials had more severe dependence than patients in U.S. trials, a factor consistent with preclinical studies showing that acamprosate has a greater effect in animals with a prolonged history of dependence. In addition, before starting medication, most patients in European trials had been abstinent longer than patients in U.S. trials.

Disulfiram (Antabuse®) interferes with degradation of alcohol, resulting in accumulation of acetaldehyde, which, in turn, produces a very unpleasant reaction including flushing, nausea, and palpitations if the patient drinks alcohol. It's available in oral form (once-daily dosing).

The utility and effectiveness of disulfiram are considered limited because compliance is generally poor when patients are given it to take at their own discretion. It is most effective when given in a monitored fashion, such as in a clinic or by a spouse. (If a spouse or other family member is the monitor, instruct both monitor and patient that the monitor should simply observe the patient taking the medication and call you if the patient stops taking it for two days.) Some patients will respond to self-administered disulfiram, however, especially if they're highly motivated to abstain. Others may use it episodically for high-risk situations, such as social occasions where alcohol is present.

How long should medications be maintained?

The risk for relapse to alcohol dependence is very high in the first 6–12 months after initiating abstinence and gradually diminishes over several years. Therefore, a minimum initial period of three months of pharmacotherapy is recommended. Although an optimal treatment duration hasn't been established, it is reasonable to continue treatment for a year or longer if the patient responds to medication during this time when the risk of relapse is highest. After patients discontinue medications, they may need to be followed more closely and have pharmacotherapy reinstated if relapse occurs.

If one medication doesn't work, should another be prescribed?

If there's no response to the first medication selected, you may wish to consider a second. This sequential approach appears to be common clinical practice, but currently there are no published studies examining its effectiveness. Similarly, there is not yet enough evidence to recommend a specific ordering of medications.

Is there any benefit to combining medications?

A large U.S. trial found no benefit to combining acamprosate and naltrexone. Naltrexone, disulfiram, and both in combination were compared with placebo in the treatment of alcohol dependence in patients with coexisting Axis I psychiatric disorders. Equivalently better outcomes were obtained with either medication, but combining them did not have any additional effect. At this time, there is no evidence supporting the combination of medications, but the number of studies examining this question is limited.

Should patients receiving medications also receive specialized alcohol counseling or a referral to mutual help groups?

Offering the full range of effective treatments will maximize patient choice and outcomes, as no single approach is universally successful or appealing to patients. The different approaches—medications for alcohol dependence, professional counseling, and mutual help groups—are complementary. They share the same goals while addressing different aspects of alcohol dependence: neurobiological, psychological, and social. The medications aren't prone to abuse, so they don't pose a conflict with other support strategies that emphasize abstinence.

Almost all studies of medications for alcohol dependence have included some type of counseling, and it's recommended that all patients taking these medications receive at least brief medical counseling. Evidence is accumulating that weekly or biweekly brief (15–20 minutes) counseling by a health professional combined with prescribing a medication is an effective treatment for many patients during early recovery. Medical counseling focuses on encouraging abstinence, adherence to the medication, and participation in community support groups.

Supporting Patients Who Take Medications for Alcohol Dependence

Pharmacotherapy for alcohol dependence is most effective when combined with some behavioral support, but this doesn't need to be specialized, intensive alcohol counseling. Nurses and physicians in general medical and mental health settings, as well as counselors, can offer brief but effective behavioral support that promotes recovery. Applying this medication management approach in such settings would greatly expand access to effective treatment, given that many patients with alcohol dependence either don't have access to specialty treatment or refuse a referral.

How can general medical and mental health clinicians support patients who take medication for alcohol dependence?

Managing the care of patients who take medication for alcohol dependence is similar to other disease management strategies, such as initiating insulin therapy in patients with diabetes mellitus. In the recent Combining Medications and Behavioral Interventions (COMBINE) clinical trial, physicians, nurses, and other health care professionals in outpatient settings delivered a series of brief behavioral support sessions for patients taking medications for alcohol dependence. The sessions promoted recovery by increasing adherence to the medication and supporting abstinence through education and referral to support groups. It was designed for easy implementation in nonspecialty settings, in keeping with the national trend toward integrating the treatment of substance use disorders into medical practice.

What are the components of medication management support?

Medication management support consists of brief, structured, outpatient sessions conducted by a health care professional. The initial session starts by reviewing with the patient the medical evaluation results as well as the negative consequences of drinking. This information frames a discussion about the diagnosis of alcohol dependence, the recommendation for abstinence, and the rationale for medication. The clinician then provides information on the medication itself and adherence strategies and encourages participation in a mutual support group such as Alcoholics Anonymous (AA).

In subsequent visits, the clinician assesses the patient's drinking, overall functioning, medication adherence, and any side effects from the medication. Session structure varies according to the patient's drinking status and treatment compliance. When a patient doesn't adhere to the medication regimen, it's important to evaluate the reasons and help the patient devise plans to address them.

Can medication management support be used with patients who don't endorse a goal of abstinence?

This medication management program has been tested only in patients for whom abstinence was recommended, as is true with most pharmacotherapy studies. It's not known whether it would also work if the patient's goal is to cut back instead of abstain. Even when patients do endorse abstinence as a goal, they often cut back without quitting. You're encouraged to continue working with those patients who are working toward recovery but haven't yet met the optimal goals of abstinence or reduced drinking with full remission of dependence symptoms. You also may find many of the techniques used in medication management support—such as linking symptoms and laboratory results with heavy alcohol use—to be helpful for managing alcohol-dependent patients in general.

Chapter 58

Alcohol Abuse Treatment: Process and Programs

Many different kinds of professionals provide treatment for substance use disorders. Most treatment programs assign patients to a treatment team of professionals. Depending on the type of treatment, teams can be made up of social workers, counselors, doctors, nurses, psychologists, psychiatrists, or other professionals.

What will happen first?

Everyone entering treatment receives a clinical assessment. A complete assessment of an individual is needed to help treatment professionals offer the type of treatment that best suits him or her. The assessment also helps program counselor(s) work with the person to design an effective treatment plan. Although clinical assessment continues throughout a person's treatment, it starts at or just before a person's admission to a treatment program.

After the assessment, a counselor or case manager is assigned to your family member. The counselor works with the person (and possibly his or her family) to develop a treatment plan. This plan lists problems, treatment goals, and ways to meet those goals. Based on the assessment, the counselor may refer your family member to a physician to decide whether he or she needs medical supervision to stop alcohol or drug use safely.

Excerpted from "What Is Substance Abuse Treatment? A Booklet for Families," Substance Abuse and Mental Health Services Administration (SAMHSA), 2004; and "FAQs: A Quick Guide to Finding Effective Alcohol and Drug Addiction Treatment," SAMHSA. Reviewed in May 2010, by Dr. David A. Cooke, MD, FACP, Diplomate, American Board of Internal Medicine.

What types of treatment programs are available?

Inpatient treatment provided in special units of hospitals or medical clinics offers both detoxification and rehabilitation services. Several years ago, many hospital-based treatment programs existed. Today, because of changes in insurance coverage, inpatient treatment is no longer as common as it used to be. People who have a mental disorder or serious medical problems as well as a substance use disorder are the ones most likely to receive inpatient treatment. Adolescents may also need the structure of inpatient treatment to make sure a full assessment of their substance use and mental disorders can be done.

Residential programs provide a living environment with treatment services. Several models of residential treatment (such as the therapeutic community) exist, and treatment in these programs lasts from a month to a year or more. The programs differ in some ways, but they are similar in many ways.

Residential programs often have phases of treatment, with different expectations and activities during each phase. For example, in the first phase, an adult's contact with family, friends, and job may be restricted. An adolescent may be able to have contact with his or her parents but not with friends or with school. This restriction helps the person become part of the treatment community and adjust to the treatment setting. In a later phase, a person may be able to start working again, going home to the facility every evening. If your loved one is in a residential treatment program, it is important that you know and understand the program rules and expectations. Often residential programs last long enough to offer general equivalency diploma (GED) preparation classes, training in job-seeking skills, and even career training. In residential programs for adolescents, the participants attend school as a part of the program. Some residential programs are designed to enable women who need treatment to bring their children with them. These programs offer child care and parenting classes.

Residential programs are best for people who do not have stable living or employment situations and/or have limited or no family support. Residential treatment may help people with very serious substance use disorders who have been unable to get and stay sober or drug free in other treatment.

Partial hospitalization or day treatment programs also may be provided in hospitals or free-standing clinics. In these programs, the person attends treatment for 4–8 hours per day but lives at home. These programs usually last for at least three months and work best for people who have a stable, supportive home environment.

Outpatient and intensive outpatient programs provide treatment at a program site, but the person lives elsewhere (usually at home). Outpatient treatment is offered in a variety of places: health clinics, community mental health clinics, counselors' offices, hospital clinics, local health department offices, or residential programs with outpatient clinics. Many meet in the evenings and on weekends so participants can go to school or work. Outpatient treatment programs have different requirements for attendance. Some programs require daily attendance; others meet only one to three times per week.

Intensive outpatient treatment programs require a person to attend 9–20 hours of treatment activities per week. Outpatient programs last from about two months to one year. People who do best in an outpatient program are willing to attend counseling sessions regularly, have supportive friends or family members, have a place to live, and have some form of transportation to get to treatment sessions (some programs will provide transportation if needed).

Opioid treatment programs (OTP), sometimes known as methadone clinics, offer medication-assisted outpatient treatment for people who are dependent on opioid drugs (such as heroin, OxyContin, or Vicodin). These programs use a medication, such as methadone, to help a person not use illicit opioids. OTP provide counseling and other services along with the medication.

What actually happens in treatment programs?

Although treatment programs differ, the basic ingredients of treatment are similar. Most programs include many or all of the following elements:

Assessment: All treatment programs begin with a clinical assessment of a person's individual treatment needs. This assessment helps in the development of an effective treatment plan.

Medical care: Programs in hospitals can provide this care on site. Other outpatient or residential programs may have doctors and nurses come to the program site for a few days each week, or a person may be referred to other places for medical care. Medical care typically includes screening and treatment for human immunodeficiency virus (HIV)/acquired immunodeficiency syndrome (AIDS), hepatitis, tuberculosis, and women's health issues.

Treatment plan: The treatment team, along with the person in treatment, develops a treatment plan based on the assessment. A treatment plan is a written guide to treatment that includes the person's goals, treatment activities designed to help him or her meet those goals, ways to tell whether a goal has been met, and a timeframe for meeting goals. The treatment plan helps both the person in treatment and treatment program staff stay focused and on track. The treatment plan is adjusted over time to meet changing needs and ensure that it stays relevant.

Group and individual counseling: At first, individual counseling generally focuses on motivating the person to stop using drugs or alcohol. Treatment then shifts to helping the person stay drug and alcohol free. The counselor attempts to help the person see the problem and become motivated to change; change his or her behavior; repair damaged relationships with family and friends; build new friendships with people who don't use alcohol or drugs; and create a recovery lifestyle.

Group counseling is different in each program, but group members usually support and try to help one another cope with life without using drugs or alcohol. They share their experiences, talk about their feelings and problems, and find out that others have similar problems. Groups also may explore spirituality and its role in recovery.

Individual assignments: People in treatment may be asked to read certain things (or listen to audiotapes), to complete written assignments (or record them on audiotapes), or to try new behaviors.

Education about substance use disorders: People learn about the symptoms and the effects of alcohol and drug use on their brains and bodies. Education groups use videotapes or audiotapes, lectures, or activities to help people learn about their illness and how to manage it.

Life skills training: This training can include learning and practicing employment skills, leisure activities, social skills, communication skills, anger management, stress management, goal setting, and money and time management.

Testing for alcohol or drug use: Program staff members regularly take urine samples from people for drug testing. Some programs are starting to test saliva instead of urine. They also may use a Breathalyzer™ to test people for alcohol use.

Relapse prevention training: Teaches people how to identify their relapse triggers, how to cope with cravings, how to develop plans for handling stressful situations, and what to do if they relapse. A trigger is anything that makes a person crave a drug. Triggers often are connected to the person's past use, such as a person he or she used drugs with, a time or place, drug use paraphernalia (such as syringes, a pipe, or a bong), or a particular situation or emotion.

Orientation to self-help groups: Participants in self-help groups support and encourage one another to become or stay drug and alcohol free. Twelve-step programs are perhaps the best known of the self-help groups. These programs include Alcoholics Anonymous (AA), Narcotics Anonymous (NA), Cocaine Anonymous, and Marijuana Anonymous. Other self-help groups include SMART (Self Management and Recovery Training) Recovery® and Women for Sobriety.

Self-help groups are very important in most people's recovery. It is important to understand, however, that these groups are not the same as treatment. There are self-help groups for family members, too, such as Al-Anon and Alateen.

Treatment for mental disorders: Many people with a substance use disorder also have emotional problems such as depression, anxiety, or posttraumatic stress disorder.

Adolescents in treatment also may have behavior problems, conduct disorder, or attention deficit/hyperactivity disorder. Treating both the substance use and mental disorders increases the chances that the person will recover. Some counselors think people should be alcohol and drug free for at least 3–4 weeks before a treatment professional can identify emotional illness correctly. The program may provide mental health care, or it may refer a person to other sites for this care. Mental health care often includes the use of medications, such as antidepressants.

Family education and counseling services: This education can help you understand the disease and its causes, effects, and treatment. Programs provide this education in many ways: lectures, discussions, activities, and group meetings. Some programs provide counseling for families or couples.

Family counseling is especially critical in treatment for adolescents. Parents need to be involved in treatment planning and followup care decisions for the adolescent. Family members also need to participate as fully as possible in the family counseling the program offers.

Medication: Many programs use medications to help in the treatment process. Although no medications cure dependence on drugs or alcohol, some do help people stay abstinent and can be lifesaving.

Follow-up care (continuing care): Even when a person has successfully completed a treatment program, the danger of returning to alcohol or drug use (called a slip or relapse) remains. The longer a person stays in treatment, including follow-up care, the more likely he or she is to stay in recovery. Once a person has completed basic treatment, a program will offer a followup care program at the treatment facility or will refer him or her to another site. Most programs recommend that a person stay in follow-up care for at least one year. Adolescents often need follow-up care for a longer period.

Follow-up care is very important to successful treatment. Once a person is back in his or her community, back in school, or back at work, he or she will experience many temptations and cravings for alcohol or drugs. In follow-up care, your family member will meet periodically with a counselor or a group to determine how he or she is coping and to help him or her deal with the challenges of recovery.

For some people, particularly those who have been in residential treatment or prison-based programs, more intensive forms of follow-up care may be helpful. Halfway houses or sober houses are alcohol- and drug-free places to live for people coming from a prison-based or residential program. People usually stay from three months to one year, and counseling is provided at the site or at an outpatient facility. Supportive living or transitional apartments provide small group living arrangements for those who need a sober and drug-free living environment. The residents support one another, and involvement in outpatient counseling and self-help groups is expected.

Why does treatment take so long?

Substance use disorders affect every part of a person's life. For that reason, treatment needs to affect every part of a person's life as well. Treatment involves more than helping someone stop drinking alcohol or using drugs. Actually, stopping alcohol use or drug use is just the beginning of the recovery process. Your family member will need to learn new ways to cope with daily life. He or she will need to relearn how to deal with stress, anger, or social situations and how to have fun without using drugs or drinking.

Learning these new skills is a lot of work. Many people enter treatment only because of pressure from the legal system, employers, parents, spouses, or other family members. The first step in treatment then is to help them see that they do have a problem and to become motivated to change for themselves. This process often takes time.

Your family member also will need time to understand and begin to use the support of the self-help groups mentioned before. These groups will be important to his or her recovery for many years to come. Remember: It can take a long time for the disease to develop and it is often chronic; therefore, it can take a long time to treat it.

Questions to Ask when Selecting a Treatment Program

- Does the program accept your insurance? If not, will they work with you on a payment plan or find other means of support for you?

- Is the program run by state-accredited, licensed, and/or trained professionals?

- Is the facility clean, organized, and well-run?

- Does the program encompass the full range of needs of the individual (medical, including infectious diseases; psychological, including co-occurring mental illness; social; vocational; legal; and so forth)?

- Does the treatment program also address sexual orientation and physical disabilities as well as provide age, gender, and culturally appropriate treatment services?

- Is long-term aftercare support and/or guidance encouraged, provided, and maintained?

- Is there ongoing assessment of an individual's treatment plan to ensure it meets changing needs?

- Does the program employ strategies to engage and keep individuals in longer-term treatment, increasing the likelihood of success?

- Does the program offer counseling (individual or group) and other behavioral therapies to enhance the individual's ability to function in the family and community?

- Does the program offer medication as part of the treatment regimen, if appropriate?

- Is there ongoing monitoring of possible relapse to help guide patients back to abstinence?

- Are services or referrals offered to family members to ensure they understand addiction and the recovery process to help them support the recovering individual?

Chapter 59

Treating Co-Occurring Drug and Alcohol Use Disorders

Chapter Contents

Section 59.1

Diagnosing Co-Occurring Drug and Alcohol Use Disorders

This section is excerpted from "Diagnosing Co-Morbid Drug Use in Patients with Alcohol Use Disorders," National Institute on Alcohol Abuse and Alcoholism (NIAAA), 2008. The complete document with references is available at http://pubs.niaaa.nih.gov/publications/arh312/148-154.pdf.

As with alcohol and other drug (AOD) use, AOD use disorders (abuse and dependence) commonly co-occur and are associated with serious consequences. Making an accurate diagnosis can be complicated, but it is an important first step toward treatment and recovery.

AOD use disorders have a high prevalence in the general population and frequently co-occur. In the 2001–2002 National Epidemiologic Survey on Alcohol and Related Conditions (NESARC), the 12-month prevalence of drug use disorders (the prevalence of those meeting the diagnosis for a drug use disorder in the previous 12 months) among those with 12-month alcohol use disorders was 13%. Conversely, the 12-month prevalence of alcohol use disorders among those with 12-month drug use disorders was 55.17%. In the general population, the 12-month prevalence of drug use disorders was 2% and the 12-month prevalence of alcohol use disorders was 8.46%. In a sample of 248 people seeking treatment for alcohol use disorders, 64% had a co-morbid drug use disorder at some point in their lifetime. Sixty-eight percent reported using one or more drugs in the past 90 days, including powder cocaine (33%), crack cocaine (29%), heroin (15%), and cannabis (24%).

Consequences of Co-Morbidity

People with both an alcohol use disorder and a co-morbid drug use disorder are more likely to have less education and a lower income and are less likely to be involved in a stable relationship than people who have an alcohol use disorder and no co-morbid drug use disorder. In addition, co-morbidity is associated with a higher prevalence of personality, mood, and anxiety disorders and is a predictor for suicide attempts. AOD use also is associated with a wide array of medical complications.

Not only are individuals at risk for complications from more than one substance (consequences of cocaine use plus consequences of alcohol use), but AODs used concurrently can interact in complex ways. For example, alcohol may enhance the pleasurable effects of cocaine and result in a larger increase in heart rate than observed with the use of either substance alone. In another example, the use of alcohol with other respiratory depressants, such as the benzodiazepines, may result in a synergistic effect and increase the risk of fatal poisoning. The use of one substance also may worsen the clinical course of the other substance used; for example, in hospitalized patients with alcohol dependence and/or cocaine dependence, post-discharge cannabis use may lead to relapse to alcohol and cocaine use and reduce the likelihood of remission. Furthermore, alcohol dependence with co-morbid drug dependence is associated with a more severe course than alcohol dependence alone. That is, such patients meet a higher number of criteria from the *Diagnostic and Statistical Manual of Mental Disorders, 4th Edition (DSM-IV),* begin drinking regularly and report being drunk for the first time at an earlier age, and have an early onset of alcohol dependence. These indicators may reflect a more heritable form of alcohol dependence.

General Guidelines for Diagnosing a Substance Use Disorder

The information necessary for the diagnosis of a substance use disorder usually is obtained from the patient (by self-report). Clinicians should ask all patients about past and present substance use. They may further screen for drug problems using validated instruments, such as the Drug Abuse Screening Test (DAST) or the CAGE-Adapted to Include Drugs (CAGE-AID), as well as obtain pertinent biological screening evaluations, such as urine testing. With a positive screen, the clinician can proceed with further history taking. A full history addresses all substances used and includes age at first use; patterns of use, including the amounts and routes of administration; related consequences; periods of abstinence; and the history of treatment.

The CAGE is a four-question instrument with each question representing a letter in the acronym (highlighted in italics in the following questions). The CAGE questions Adapted to Include Drugs (CAGE-AID) are: Have you felt you ought to *cut* down on your drinking or drug use? Have people *annoyed* you by criticizing your drinking or drug use? Have you felt bad or *guilty* about your drinking or drug use? Have you ever had a drink or used drugs first thing in the morning to steady your nerves or to get rid of a hangover (an *eye-opener*)? Substance use problems also should be assessed in an orderly sequence. This can be done by either asking the patient to identify the drug that currently is causing him or her the most problems or by assessing the quantity and frequency of each drug being used and establishing a sequential hierarchy to guide the interview. The clinician then can arrive at diagnoses for each category of drug used in a systematic, step-by-step fashion. Evaluating the patient for intoxication and withdrawal is a crucial component of every assessment, as both may require urgent medical or psychiatric care. The diagnosis of AOD use disorders must be made within the context of a larger clinical picture. The full assessment also includes the patient's psychiatric history, medical history, family history, and social and developmental history. The clinician also should obtain a physical and mental status examination, followed by relevant laboratory and imaging tests. Clinicians may supplement these assessments using structured diagnostic interviews—reliable, albeit time-consuming, instruments for diagnosing AOD use disorders—such as the Structured Clinical Interview for DSM-IV Axis I Disorders, Clinician Version (SCID-CV), the Semi-Structured Assessment for the Genetics of Alcoholism (SSAGA), and the Semi-Structured Assessment for Drug Dependence and Alcoholism (SSADDA). After obtaining signed patient consent, access to previous records and information from family and friends also can provide valuable information.

Meeting DSM-IV-TR Criteria

DSM-IV and its text revision (*DSM-IV-TR*) (American Psychiatric Association 1994 and 2000, respectively) identify substance use disorders as substance dependence or substance abuse and define diagnostic criteria that apply to all substances of abuse.

Substance Dependence

Substance dependence is defined as a maladaptive pattern of substance use leading to clinically significant impairment or distress, as manifested by the presence of at least three of seven criteria within the same 12-month period. Two of the criteria reflect physiological dependence, defined as tolerance or withdrawal. The remaining five criteria reflect loss of control and adverse consequences:

- Use in larger amounts or over a longer period than was intended

- A persistent desire or unsuccessful efforts to cut down or control use

- A great deal of time spent on activities necessary to obtain the substance, use it, or recover from its effects

- Giving up or reducing important social, occupational, or recreational activities because of use

- Continued use despite having a persistent or recurrent physical or psychological problem that is likely to have been caused or exacerbated by the substance

In addition, *DSM-IV-TR* identifies six criteria for substance dependence that are meant to aid in the identification of different subgroups of patients. Four of these course specifiers define types of disorder remission (early full remission, early partial remission, sustained full remission, and sustained partial remission), and two additional specifiers are applied if the patient is receiving a prescribed medication that mimics the substance of abuse (agonist therapy) or is currently living in a controlled treatment environment.

Substance Abuse

Substance abuse is defined as a maladaptive pattern of substance use leading to clinically significant impairment or distress, as manifested by the presence of at least one of four of the following criteria within a 12-month period:

- Failure to fulfill major role obligations

- Recurrent use in situations in which it is physically hazardous

- Recurrent substance-related legal problems

- Continued use despite having persistent or recurrent social or interpersonal problems caused or exacerbated by the effects of the substance

If criteria for both substance abuse and substance dependence are met, the diagnosis of substance dependence should be given. If criteria for more than one substance use disorder are met, all individual diagnoses should be documented (alcohol dependence, cocaine dependence, heroin dependence, and phencyclidine abuse). However, if a patient repeatedly uses at least three groups of substances (not including caffeine and nicotine), with no single substance predominating, and the criteria for substance dependence are met for these substances as a group but not for any specific substance, the patient is diagnosed with polysubstance dependence. The commonly used term polysubstance abuse is not a valid *DSM-IV-TR* diagnosis.

Barriers to Accurate Diagnosis of Substance Use Disorders

Although accurate identification facilitates timely intervention, substance use disorders often go undetected, and establishing an accurate diagnosis can be challenging. Issues that can complicate an accurate diagnosis include (1) patient misreport, (2) clinician misrecognition, and (3) challenges related to use of the *DSM-IV-TR*. Naturally, this distinction is arbitrary, and there is considerable overlap between these three areas. It is our intention here, however, to describe the interplay between the three components of the diagnostic interaction: the patient, the clinician, and the diagnostic system used.

Challenges Related to DSM-IV-TR

Diagnosing substance use disorders based on the *DSM-IV-TR* criteria poses challenges that may hamper accurate diagnosis or assessment. For example, deciding between a diagnosis of substance abuse or substance dependence can be difficult, as some of the criteria overlap. Another challenge lies in distinguishing between physiological dependence (tolerance and withdrawal) and the *DSM-IV-TR* diagnosis of substance dependence. Because the *DSM-IV-TR* requires the presence of three out of seven criteria, physiological dependence alone is not sufficient for a diagnosis of substance dependence. For example, a patient on long-term opioid therapy for chronic pain will have developed physiological dependence but does not meet criteria for the *DSM-IV-TR* diagnosis of substance dependence unless at least one additional criterion of substance dependence is present. Conversely, physiological dependence is not necessary for a *DSM-IV-TR* diagnosis of substance dependence. As an example, the use of hallucinogens or binge drinking of alcohol may not lead to tolerance or withdrawal, but the presence of any other three out of seven criteria establishes the diagnosis of substance dependence. Nevertheless, the presence of tolerance and withdrawal should alert the clinician that the patient may have a *DSM-IV-TR* substance dependence diagnosis, in which case the disorder is associated with greater severity.

Additional challenges lie in assessing patients whose substance use is hazardous or harmful but does not meet the criteria for a *DSM-IV-TR* diagnosis of substance abuse or dependence. For example, a patient who has used cocaine several times might not have developed clinically significant impairment or distress to qualify for a *DSM-IV-TR* diagnosis. This should not prevent the clinician from thoroughly evaluating the patient, providing preventive measures and early intervention, and following the course of use over time. The clinician should be especially concerned when a patient reports beginning substance use at an early age, which is a predictor of developing a substance use disorder as well as a predictor of higher disorder severity. Further, substance use disorders change over time, so clinicians should remain flexible and make diagnostic revisions when necessary.

Classification systems other than the *DSM-IV-TR* also may be used in diagnosing substance use disorders. For example, the *10th Revision of the International Statistical Classification of Diseases and Related Health Problems (ICD-10)* (World Health Organization 1992) is widely used in many countries and often corresponds to the *DSM-IV-TR*. Other medical specialties may use different language and criteria to define and diagnose substance use disorders. At the same time, knowledge of *DSM-IV-TR* criteria is important, as these indicators continue to be the standard in diagnosing substance use disorders in the United States, especially by mental health professionals.

Special Considerations in Patients with Alcohol Use Disorders

Patients with alcohol use disorders and other co-occurring substance use may experience adverse consequences in a wide range of areas, affecting social, mental, and physical functions. It can be difficult to determine whether that loss of function is related to all or some of the substances being used. For example, a patient may attribute his or her problems to the continued use of alcohol and heroin but may deny or not recognize the adverse consequences related to his or her biweekly cocaine use. The clinician certainly should address the patient's use of cocaine, but deciding whether it technically qualifies for a *DSM-IV-TR* diagnosis and, if so, whether it is cocaine abuse or dependence may not be a central issue. Instead, clinicians should document diagnostic dilemmas and use good clinical judgment to address all used substances, while at the same time following the course of illness over time, making diagnostic revisions, and providing adequate treatment or referral.

Section 59.2

Integrated Treatments for Co-Occurring Drug and Alcohol Use Disorders

This section is excerpted from "Treatment of Co-Occurring Alcohol and Other Drug Use Disorders," National Institute on Alcohol Abuse and Alcoholism (NIAAA), 2008. The complete document with references is available at http://pubs.niaaa.nih.gov/publications/arh312/155-167.htm.

An estimated 1.1% of the United States (U.S.) population has an alcohol use disorder with a co-occurring drug use disorder (DUD). This type of co-morbidity is sometimes referred to as homotypic co-morbidity or dual dependence. To be consistent this document refers to people with this combination of disorders as having alcohol and other drug (AOD) use disorders (AODUDs). Many people with alcohol use disorders use other substances at some point in their lives. This section focuses on the following AOD combinations: alcohol and cocaine, alcohol and cannabis, opioids and cocaine, and alcohol and cocaine with methadone maintenance. The drug that most commonly is combined with AODs is nicotine, which is discussed in Chapter 41, Section 41.1 of this book.

Assessment, Placement, and Treatment Matching

In general, patients with AODUDs have a greater severity of substance dependence than patients with only an alcohol use disorder or a DUD. People with AODUDs are at least as likely to have co-occurring psychiatric disorders as those who have only DUDs and are more likely to have such disorders than those with only alcohol use disorders. In addition, people with AODUDs are more likely than those with either drug or alcohol use disorders alone to seek treatment. Thus, patients with AODUDs are perhaps best evaluated for treatment planning by a practitioner with specialized expertise in addictive disorders. Although many factors dictate the initial placement and treatment of the AODUD patient (for example, co-occurring pregnancy or the need for medical detoxification), general guidelines are available. Treatment that integrates AODUDs and psychiatric care probably is optimal for most AODUD patients, particularly those with greater severity of psychiatric co-morbidity. Effective, integrated, dual-diagnosis programs emphasize the combination of multiple treatment modalities delivered in a format that acknowledges the limitations and nature of co-occurring psychiatric illness and is delivered by a staff skilled in the treatment of both addictive and psychiatric disorders.

Evidence-Based Treatments for Individual SUDs

Although a complete review of the behavioral and pharmacologic treatment literature for specific addictive disorders is beyond the scope of this chapter, this section provides a brief summary of the major treatment modalities that currently are in use. In general, an approach that combines behavioral and pharmacologic treatments is optimal for most patients. However, recent findings from studies of the pharmacotherapy of alcohol dependence have shown that some patients may do well when medication is combined with a minimal behavioral approach focusing on medication adherence. In addition, among alcohol-dependent patients, those with a goal of abstinence from alcohol likely have better treatment outcomes. However, because some patients do not subscribe to such a goal, it often is necessary to negotiate a harm reduction approach with them, with the option of modifying the goal if their efforts to reduce their drinking substantially are not successful. In drug dependence treatment, behavioral therapies often are considered primary and medications secondary, except in the case of patients receiving opioid agonist maintenance therapy. In opioid agonist therapy, patients receive a drug, such as methadone or buprenorphine, that is chemically similar to opioid drugs.

Behavioral Therapies

Table 59.1 lists the research-based behavioral therapies for different SUDs, with a general description of the level of research evidence supporting each of the treatments. Because people with substance dependence often are ambivalent about changing their behavior, some experts consider motivational enhancement therapy (MET) to be an essential element of addictions treatment, although the evidence supporting its use may be strongest in the treatment of alcohol use disorders. MET aims to engage in treatment patients who are resistant to behavioral change and may be the most acceptable therapeutic approach when patients are new to treatment for

531

AODUDs. MET can help to build a working alliance between the patient and practitioner and provide a foundation on which other useful therapies, including medications, may be added. Cognitive-behavioral therapy (CBT) and MET are effective in the treatment of cannabis dependence. Contingency management interventions also have proven to be effective in treating SUDs, including reducing both drug use and drinking in alcohol-dependent patients. Contingency management is the systematic reinforcement of desired behaviors and the withholding of reinforcement or punishment of undesired behaviors. In addition to the therapies shown in Table 59.1, an intensive outreach counseling program may be helpful in reducing illicit drug use and returning to treatment patients who drop out from methadone maintenance.

A variety of behavioral approaches have shown efficacy in the treatment of alcohol use disorders.

Table 59.1. Summary of Research on Behavioral Therapies for Specific Substance Use Disorders

	Alcohol	Cocaine	Opioid	Marijuana
Cognitive-behavioral therapy	++ (A)	++ (A)		+ (B)
Motivational enhancement therapy	++ (A)	+/- (B)	+/- (B)	+ (B)
Contingency management	++ (A)	+ (A)	+ (A)	+ (B)
Brief intervention	++ (A)			
Twelve-step facilitation	+ (A)	+/- (B)	+/- (B)	
Cue exposure therapy	+ (B)			
Brief couples therapy	+ (B)			
Community reinforcement approach	++ (A)			

For level of evidence supporting the use of therapies: (-) indicates that the treatment appears not to be efficacious, (+/-) indicates conflicting results or preliminary evidence of efficacy, (+) indicates evidence of efficacy from randomized controlled trials, and (++) indicates evidence of efficacy from multiple trials and/or meta-analyses.

Evidence-based strength of recommendation taxonomy: (A) recommendation based on consistent and good-quality patient-oriented evidence; (B) recommendation based on inconsistent or limited-quality patient-oriented evidence; (C) recommendation based on consensus, usual practice, opinion, disease-oriented evidence, or case series for studies of diagnosis, treatment, prevention, or screening.

Treatment of AODUDs

Most studies have focused on the treatment of individual SUDs rather than co-occurring disorders. Although studies conducted specifically in AODUD populations are limited, the evidence to date suggests that approaches similar to those used to treat the individual SUDs may be effective. As with the treatment of dependence on individual substances, behavioral therapies provide the backbone or main component of treatment for patients with AODUDs. In addition, because the studies evaluating pharmacotherapies in AODUD patients almost always include at least one behavioral therapy component, this review does not examine these types of therapy separately. Table 59.2 summarizes the evidence for various individual treatments for AODUDs.

Table 59.2. Summary of Research on Treatments for AODUDs

	Alcohol/ Cocaine	Alcohol/ Opioid	Cocaine/ Opioid
Disulfiram	+/- (B)	+/- (B)**	+ (B)
Naltrexone	+/- (B)	* (C)	* (C)
Buprenorphine			+ (B)
Methadone		+/- (C)	+ (B)
Desipramine			+ (B)
Topiramate	* (C)		
Baclofen	* (C)		
Tiagabine		+/- (B)	
Cognitive-behavioral therapy	+ (B)		+ (B)
Contingency management	+/- (B)	+ (B)	+ (B)
Twelve-step facilitation	+/- (B)		

Notes: AODUDs = Alcohol and other drug use disorders.

* = Recommendation synthesized from studies performed in primarily alcohol or cocaine dependent subjects, not specifically in the dually dependent group.

** = May only be effective when continued opioid agonist therapy is made contingent on disulfiram ingestion.

For level of evidence supporting the use of therapies: (-) indicates that the treatment appears to be ineffective, (+/-) indicates conflicting results or preliminary evidence of efficacy, (+) indicates evidence of efficacy from randomized controlled trials, (++) indicates evidence of efficacy from multiple trials and/or meta-analyses.

Evidence-based strength of recommendation taxonomy: (A) recommendation based on consistent and good-quality patient-oriented evidence; (B) recommendation based on inconsistent or limited-quality patient-oriented evidence; (C) recommendation based on consensus, usual practice, opinion, disease-oriented evidence, or case series for studies of diagnosis, treatment, prevention, or screening.

Contingency management has been shown to increase treatment retention and improve outcomes across a spectrum of addictive disorders, irrespective of psychiatric severity. Hence, contingency management may serve effectively as a platform for the treatment of AODUDs. A review of treatments for alcoholic methadone patients suggested that making methadone treatment contingent on disulfiram ingestion may effectively reduce drinking and alcohol-related adverse outcomes. Along similar lines, contingency management using both prizes and vouchers has been shown to be beneficial for co-occurring opioid and cocaine/stimulant use disorders, as well as other co-occurring substance dependence disorders, including alcohol dependence.

Treatment Recommendations for Patients with AODUDs

For patients with alcohol and cocaine dependence, disulfiram has better empirical support than any other medication. Less compelling evidence exists for the use of either naltrexone or topiramate, but these also should be considered for treatment of these co-occurring disorders. A daily dose of more than 50 milligrams (mg) of naltrexone is needed to treat these disorders but may not be efficacious for women with co-occurring alcohol and cocaine dependence. Topiramate has not yet been studied in AODUD patients, but its safety and efficacy have been demonstrated in patients with alcohol or cocaine dependence. Although the optimal dosage has not yet been determined, preliminary findings suggest that 200 to 300 mg per day, increased gradually over 6–8 weeks, is required. Second-line therapies may be effective in patients with cocaine dependence but not alcohol dependence (modafinil and tiagabine) or vice versa (acamprosate). Baclofen also could be considered for use in select patients based on evidence of its efficacy in alcohol or cocaine dependence. In addition to an absence of data on the efficacy of these medications in co-occurring cocaine and alcohol dependence, it is unclear whether these medications should be used alone or combined with first-line or other second-line agents. There is limited evidence to support combining disulfiram and naltrexone to treat co-occurring alcohol and cocaine dependence; further research on the combination is needed before it can be recommended as offering an advantage over the use of either medication alone.

For alcohol-dependent patients on methadone maintenance, optimizing the dosage of methadone may help to reduce drinking. Stabilizing opioid withdrawal symptoms and illicit opioid use with methadone or buprenorphine in qualifying patients is an appropriate first step. For patients who continue to drink while receiving opioid maintenance therapy, the first-line alcohol treatments (with the exception of naltrexone) should be considered. Disulfiram may be the medication of choice for such patients, because they also may have a cocaine use disorder. To increase adherence to disulfiram treatment in this patient population, it is probably necessary to require that the patient submit to observed disulfiram ingestion as a condition of continued opioid agonist treatment. Topiramate may be an option in this population as well, though there are no published reports to guide this approach.

For patients dependent on opioids and cocaine, adequate dosing of buprenorphine and methadone may reduce use of both substances. This approach should be considered as a first-line therapy for such patients, as long as the severity of their opioid dependence warrants opioid agonist therapy. If monotherapy with buprenorphine or methadone is inadequate to control co-occurring cocaine use, adding disulfiram to either agonist treatment should be considered. Research also suggests that adding desipramine or high-dose tiagabine to an opioid agonist maintenance regimen can be helpful. However, caution is necessary in prescribing medications to patients with co-occurring opioid and cocaine dependence as they may have significant medical co-morbidity, including cardiac and liver disease. This strategy also has the potential to cause drug-drug interactions. As is true for the treatment of patients with other combinations of AODUDs, pharmacotherapy in this patient group should be combined with behavioral therapies, such as contingency management, which may be particularly useful in combination with desipramine.

Summary of General Treatment Recommendations

Although the treatment literature is rapidly growing for individual SUDs, there is a paucity of systematic research on treatments for AODUDs. The existing literature shows that, as with DUDs alone, combined behavioral and psychopharmacological treatments for patients with AODUDs are likely to be optimal. At a minimum, patients should be encouraged to participate in a 12-step program and are likely to benefit from the addition of group or individual therapies that use motivational enhancement and cognitive-behavioral techniques. When available, the use of contingency management is likely to enhance outcomes for patients with AODUDs. The use of medications to improve outcomes in AODUD patients has shown initial promise, particularly for co-occurring alcohol and cocaine dependence.

Treatment planning for patients with AODUDs should include medical and psychiatric evaluations and integrated treatment to address co-occurring substance use and psychiatric disorders. Given the burden of psychopathology, patients with AODUDs often may require a higher level of care (inpatient rehabilitation, psychiatric partial hospital or intensive outpatient dual diagnosis programs) for initial stabilization. Medications with beneficial effects on drinking behavior and other drug use should be used in combination with behavioral interventions. In short, treatment for patients with AODUDs should start with a motivational intervention, with a focus on developing a therapeutic alliance. In these efforts, the clinician should be mindful of the patient's stage of change and level of motivation, utilize empathic listening and expression, address the patient's goals and needs, emphasize and promote self-regulation skills, utilize multiple treatment modalities, actively address co-occurring medical and psychiatric illness, and promote adherence to the treatment program.

Chapter 60

Recovery from Co-Occurring Mental Illness and Alcohol Abuse

Dual disorders refers to the presence of both a severe mental illness and a substance use disorder. Integrated dual disorders treatment has been shown to work effectively for consumers with both disorders. In this treatment model, one clinician or treatment team provides both mental health and substance abuse treatment services.

Recovery from mental illness and substance use: People with mental illnesses are also prone to develop problems with alcohol and drug use, tending to use drugs and alcohol for the same reasons that people without a mental illness do, but are often more sensitive to the negative effects of alcohol and drugs. The result is that one of every two individuals with severe mental illness has the additional problem of substance use disorder, (which means abuse or dependence related to alcohol or other drugs). However, there is good news.

Most of individuals with dual disorders can achieve recovery. And lives are much better when impacted individuals are in recovery. Building a satisfying and meaningful life without drugs or alcohol requires time, support, education, courage, and learning new skills.

"Evidence-Based Practices: Shaping Mental Health Services Toward Recovery," Substance Abuse and Mental Health Services Administration (SAMHSA), 2003. Reviewed in May 2010, by Dr. David A. Cooke, MD, FACP, Diplomate, American Board of Internal Medicine.

How can people with dual disorders achieve recovery from both mental illness and substance abuse?

- Most people with dual disorders are able to achieve recovery. The chance of recovery improves when people receive integrated dual disorders treatment, which means combined mental health and substance abuse treatment from the same clinician or treatment team.

- Relapses do happen, but most people are able to recover from relapses relatively quickly and get back to where they were before they relapsed.

- Families and clinicians cannot force people to give up alcohol and drugs. Family and other supporters can help by providing support and hope, but recovery must be a person's own choice. It may take a long time for some people to achieve recovery.

- People with dual disorders can learn from peers who are in recovery. Some may benefit from self-help groups like Alcoholics Anonymous, Narcotics Anonymous, and Dual Recovery Anonymous. It is a matter of personal preference.

What is integrated dual disorders treatment?

Integrated dual disorders treatment occurs when a person receives combined treatment for mental illness and substance use from the same clinician or treatment team. It helps people develop hope, knowledge, skills, and the support they need to manage their problems and to pursue meaningful life goals. You will know if you are receiving integrated treatment because your clinician or treatment team will do several things at the same time, including the following:

- Help you think about the role that alcohol and other drugs play in your life. This should be done confidentially, without any negative consequences. People feel free to discuss these issues when the discussion is confidential, nonjudgmental, and not tied to legal consequences.

- Offer you a chance to learn more about alcohol and drugs, to learn about how they interact with mental illnesses and with medications, and to discuss your own use of alcohol and drugs.

- Help you become involved with supported employment and other services that may help your process of recovery.

- Help you identify and develop your own recovery goals. If you decide that your use of alcohol or drugs may be a problem, a counselor trained in integrated dual disorders treatment can help you identify and develop your own recovery goals. This process includes learning about steps toward recovery from both illnesses.

- Provide special counseling specifically designed for people with dual disorders. If you decide that your use of alcohol or drugs may be a problem, a trained counselor can provide special counseling specifically designed for people with dual disorders. This can be done individually, with a group of peers, with your family, or with a combination of these.

If you are a person with dual disorders, participating in integrated dual disorders treatment is extremely important. Effective treatment will help reduce the risk for many additional problems, such as increased symptoms of a mental illness, hospitalizations, financial problems, family problems, homelessness, suicide, violence, sexual and physical victimization, incarceration, serious medical illnesses, such as human immunodeficiency virus (HIV) and hepatitis B and C, and sometimes even early death.

What can you, as a consumer with dual disorders, do?

- Get more information and support about what having dual disorders means and how it affects your recovery process.

- Do everything you can to build a positive life for yourself without alcohol and drugs. For most people recovery includes meaningful activities, like a job, friendships with people who do not use alcohol or drugs, a safe place to live, and enjoying leisure activities that are fun and relaxing. This all takes time. Don't give up.

- If you are having trouble with your mental illness as well as with substance abuse, it is important to talk with mental health professionals about how to get your symptoms under better control, and how to improve your recovery process.

Chapter 61

The Role of Mutual Support Groups in Alcohol Abuse Recovery

Mutual Support Groups Aid Recovery from Substance Use Disorders

Mutual support (also called self-help) groups are an important part of recovery from substance use disorders (SUDs). Mutual support groups exist both for persons with an SUD and for their families or significant others and are one of the choices an individual has during the recovery process.

Mutual support groups are nonprofessional groups comprising members who share the same problem and voluntarily support one another in the recovery from that problem. Although mutual support groups do not provide formal treatment, they are one part of a recovery-oriented systems-of-care approach to substance abuse recovery. By providing social, emotional, and informational support for persons throughout the recovery process, mutual support groups help individuals take responsibility for their alcohol and drug problems and for their sustained health, wellness, and recovery. The most widely available mutual support groups are twelve-step groups, such as Alcoholics Anonymous (AA), but other mutual support groups such as Women for Sobriety (WFS), SMART Recovery®, and Secular Organizations for Sobriety/Save Our Selves (SOS) are also available.

This chapter includes text from "Substance Abuse in Brief Fact Sheet, Vol. 5, Issue 1: An Introduction to Mutual Support Groups for Alcohol and Drug Abuse," Substance Abuse and Mental Health Services Administration (SAMHSA), Spring 2008; and, "Participation in Self-Help Groups for Alcohol and Illicit Drug Use: 2006 and 2007," SAMHSA, November 13, 2008.

Twelve-Step Groups

Twelve-step groups emphasize abstinence and have 12 core developmental steps to recovering from dependence. Other elements of twelve-step groups include taking responsibility for recovery, sharing personal narratives, helping others, and recognizing and incorporating into daily life the existence of a higher power. Participants often maintain a close relationship with a sponsor, an experienced member with long-term abstinence, and lifetime participation is expected.

AA is the oldest and best known twelve-step mutual support group. There are more than 100,000 AA groups worldwide and nearly two million members. The AA model has been adapted for people with dependence on drugs and for their family members. Some groups, such as Narcotics Anonymous (NA) and Chemically Dependent Anonymous, focus on any type of drug use. Other groups, such as Cocaine Anonymous and Crystal Meth Anonymous, focus on abuse of specific drugs. Groups for persons with co-occurring substance use and mental disorders also exist (Double Trouble in Recovery; Dual Recovery Anonymous). Other twelve-step groups—Families Anonymous, Al-Anon/Alateen, Nar-Anon, and Co-Anon—provide support to significant others, families, and friends of persons with SUDs.

Twelve-step meetings are held in locations such as churches and public buildings. Metropolitan areas usually have specialized groups, based on such member characteristics as gender, length of time in recovery, age, sexual orientation, profession, ethnicity, and language spoken. Attendance and membership are free, although people usually give a small donation when they attend a meeting.

Meetings can be open or closed, that is, anyone can attend an open meeting, but attendance at closed meetings is limited to people who want to stop drinking or using drugs. Although meeting formats vary somewhat, most twelve-step meetings have an opening and a closing that are the same at every meeting, such as a twelve-step reading or prayer. The main part of the meeting usually consists of members sharing their stories of dependence, its effect on their lives, and what they are doing to stay abstinent; the study of a particular step or other doctrine of the group; or a guest speaker.

Twelve-step groups are not necessarily for everyone. Some people are uncomfortable with the spiritual emphasis and prefer a more secular approach. Others may not agree with the twelve-step philosophy that addiction is a chronic disease, thinking that this belief can be a self-fulfilling prophesy that weakens the ability to remain abstinent. Still others may prefer gender specific groups.

Mutual support groups that are not based on the twelve-step model typically do not advocate sponsors or lifetime membership. These support groups offer an alternative to traditional twelve-step groups, but the availability of in-person meetings is more limited than that of twelve-step programs. However, many offer literature, discussion boards, and online meetings.

Women for Sobriety (WFS)

WFS is the first national self-help group solely for women wishing to stop using alcohol and drugs. The program is based on *Thirteen Statements* that encourage emotional and spiritual growth, with abstinence as the only acceptable goal. Although daily meditation is encouraged, WFS does not otherwise emphasize God or a higher power. The nearly 300 meetings held weekly are led by experienced, abstinent WFS members and follow a structured format which includes reading the *Thirteen Statements*, an introduction of members, and a moderated discussion.

SMART Recovery

SMART Recovery helps individuals become free from dependence on any substance. Dependence is viewed as a learned behavior that can be modified using cognitive-behavioral approaches. Its four principles are to: (1) enhance and maintain motivation to abstain; (2) cope with urges; (3) manage thoughts, feelings, and behaviors; and (4) balance momentary and enduring satisfactions. At the approximately 300 weekly group meetings held worldwide, attendees discuss personal experiences and real-world applications of these SMART Recovery principles. SMART Recovery has online meetings and a message board discussion group on its website.

Secular Organization for Sobriety/Save Our Selves (SOS)

SOS considers recovery from alcohol and drugs an individual responsibility separate from spirituality and emphasizes a cognitive approach to maintaining lifelong abstinence. Meetings typically begin with a reading of the SOS *Guidelines for Sobriety* and introductions, followed by an open discussion of a topic deemed appropriate by the members. However, because each of the approximately 500 SOS groups is autonomous, the meeting format may differ from group to group. SOS also has online support groups, such as the SOS International E-Support Group.

LifeRing Secular Recovery

Originally part of SOS, LifeRing is now a separate organization for people who want to stop using alcohol and drugs. The principles of Life-Ring are sobriety, secularity, and self-help. LifeRing encourages participants to develop a unique path to abstinence according to their needs and to use the group meetings to facilitate their personal recovery plan. LifeRing meetings are relatively unstructured; attendees discuss what has happened to them in the past week, but some meetings focus on helping members create a personal recovery plan. Although there are fewer than 100 meetings worldwide, LifeRing has a chat room, e-mail lists, and an online forum that provide additional support to its members.

The Effectiveness of Mutual Support Groups

Research on mutual support groups indicates that active participation in any type of mutual support group significantly increases the likelihood of maintaining abstinence. Previous research has shown that participating in twelve-step or other mutual support groups is related to abstinence from alcohol and drug use. An important finding is that these abstinence rates increase with greater group participation. Persons who attend mutual support groups have also been found to have lower levels of alcohol- and drug-related problems.

Another benefit of mutual support group participation is that "helping helps the helper." Helping others by sharing experiences and providing support increases involvement in twelve-step groups, which in turn increases abstinence and lowers binge drinking rates among those who have not achieved abstinence.

Facilitating Mutual Support Group Participation

If a health care or social service provider suspects that a patient or client has an substance use disorder (SUD), the provider should ensure that the client receives formal treatment. Once the client receives formal treatment—or if he or she refuses or cannot afford treatment—the provider's next step is to facilitate involvement in a mutual support group. Matching clients to treatment based solely on gender, motivation, cognitive impairment, or other such characteristics has not been proven to be effective. Clients who are philosophically well-matched to a mutual support group are more likely to actively participate in that group. Thus, the best way to help a client benefit from mutual support groups is to encourage increased participation in his or her chosen group.

Understanding the needs and beliefs of clients with SUDs helps providers make informed referrals. Providers should find out clients' experiences with mutual support groups, their concerns and misconceptions about mutual support groups, and their personal beliefs. Persons who agree with the group's belief system are more likely to participate and, thus, more likely to have better outcomes.

Participation in Self-Help Groups for Alcohol and Illicit Drug Use: 2006 and 2007

Participation in self-help groups, such as Alcoholics Anonymous and Narcotics Anonymous, is an important adjunct to formal treatment for substance use problems, and it provides valuable peer support throughout the recovery process. The National Survey on Drug Use and Health (NSDUH) includes a question for persons aged 12 or older about their participation in the past 12 months in a self-help group for substance use (alcohol use, illicit drug use, or both). NSDUH also asks questions about past year receipt of treatment for substance use problems in a specialty treatment facility.

Who attended self-help groups for substance use?

An annual average of 5.0 million persons aged 12 or older (2.0% of the population in that age group) attended a self-help group in the past year because of their use of alcohol or illicit drugs. The majority of people who attended a self-help group for their substance use in the past year were male (66.1%). Most attendees (80.2%) were over the age of 25, two-thirds (67.7%) were White, a majority (55.6%) lived in a large metropolitan area, and over two-thirds (68.1%) had a total family income of under $50,000 per year.

Among persons aged 12 or older who attended a self-help group in the past year, 45.3% attended a group because of their alcohol use only, and 21.8% attended a group because of their illicit drug use only. One-third (33.0%) attended a group because of their use of both alcohol and illicit drugs.

How many attendees had stopped using substances, and how many continued to use?

Among past year self-help group participants aged 12 or older, 45.1% abstained from substance use in the past month, and the remaining 54.9% continued to use substances. Rates of abstinence differed depending on the substance(s) for which individuals were attending

Table 61.1. Percent distribution of persons aged 12 or older who attended a self-help group in the past year because of their alcohol or illicit drug use* and of total population aged 12 or older, by sociodemographic characteristics: 2006 and 2007

Sociodemographic Characteristic	Percent of Self-Help Group Participants	Percent** of Total Population
Total	100.0%	100.0%
Gender		
Male	66.1%	48.5%
Female	33.9%	51.5%
Age Group in Years		
12 to 17	4.6%	10.3%
18 to 25	15.3%	13.3%
26 to 49	57.4%	40.6%
50 or Older	22.8%	35.9%
Race/Ethnicity		
White	67.7%	68.3%
Black or African American	15.8%	11.8%
Hispanic or Latino	12.9%	13.7%
American Indian or Alaska Native	1.2%	0.5%
Native Hawaiian or Other Pacific Islander	0.3%	0.3%
Asian	0.7%	4.2%
Two or more races	1.4%	1.1%
County Type		
Large metropolitan	55.6%	53.7%
Small metropolitan	28.9%	29.4%
Non-metropolitan	15.4%	16.8%
Family Income		
Less than $20,000	30.5%	18.6%
$20,000 to $49,999	37.6%	33.7%
$50,000 to $74,999	13.4%	17.9%
$75,000 or more	18.5%	29.8%

*These data include respondents who reported attendance at a self-help group, but did not report for which substance(s) (alcohol, illicit drugs, or both) they attended.
**Due to rounding, percentages do not total 100%.
Source: SAMHSA, 2006 and 2007 NSDUHs.

self-help groups. For example, past month abstinence from alcohol and illicit drug use was reported by 33.3% of those who attended a self-help group for their illicit drug use only. This compares with 47.3% of those who attended a self-help group for their alcohol use only and 52.5% of those who attended a self-help group for their use of both alcohol and illicit drugs.

How many attendees received specialty treatment for alcohol or illicit drugs?

Almost one-third (32.7%) of individuals aged 12 or older who attended a self-help group for their substance use in the past year also received specialty treatment for substance use in the past year. About one-quarter (26.1%) of persons who attended a self-help group for their alcohol use only also received specialty treatment for any substance use, compared with 43.4% of those who attended a self-help group because of their illicit drug use only and 32.2% of those who attended a self-help group for their use of both alcohol and illicit drugs.

Two-thirds (66.0%) of persons aged 12 or older who received any alcohol or illicit drug use specialty treatment in the past year also attended a self-help group in the same time frame. Three-fourths (75.6%) of the persons who received specialty treatment for both alcohol and illicit drug use also attended a self-help group compared with 65.8% of those who received specialty treatment for illicit drug use only and 63.6% of those who received specialty treatment for alcohol use only.

Recovery from problem substance use and abuse is an ongoing life event that requires long-term support and treatment. A substantial body of research has found that attendance at self-help groups improves substance use outcomes, mainly in the form of reductions in the amount used and increases in rates of abstinence. Self-help groups often are used in conjunction with specialty treatment and also continue beyond treatment as people go through the recovery process.

Part Eight

Additional Help
and Information

Chapter 62

Glossary of Terms Related to Alcohol Use and Abuse

abstinence: Not drinking any alcoholic beverage, including beer, wine, and hard liquor. It is recommended that all pregnant women abstain from alcohol to avoid fetal damage.

abuser: A person who uses alcohol or other drugs in ways that threaten his health or impair his social or economic functioning.[1]

addiction: A state of dependence caused by habitual use of drugs, alcohol, or other substances. It is characterized by uncontrolled craving, tolerance, and symptoms of withdrawal when access is denied. Habitual use produces changes in body chemistry, and treatment must be geared to a gradual reduction in dosage.

alcohol: A drink containing the substance ethanol.

alcohol dependence: A diagnosis of a maladaptive pattern of substance use as shown by three of the following criteria, noted in a 12-month period: tolerance; withdrawal or use of alcohol to avoid withdrawal; use in larger amounts or for longer than intended; unsuccessful efforts to decrease or discontinue use or a persistent desire to do so; alcohol use as a major focus of time and life; abandonment of

---

Terms in this chapter are excerpted from "SAMHSA Fetal Alcohol Spectrum Disorders Center for Excellence. Curriculum for Addictions Professionals: Level 1." Center for Substance Abuse Prevention, Substance Abuse and Mental Health Services Administration (SAMHSA), 2007. Terms marked with a [1] are excerpted from "Glossary of Terms," U.S. Department of Labor, March 12, 2009.

social, occupational, or recreational activities; continued use despite recognized psychological or physical consequences.

alcohol metabolism: Refers to the body's process of converting ingested alcohol to other compounds. Metabolism results in some substances becoming more or less toxic than those originally ingested. Metabolism involves a number of processes, one of which is oxidation. Through oxidation, alcohol is detoxified and removed from the blood, preventing the alcohol from accumulating and destroying cells and organs. A minute amount of alcohol escapes metabolism and is excreted unchanged in the breath and in urine. Until all the alcohol consumed has been metabolized, it is distributed throughout the body, affecting the brain and other tissues.

alcohol screening: A question-based method for identifying individuals with alcohol problems and assessing the severity of use.

alcoholism: A treatable illness brought on by harmful dependence upon alcohol which is physically and psychologically addictive. As a disease, alcoholism is primary, chronic, progressive, and fatal.[1]

alcohol-related birth defects (ARBD): A term used to describe individuals with confirmed maternal alcohol use and one or more congenital defects, including heart, bone, kidney, vision, or hearing abnormalities.

alcohol-related neurodevelopmental disorder (ARND): A term used to describe individuals with confirmed maternal alcohol use, neurodevelopmental abnormalities, and a complex pattern of behavioral or cognitive abnormalities inconsistent with developmental level and not explained by genetic background or environment. Problems may include learning disabilities, school performance deficits, inadequate impulse control, social perceptual problems, language dysfunction, abstraction difficulties, mathematics deficiencies, and judgment, memory, and attention problems.

Alcohol Use Disorders Identification Test (AUDIT): A simple ten-question test developed by the World Health Organization (WHO) to determine if a person's alcohol consumption is excessive. WHO designed the test for international use and it was validated in a six-country study. Questions 1–3 deal with alcohol consumption, 4–6 relate to alcohol dependence and 7–10 consider alcohol related problems. A score of eight or more in men (seven in women) indicates a strong likelihood of hazardous or harmful alcohol consumption. A score of 13 or more is suggestive of alcohol-related harm.

binge drinking: Refers to the consumption of four or more drinks in about two hours. Binge drinking during pregnancy can result in fetal alcohol spectrum disorders (FASD).

birth defect: Physical or biochemical defect (for example: Down syndrome, fetal alcohol syndrome [FAS], cleft palate) that is present at birth and may be inherited or environmentally induced.

blood alcohol concentration (BAC): The amount of alcohol in the bloodstream measured in percentages. A BAC of 0.10% means that a person has one part alcohol per 1,000 parts blood in the body.[1]

brief intervention: Approximately one to four therapy sessions delivered to individuals with problem drinking and other problematic behaviors. The intervention may include advice to abstain from alcohol use or decrease alcohol consumption to below risk drinking levels, brief counseling, goal setting, and development of action plans.

CAGE: A screening tool for identifying risk drinkers. Each positive answer is scored as one point. A score of two or more points is considered evidence of possible risk drinking. The CAGE has been used effectively to identify alcoholic clients, but it may not be as sensitive as other brief scales with female populations. The acronym stands for:

C   Have you ever felt you ought to Cut Down on your drinking?

A   Have people ever Annoyed you by criticizing your drinking?

G   Have you ever felt bad or Guilty about your drinking?

E   Have you ever had a drink first thing in the morning to steady your nerves or get rid of a hangover (Eye-Opener)?

cognitive-behavioral therapy: In the field of substance abuse treatment, cognitive-behavioral therapy is an approach that includes self-management and relapse prevention strategies. It is designed to help individuals stop or reduce alcohol consumption by observing their drinking behavior, setting behavioral objectives, or training in skills to handle conflicts or stress without resorting to drinking.

congenital defects: Imperfections with which a person is born, acquired during development in the uterus. The defects may be due to genetics or to fetal injury or insult (maternal alcohol use or infection).

co-occurring: Simultaneous existence of a disorder (for example: alcoholism) interacting with one or more independent disorders (such as depression, schizophrenia) or disabilities. The disorder/disability is of a type and severity that exacerbates the other conditions, complicates treatment, or interferes with functioning in age-appropriate social roles. In substance abuse, it is typically used to describe persons who have both mental illness and a substance abuse/dependence disorder.

depression: Major depressive disorder is marked by a depressed mood or a loss of interest or pleasure in daily activities consistently for at least two weeks. This mood must represent a change from the person's normal mood; social, occupational, educational, or other important functioning must also be negatively impaired by the change in mood.

diagnosis: The process of determining disease status through the study of symptom patterns and the factors responsible for producing them.

enabling: Allowing irresponsible and destructive behavior patterns to continue by taking responsibility for others, not allowing them to face the consequences of their own actions.[1]

ethyl alcohol: Ethanol is the member of the alcohol series of chemicals which is used in alcoholic beverages. It is less toxic than other members of this series, but it is a central nervous system depressant and has a high abuse potential.[1]

ethnicity, ethnic background: Refers to racial, national, tribal, religious, linguistic, or cultural origin or background.

fetal alcohol spectrum disorders (FASD): An umbrella term describing the range of effects that can occur in an individual whose mother drank alcohol during pregnancy. These effects may include physical, mental, behavioral, and/or learning disabilities with possible lifelong implications. The term FASD is not intended for use as a clinical diagnosis.

fetal alcohol spectrum disorders (FASD) screening: A technique that uses a variety of tools to identify individuals who show signs of an FASD in infancy and early childhood or who are known to have had prenatal alcohol exposure. It can also be used to identify adolescents and adults who may have the disorder and have not been previously diagnosed.

fetal alcohol syndrome (FAS): Describes individuals with documented prenatal exposure to alcohol and (1) prenatal and postnatal growth retardation, (2) characteristic facial features, and (3) central nervous system problems.

genetic disorders: Caused by a disturbance of one gene or several genes or chromosomes. They may be inherited or caused by environmental factors. Genetic disorders may cause various diseases and disorders.

heavy drinking: Refers to the consumption of five or more drinks on the same occasion on five or more days in the past month.

indicated prevention: Targets high-risk individuals who have signs or symptoms of a condition or have biologic markers indicating predisposition. Targets of indicated prevention include women who abuse alcohol, such as women who binge drink while pregnant, particularly pregnant or preconceptional women who drink alcohol and have already given birth to children with an FASD. Substance abuse treatment for pregnant women is a form of indicated prevention.

motivational interviewing (MI): A structured brief intervention procedure for people with alcohol or other substance use problems. It includes clinician empathy and advice, feedback, establishment of client responsibility, determination of options, and encouragement of the client's self-efficacy in changing behavior.

neurodevelopmental abnormalities: Central nervous system abnormalities, such as small head size at birth, and structural brain abnormalities leading to impaired fine motor skills, hearing loss, gait problems, and poor eye-hand coordination.

palpebral fissures: Refers to eye openings. People with FAS have short palpebral fissures. The palpebral fissure is measured from the inner canthus (corner) of the eye to the outer canthus of the eye.

philtrum: The vertical groove between the nose and the middle part of the upper lip. Individuals diagnosed with fetal alcohol syndrome have a flattening of the philtrum.

prenatal exposure to alcohol (PEA), prenatal alcohol exposure: Refers to the exposure of a fetus to alcohol through maternal drinking during pregnancy.

prevalence: The number of instances of the disorder in a given population at a designated time, for example: the prevalence of fetal alcohol spectrum disorders is estimated to be at least ten per 1,000 live births.

prevention: The protection of health through personal and community efforts.

problem drinking: An individual with problem drinking has issues concerning alcohol use and may require treatment to manage the problem.

residential treatment: A living setting designed for individuals who have difficulty living with family or on their own due to alcohol abuse, alcoholism, physical problems, developmental disabilities, or mental illness. It provides adult supervision, therapy, and skills training in a large or small group setting.

standard drink: Because alcoholic beverages vary in alcohol concentration, drinks are designated by a standard drink conversion. One standard drink is 12 ounces (oz.) of beer, 5 oz. of wine, or 1.5 oz. of hard liquor. All have the same equivalency of 0.48 oz. of absolute alcohol.

substance abuse treatment: A therapeutic program, staffed by addiction professionals, for individuals with alcohol or drug problems. It may involve inpatient or outpatient care.

T-ACE: A screening tool for identifying pregnant women with alcohol problems. The tolerance question is scored as two points if the respondent reports needing more than two drinks to get high. A positive response to A, C, or E is scored as one point each. A score of two or more indicates likely drinking during pregnancy. The T-ACE has been found to be effective in identifying pregnant women who consumed sufficient amounts of alcohol to endanger a fetus. The acronym stands for:

T   Tolerance: How many drinks does it take you to feel high?

A   Annoyed: Have people annoyed you by criticizing your drinking?

C   Cut Down: Have you ever felt you ought to cut down on your drinking?

E   Eye-opener: Have you ever had a drink first thing in the morning to steady your nerves or get rid of a hangover?

teratogen, teratogenic: Any substance, such as alcohol, or condition, such as measles, that can cause damage to a fetus, resulting in deformed fetal structures. Alcohol causes birth defects and brain damage, resulting in neurobehavioral problems in exposed offspring.

tolerance: A state in which the body's tissue cells adjust to the presence of a drug, a state in which the body becomes used to the presence of a drug in given amounts and eventually fails to respond to ordinarily effective dosages. Hence, increasingly larger doses are necessary to produce desired effects.[1]

TWEAK: A screening tool for identifying pregnant women with alcohol problems. On the tolerance question, two points are given if a woman reports that she can consume more than five drinks without falling asleep or passing out. A positive response to the worry question yields two points and positive responses to the last three questions yield one point each. A score of two signals an at-risk drinker. TWEAK has been found to be highly sensitive in identifying women who are at-risk drinkers. The acronym stands for:

T   Tolerance: How many drinks can you hold?

W   Have close friends or relatives Worried or complained about your drinking in the past?

E   Eye-opener: Do you sometimes take a drink in the morning?

A   Amnesia: Has a friend or family member ever told you about things you said or did while you were drinking that you could not remember?

K(c) Do you sometimes feel the need to Cut Down on your drinking?

universal prevention: Strives to ensure that all members of society understand that a behavior, such as drinking alcohol during pregnancy, can have hazardous consequences. Mass media campaigns to the general public over radio and television are examples of universal prevention.

withdrawal: Symptoms that appear during the process of stopping the use of a drug that has been taken regularly.[1]

Chapter 63

Directory of Support Groups for Alcohol-Related Concerns

Mutual-Help Groups

Alcoholics Anonymous (AA)
AA World Services, Inc.
P.O. Box 459
New York, NY 10163
Phone: 212-870-3400
Website: http://www.aa.org

AA Online Intergroup
http://www.aa-intergroup.org

Moderation Management Network, Inc.
22 W. 27th St., 5th Fl.
New York, NY 10001
Phone: 212-871-0974
Website: http:www.moderation
.org
E-mail: mm@moderation.org

SMART Recovery
7304 Mentor Ave.
Suite F
Mentor, OH 44060
Toll-Free: 866-951-5357
Phone: 440-951-5357
Fax: 440-951-5358
Website: http://www
.smartrecovery.org

Women for Sobriety, Inc.
P.O. Box 618
Quakertown, PA 18951
Phone: 215-536-8026
Website: http://www
.womenforsobriety.org

This list is not inclusive of available support groups for individuals seeking assistance for alcohol-related concerns. All contact information was current in May 2010.

Groups for People with Co-Occurring Disorders

Double Trouble in Recovery, Inc.
P.O. Box 245055
Brooklyn, NY 11224
Phone: 718-373-2684
Website: http://www
.doubletroubleinrecovery.org
E-mail: information@
doubletroubleinrecovery.org

Dual Recovery Anonymous World Network, Inc.
P.O. Box 8107
Prairie Village, KS 66208
Phone: 913-991-2703
Website: http://www
.dualrecovery.org

Groups for Family and Friends

Al-Anon/Ala-Teen
1600 Corporate Landing Pkwy.
Virginia Beach, VA 23454
Phone: 757-563-1600
Fax: 757-563-1655
Website: http://www.al-anon
.alateen.org
E-mail: wso@al-anon.org

Adult Children of Alcoholics
World Service Organization
P.O. Box 3216
Torrance, CA 90510
Phone: 562-595-7831
Website: http://www
.adultchildren.org
E-mail: info@adultchildren.org

Co-Anon Family Groups World Services
P.O. Box 12722
Tucson, AZ 85732
Toll-Free National Referral Line:
800-347-8998
Toll-Free: 800-898-9985
Phone: 520-513-5028
Website: http://www.co-anon.org
E-mail: info@co-anon.org

National Association for Children of Alcoholics
11426 Rockville Pike, Suite 301
Rockville, MD 20852
Toll-Free: 888-554-2627
Phone: 301-468-0985
Fax: 301-468-0987
Website: http://www.nacoa.net
E-mail: nacoa@nacoa.org

Chapter 64

Directory of State Agencies for Substance Abuse Services

Alabama
Substance Abuse Services Div.
P.O. Box 301410
100 N. Union St.
Montgomery, AL 36130
Toll-Free: 800-367-0955
Phone: 334-242-3454
Fax: 334-242-0725
Website: http://www.mh
.alabama.gov

Alaska
Div. of Behavioral Health
Dept. of Health and Social
Services
350 Main St., Suite 214
P.O. Box 110620
Juneau, AK 99811
Phone: 907-465-3370
Fax: 907-465-2668
Website: http://www.hss.state
.ak.us

American Samoa
American Samoa Government
Dept. of Human and Social
Services
P.O. Box 997534
Pago Pago, AS 96799
Phone: 684-633-2609
Fax: 684-633-7449

Arizona
Div. of Behavioral Health
Services
Dept. of Health Services
150 N. 18th Ave., 2nd Fl.
Phoenix, AZ 85007
Toll-Free: 800-867-5808
Phone: 602-542-1025
Fax: 602-364-4558
Website: http://www.azdhs.gov

Excerpted from "Facility Locator," Substance Abuse and Mental Health Services Administration (SAMHSA). All contact information was verified as current in May 2010.

Arkansas
Office of Alcohol and Drug Abuse
Prevention
Div. of Behavioral Health
Services
305 S. Palm St.
Little Rock, AR 72205
Phone: 501-686-9866
Website: http://www.arkansas
.gov/dhs/dmhs/alco_drug_abuse
_prevention.htm

California
Dept. of Alcohol and Drug
Programs
1700 K Street
Sacramento, CA 95811
Toll-Free: 800-879-2772
Website: http://www.adp.ca
.gov/default.asp
E-mail: ResourceCenter
@adp.ca.gov

Colorado
Div. of Behavioral Health
Dept. of Human Services
3824 W. Princeton Circle
Denver, CO 80236
Phone: 303-866-7400
Fax: 303-866-7481
Website: http://www.cdhs.state
.co.us/adad

Connecticut
410 Capitol Ave.
P.O. Box 341431
Hartford, CT 06134
Toll-Free: 800-446-7348
Phone: 860-418-7000
TTY: 860-418-6707
Website: http://www.ct.gov/dmhas

Delaware
Alcohol and Drug Services
Div. of Substance Abuse and MH
1901 N. DuPont Hwy., Main Bldg.
New Castle, DE 19720
Phone: 302-255-9399
Fax: 302-255-4427
Website: http://www.dhss
.delaware.gov/dsamh/index.html

District of Columbia
Addiction, Prevention, and
Recovery Administration
1300 First St., NE
Washington, DC 20002
Phone: 202-727-8857
Fax: 202-777-0092
Website: http://www.dchealth
.dc.gov/doh

Florida
Substance Abuse Program Office
Dept. of Children and Families
1317 Winewood Blvd.
Building 1, Rm. 202
Tallahassee, FL 32399
Phone: 850-487-1111
Fax: 850-922-4996
Website: http://www.dcf.state.fl
.us/mentalhealth/sa

Georgia
Addictive Diseases Services
Two Peachtree St., NW
22nd Fl., Suite 22-273
Atlanta, GA 30303
Toll-Free: 800-715-4225
Phone: 404-657-2331
Fax: 404-657-2256
Website: http://mhddad.dhr
.georgia.gov

Guam

Drug and Alcohol Treatment
Services
Dept. of Mental Health and
Substance Abuse
790 Governor Carlos Camacho Rd.
Tamuning, GU 96913
Phone: 671-647-5330
Fax: 671-649-6948

Hawaii

Alcohol and Drug Abuse Division
Dept. of Health
601 Kamokila Blvd., Rm. 360
Kapolei, HI 96707
Phone: 808-692-7506
Fax: 808-692-7521
Website: http://hawaii.gov/health
/substance-abuse

Idaho

Div. of Behavioral Health
Dept. of Health and Welfare
450 W. State St., 3rd Fl.
P.O. Box 83720
Boise, ID 83720
Toll-Free: 800-926-2588
Phone: 208-334-5935
Fax: 208-332-7305
Website: http://
healthandwelfare.idaho.gov

Illinois

Div. of Alcoholism and Substance
Abuse
Dept. of Human Services
401 S. Clinton St.
Chicago, IL 60607
Toll-Free: 800-843-6154
Toll-Free TTY: 800-447-6404
Website: http://www.dhs.state.il
.us/page.aspx?item=29725

Indiana

Div. of Mental Health and
Addiction
Family and Social Services
Administration
402 W. Washington St., Rm. W353
Indianapolis, IN 46204
Toll-Free: 800-457-8283
Phone: 317-232-7895
Fax: 317-233-3472
Website: http://www.in.gov/fssa
/dmha/index.htm

Iowa

Div. of Behavioral Health
Dept. of Public Health
Lucas State Office Bldg.
321 East 12th St.
Des Moines, IA 50319
Toll-Free: 866-227-9878
Phone: 515-281-7689
Website: http://www.idph.state
.ia.us/bh/substance_abuse.asp

Kansas

Addiction and Prevention
Services
Dept. of Social and Rehab
Services
915 Harrison St.
Topeka, KS 66612
Phone: 785-296-6807
Website: http://www.srskansas
.org/hcp/AAPSHome.htm

Kentucky
Div. of Mental Health and
Substance Abuse
Dept. for MH/MR Services
100 Fair Oaks Lane, 4E-D
Frankfort, KY 40621
Phone: 502-564-4456
Fax: 502-564-9010
Website: http://mhmr.ky.gov
/mhsas

Louisiana
Office for Addictive Disorders
The Bienville Bldg.
628 N. 4th Street
P.O. Box 2790, Bin 18
Baton Rouge, LA 70821
Toll-Free: 877-664-2248
Phone: 225-342-6717
Fax: 225-342-3875
Website: http://www.dhh
.louisiana.gov/offices/?ID=23

Maine
Maine Office of Substance Abuse
41 Anthony Ave.
#11 State House Station
Augusta, ME 04333
Toll-Free (ME only): 800-499-0027
Toll-Free TTY: 800-606-0215
Phone: 207-287-2595
Fax: 207-287-8910
Website: http://www.maine.gov
/dhhs/osa
E-mail: osa.ircosa@maine.gov

Maryland
Alcohol and Drug Abuse
Administration
Dept. of Health and Mental
Hygiene
55 Wade Ave.
Catonsville, MD 21228
Phone: 410-402-8600
Website: http://dhmh.maryland
.gov/adaa
E-mail: adaainfo@dhmh.state
.md.us

Massachusetts
Bureau of Substance Abuse
Services
Dept. of Public Health
250 Washington St.
Boston, MA 02108
Toll-Free: 800-327-5050
Toll-Free TTY: 888-448-8321
Website: http://www.mass.gov
/dph/bsas

Michigan
Bureau of Substance Abuse and
Addiction Services
320 S. Walnut
Lansing, MI 48913
Phone: 517-373-4700
TTY: 571-373-3573
Fax: 517-335-2121
Website: http://www.michigan
.gov/mdch-bsaas
E-mail: MDCH-BSAAS@
michigan.gov

Minnesota
Alcohol and Drug Abuse Division
Dept. of Human Services
P.O. Box 64977
Saint Paul, MN 55164
Toll-Free Disability Linkage
Line: 866-333-2466
Phone: 651-431-2460
Fax: 651-431-7449
Website: http://www
.minnesotahelp.info/public
(online access to state resources)
Website: http://www.dhs.state
.mn.us (click Disabilities, then
Alcohol and Drug Abuse)
E-mail: dhs.adad@state.mn.us

Mississippi
Bureau of Alcohol and Drug
Abuse
Dept. of Mental Health
1101 Robert E Lee Bldg.
239 N. Lamar St.
Jackson, MS 39201
Toll-Free: 877-210-8513
Phone: 601-359-1288
Fax: 601-359-6295
TDD: 601-359-6230
Website: http://www.dmh.state
.ms.us/substance_abuse.htm

Missouri
Div. of Alcohol and Drug Abuse
Missouri Dept. of Mental Health
1706 East Elm St.
P.O. Box 687
Jefferson City, MO 65102
Toll-Free: 800-364-9687
Phone: 573-751-4122
TTY: 573-526-1201
Fax: 573-751-8224
Website: http://www.dmh
.missouri.gov/ada/adaindex.htm
E-mail: dmhmail@dmh.mo.gov

Montana
Addictive and Mental Disorders
Division
Dept. of PH and HS
555 Fuller Ave.
P.O. Box 202905
Helena, MT 59620
Phone: 406-444-3964
Fax: 406-444-4435
Website: http://www.dphhs.mt
.gov/amdd

Nebraska
DHHS Division of Behavioral
Health
P.O. Box 95026
Lincoln, NE 68509
Substance Abuse Hotline:
402-473-3818
Phone: 402-471-7818
Fax: 402-471-7859
Website: http://www.dhhs.ne.gov
/sua/suaindex.htm
E-mail: BHDivision@dhhs.ne.gov

Nevada
DHHS Mental Health and
Developmental Services
4126 Technology Way, 2nd Floor
Carson City, NV 89706
Phone: 775-684-5943
Fax: 775-684-5964
Website: http://mhds.state.nv.us

New Hampshire
DHHS Bureau of Drug and
Alcohol Services
105 Pleasant St.
Concord, NH 03301
Phone: 603-271-6110
Website: http://www.dhhs.state
.nh.us/dhhs/atod/a1-treatment

New Jersey
Div. of Addiction Services
P.O. Box 1004
Williamstown, NJ 08094
NJ Addictions Hotline:
800-238-2333
Website: http://www
.njdrughotline.org
E-mail: contact@
addictionshotlineofnj.org

New Mexico
Behavioral Health Services Div.
Dept. of Health
37 Plaza la Prensa
Santa Fe, NM 87507
Toll-Free Consumer Hotline:
866-660-7185
Toll-Free TTY Hotline:
800-855-2881
Website: http://www.bhc.state
.nm.us
Website for Consumer
Assistance: http://www
.optumhealthnewmexico.com

New York
Office of Alcoholism and
Substance Abuse Services
1450 Western Ave.
Albany, NY 12203
Phone: 518-473-3460
Website: http://www.oasas.state
.ny.us/index.cfm
E-mail: communications@oasas
.state.ny.us

North Carolina
Community Policy Management
Div. of MH/DD/SA Services
325 N. Salisbury St., Suite 679-C
3007 Mail Service Center
Raleigh, NC 27699
Toll-Free: 800-662-7030
Phone: 919-733-4670
Fax: 919-733-4556
Website: http://www.dhhs.state
.nc.us/mhddsas
E-mail: contactdmh@ncmail.net

North Dakota

Div. of MH and SA Services
Dept. of Human Services
600 E. Blvd. Ave., Dept. 325
Bismarck, ND 58505
Toll-Free (ND only):
800-472-2622
Phone: 701-328-2310
Fax: 701-328-2359
Website: http://www.nd.gov/dhs
/services/mentalhealth
E-mail: dhseo@nd.gov

Ohio

Dept. of Alcohol and Drug
Addiction Services
280 Plaza
280 N. High St., 12th Fl.
Columbus, OH 43215
Toll-Free: 800-788-7254
Phone: 614-466-3445
Fax: 614-752-8645
Website: http://www.ada.ohio
.gov/public
E-mail: info@ada.ohio.gov

Oklahoma

ODMHSAS
1200 NE 13th St.
P.O. Box 53277
Oklahoma City, OK 73152
Toll-Free: 800-522-9054
Phone: 405-522-3908
TDD: 405-522-3851
Fax: 405-522-3650
Website: http://www.odmhsas
.org

Oregon

Addictions and Mental Health
Div.
Dept. of Human Services
500 Summer St. NE E86
Salem, OR 97301
Toll-Free: 800-544-7078
Toll-Free TTY: 800-375-2863
Phone: 503-945-5763
Fax: 503-378-8467
Website: http://www.oregon.gov
/DHS/addiction/index.shtml
E-mail: omhas.web@state.or.us

Pennsylvania

Bureau of Drug and Alcohol
Programs
Pennsylvania Dept. of Health
02 Kline Plaza, Suite B
Harrisburg, PA 17104
Toll-Free: 877-724-3258
Phone: 717-783-8200
Fax: 717-787-6285
Website: http://www.portal
.state.pa.us/portal/server.pt
/community/drug___alcohol
/14221

Puerto Rico

Mental Health and
Anti-Addiction Services
Administration
P.O. Box 21414
San Juan, PR 00928
Toll-Free 800-981-0023
Phone: 787-763-7575
Fax: 787-765-5888
Website: http://www.gobierno
.pr/assmca/inicio

Rhode Island

Div. of Behavioral Health
14 Harrington Rd.
Cranston, RI 02920
Phone: 401-462-4680
Fax: 401-462-6078
Website: http://www.mhrh.ri
.gov/SA

South Carolina

SC Dept. of Alcohol and Other
Drug Abuse Services
101 Executive Ctr. Dr., Suite 215
Columbia, SC 29210
Phone: 803-896-5555
Fax: 803-896-5557
Website: http://www.daodas.state
.sc.us

South Dakota

DHS Div. of Alcohol and Drug
Abuse
3800 E. Hwy. 34, Hillsview Plaza
500 E. Capitol Ave.
Pierre, SD 57501
Toll-Free: 800-265-9684
Phone: 605-773-3123
Fax: 605-773-7076
Website: http://dhs.sd.gov
E-mail: infodada@dhs.state.sd.us

Tennessee

Dept. of Mental Health and DD
TN Dept. of Health
425 Fifth Ave. N.
Cordell Hull Bldg., 1st Fl
Nashville, TN 37243
Toll-Free Crisis: 800-809-9957
Phone: 615-741-3111
Website: http://health.state.tn
.us/index.htm
E-mail: tn.health@tn.gov

Texas

DSHS Substance Abuse Services
P. O. Box 149347
Austin, TX 78714
Toll-Free: 866-378-8440
Toll-Free Hotline: 877-966-3784
Phone: 512-206-5000
Fax: 512-206-5714
Website: http://www.dshs.state.tx
.us/sa/default.shtm
E-mail: contact@dshs.state.tx.us

Utah

Div. of Substance Abuse and
Mental Health
Utah Dept. of Human Services
195 N. 1950 W.
Salt Lake City, UT 84116
Phone: 801-538-3939
Fax: 801-538-9892
Website: http://www.dsamh.utah
.gov
E-mail: dsamhwebmaster@utah
.gov

Vermont

Alcohol and Drug Abuse
Programs
Dept. of Health
108 Cherry St.
Burlington, VT 05402
Toll-Free (VT only):
800-464-4343
Phone: 802-863-7200
Fax: 802-865-7754
Website: http://healthvermont
.gov/adap/adap.aspx
E-mail: vtadap@vdh.state.vt.us

Virginia
Office of Substance Abuse
Services
Dept. of MH, MR, and SAS
P.O. Box 1797
Richmond, VA 23218
Phone: 804-786-3921
TTY: 804-786-1587
Fax: 804-371-6638
Website: http://www.dbhds
.virginia.gov/OSAS-default.htm

Virgin Islands
Div of MH, Alcoholism, and Drug
Dependency Services
Dept. of Health
Barbel Plaza, 2nd Fl.
Christiansted, VI 00820
Phone: 340-774-4888
Fax: 340-774-4701

Washington
Div. of Alcohol and Substance
Abuse
Dept. of Social and Health
Services
P.O. Box 45130
Olympia, WA 98504
Toll-Free (WA only):
800-737-0617
Phone: 877-301-4557
Website: http://www.dshs.wa
.gov/DASA
E-mail: DASAInformation@
shs.wa.gov

West Virginia
Bureau for Behavioral Health
and Health Facilities
350 Capitol St., Rm. 350
Charleston, WV 25301
Phone: 304-558-0627
Fax: 304-558-1008
Website: http://www.wvdhhr
.org/bhhf/ada.asp
E-mail: obhs@wvdhhr.org

Wisconsin
Bureau of Prevention,
Treatment, and Recovery
1 W. Wilson St.
P.O. Box 7851
Madison, WI 53707
Phone: 608-266-1865
Toll-Free TTY: 888-701-1251
Fax: 608-266-1533
Website: http://dhs.wisconsin.gov
/substabuse/INDEX.HTM

Wyoming
Mental Health and Substance
Abuse Services Division
6101 Yellowstone Rd., Suite 220
Cheyenne, WY 82002
Toll-Free: 800-535-4006
Phone: 307-777-6494
Fax: 307-777-5849
Website: http://wdh.state.wy.us
/mhsa/index.html

Chapter 65

Directory of Organizations with Information about Alcohol Use and Abuse

Government Organizations

Alcohol Policy Information System (NIAAA)
Website: http://www
.alcoholpolicy.niaaa.nih.gov

Center for Substance Abuse Treatment (SAMHSA)
Toll-Free: 800-662-4357
Toll-Free TDD: 800-487-4889
Phone: 240-276-2750
Website: http://csat.samhsa.gov

Centers for Disease Control and Prevention (CDC)
1600 Clifton Rd.
Atlanta, GA 30333
Toll-Free: 800-CDC-INFO
(232-4636)
Toll-Free TTY: 888-232-6348
Website: http://www.cdc.gov
E-mail: cdcinfo@cdc.gov

Division of Workplace Programs (SAMHSA)
Toll-Free: 800-843-4971
Website: http://www.workplace
.samhsa.gov

Resources in this chapter were compiled from several sources deemed reliable; all contact information was verified and updated in May 2010.

FASD Center for Excellence (SAMHSA)
2101 Gaither Rd., Suite 600
Rockville, MD 20850
Toll-Free: 866-STOPFAS
(786-7327)
Website: http://www.fasdcenter
.samhsa.gov
E-mail: fasdcenter@samhsa.hhs
.gov

Health Information Network (SAMHSA)
P.O. Box 2345
Rockville, MD 20847
Toll-Free: 877-726-4727
Toll-Free TTY: 800-487-4889
Fax: 240-221-4292
Website: http://www.samhsa.gov
/shin
E-mail: SHIN@samhsa.hhs.gov

National Clearinghouse for Alcohol and Drug Information (NCADI)
Toll-Free: 800-729-6686
Toll-Free TDD: 800-487-4889
Website: http://ncadi.samhsa.gov

National Digestive Diseases Information Clearinghouse
2 Information Way
Bethesda, MD 20892
Toll-Free: 800-891-5389
Toll-Free TTY: 866-569-1162
Fax: 703-738-4929
Website: http://digestive.niddk
.nih.gov
E-mail: nddic@info.niddk.nih.gov

National Drug and Treatment Referral Routing Service
Toll-Free: 800-662-4357

National Heart, Lung, and Blood Institute (NHLBI)
Health Information Center
P.O. Box 30105
Bethesda, MD 20824
Phone: 301-592-8573
TTY:240-629-3255
Fax: 240-629-3246
Website: http://nhlbi.nih.gov
E-mail: nhlbiinfo@nhlbi.nih.gov

National Highway Traffic Safety Administration (NHTSA)
1200 New Jersey Ave., SE
West Building
Washington, DC 20590
Toll-Free: 888-327-4236
Toll-Free TTY: 800-424-9153
Website: http://www
.stopimpaireddriving.org

National Institute of Arthritis and Musculoskeletal and Skin Diseases (NIAMS)
1 AMS Circle
Bethesda, MD 20892
Toll Free: 877-22-NIAMS
(226-4267)
Phone: 301-495-4484
TTY: 301-565-2966
Fax: 301-718-6366
Website: http://www.niams.nih
.gov
E-mail: NIAMSinfo@mail.nih.gov

National Institute of Environmental Health Sciences (NIEHS)

P.O. Box 12233, MD K3-16
Research Triangle Park
NC 27709
Phone: 919-541-3345
Fax: 919-541-4395
Website: http://www.niehs.nih.gov

National Institute of Neurological Disorders and Stroke (NINDS)

P.O. Box 5801
Bethesda, MD 20824
Toll-Free: 800-352-9424
Phone: 301-496-5751
TTY: 301-468-5981
Website: http://www.ninds.nih
.gov

National Institute on Alcohol Abuse and Alcoholism (NIAAA)

5635 Fishers Ln., MSC 9304
Bethesda, MD 20892
Phone: 301-443-3860
Website: http://www.niaaa.nih.gov
E-mail: niaaaweb-r@exchange
.nih.gov

National Institute on Drug Abuse (NIDA)

6001 Executive Blvd., Rm. 5213
Bethesda, MD 20892
Phone: 301-443-1124
Fax: 301-443-7397
Websites: http://www.nida.nih
.gov; and http://www.drugabuse
.gov
E-mail: information@nida.nih.gov

National Mental Health Information Center

Substance Abuse and Mental
Health Services Administration
P.O. Box 2345
Rockville, MD 20847
Toll-Free: 800-789-2647
Toll-Free TDD: 866-889-2647
Phone: 240-221-4021
Fax: 240-221-4295
Website: http://mentalhealth
.samhsa.gov
E-mail: info@mentalhealth.org

Office of Applied Studies (OAS) (SAMHSA)

Phone: 240-276-1212
Website: http://www.oas.samhsa
.gov
E-mail: oaspubs@samhsa.hhs
.gov

Office of National Drug Control Policy (ONDCP)

Drug Policy Information
Clearinghouse
P.O. Box 6000
Rockville, MD 20849
Toll-Free: 800-666-3332
Fax: 301-519-5212
Website: http://www
.whitehousedrugpolicy.gov
E-mail: ondcp@ncjrs.gov

Stop Underage Drinking Portal of Federal Resources

Website: http://www
.stopalcoholabuse.gov

Substance Abuse and Mental Health Services Administration (SAMHSA)
1 Choke Cherry Rd.
Rockville, MD 20857
Phone: 240-276-2130
Websites: http://www
.samhsa.gov; http://www
.underagedrinking.samhsa
.gov/default.aspx

Substance Abuse Treatment Facility Locator
Toll-Free: 800-662-4357
Toll-Free TDD: 800-487-4889
Website: http://dasis3.samhsa
.gov

U.S. Food and Drug Administration (FDA)
10903 New Hampshire Ave.
Silver Spring, MD 20993
Toll-Free: 888-INFO-FDA
(463-6332)
Website: http://www.fda.gov

Private Organizations

ADDICTIONSand RECOVERY.org
208 Bloor St. W., Suite 702
Toronto, ON
Canada, M5S 3B4
Phone: 416-920-2982
Website: http://www
.addictionsandrecovery.org

Adult Children of Alcoholics
World Service Organization
P.O. Box 3216
Torrance, CA 90510
Phone: 562-595-7831
Website: http://www
.adultchildren.org
E-mail: info@adultchildren.org

Alcoholics Anonymous (AA)
AA World Services, Inc.
P.O. Box 459
New York, NY 10163
Phone: 212-870-3400
Website: http://www.aa.org

Al-Anon/Ala-Teen
1600 Corporate Landing Pkwy.
Virginia Beach, VA 23454
Phone: 757-563-1600
Fax: 757-563-1655
Website: http://www.al-anon
.alateen.org
E-mail: wso@al-anon.org

American Heart Association
7272 Greenville Ave.
Dallas, TX 75231
Toll-Free: 800-242-8721
Website: http://www.heart.org

American Institute for Cancer Research

1759 R St., NW
Washington, DC 20009
Toll-Free: 800-843-8114
Phone: 202-328-7744
Fax: 202-328-7226
Website: http://www.aicr.org
E-mail: aicrweb@aicr.org

American Liver Foundation

75 Maiden Lane, Suite 603
New York, NY 10038
Phone: 212-668-1000
Fax: 212-483-8179
Website: http://www
.liverfoundation.org

Anxiety Disorders Association of America

8730 Georgia Ave.
Silver Spring, MD 20910
Phone: 240-485-1001
Website: http://www.adaa.org

Center of Alcohol Studies

Rutgers, the State University of
New Jersey
607 Allison Rd.
Piscataway, NJ 08854
Phone: 732-445-2190
Fax: 732-445-5300
Website: http://www
.alcoholstudies.rutgers.edu

Center on Alcohol Marketing and Youth (CAMY)

Johns Hopkins University
Rm. 292
624 N. Broadway
Baltimore, MD 21205
Phone: 410-502-6579
Website: http://camy.org
E-mail: info@camy.org

Co-Anon Family Groups World Services

P.O. Box 12722
Tucson, AZ 85732
Toll-Free National Referral Line:
800-347-8998
Toll-Free: 800-898-9985
Phone: 520-513-5028
Website: http://www.co-anon.org
E-mail: info@co-anon.org

Do It Now Foundation

P.O. Box 27568
Tempe, AZ 85285
Phone: 480-736-0599
Fax: 480-736-0771
Website: http://www.doitnow.org
E-mail: email@doitnow.org

Higher Education Center for Alcohol and Other Drug Abuse and Violence Prevention

Education Development Center,
Inc.
55 Chapel St.
Newton, MA 02458
Toll-Free: 800-676-1730
Fax: 617-928-1537
Website: http://www
.higheredcenter.org
E-mail: HigherEdCtr@edc.org

International Center for Alcohol Policies (ICAP)
1519 New Hampshire Ave., NW
Washington, DC 20036
Phone: 202-986-1159
Fax: 202-986-2080
Website: http://www.icap.org
E-mail: info@icap.org

Marin Institute
24 Belvedere St.
San Rafael, CA 94901
Phone: 415-456-5692
Fax: 415-456-0491
Website: http://www
.MarinInstitute.org

Mothers Against Drunk Driving (MADD)
National Office
511 E. John Carpenter Fwy.
Suite 700
Irving, TX 75062
Toll-Free: 800-GET-MADD
(438-6233)
Phone: 214-744-6233
Victim Services 24-Hour Help
Line: 877-MADD-HELP
(623-3435)
Fax: 972-869-2206
Website: http://www.madd.org

National Association for Children of Alcoholics
11426 Rockville Pike, Suite 301
Rockville, MD 20852
Toll-Free: 888-554-2627
Phone: 301-468-0985
Fax: 301-468-0987
Website: http://www.nacoa.net
E-mail: nacoa@nacoa.org

National Association of Addiction Treatment Providers
313 W. Liberty St., Suite 129
Lancaster, PA 17603
Phone: 717-392-8480
Fax: 717-392-8481
Website: http://www.naatp.org
E-mail: rhunsicker@naatp.org

National Center on Addiction and Substance Abuse at Columbia University (CASA)
633 Third Ave., 19th Fl.
New York, NY 10017
Phone: 212-841-5200
Fax: 212-956-8020
Website: http://www
.casacolumbia.org

National Council on Alcoholism and Drug Dependence
244 East 58th St., 4th Fl.
New York, NY 10022
Toll-Free Hope Line: 800-NCA-CALL (622-2255)
Phone: 212-269-7797
Fax: 212-269-7510
Website: http://www.ncadd.org
E-mail: national@ncadd.org

National Organization on Fetal Alcohol Syndrome (NOFAS)

1200 Eton Ct., NW, Third Floor
Washington, DC, 20007
Toll-Free: 800-66-NOFAS (66327)
Phone: 202-785-4585
Fax: 202-466-6456
Website: http://nofas.org
E-mail: information@nofas.org

National Parents Resource Institute for Drug Education (PRIDE)

PRIDE Youth Programs
4 W. Oak St.
Fremont, MI 49412
Toll-Free: 800-668-9277
Phone: 231-924-1662
Fax: 231-924-5663
Website: http://www
.prideyouthprograms.org
E-mail: info@pridyouthprograms
.org

Nemours Foundation

1600 Rockland Rd.
Wilmington, DE 19803
Phone: 302-651-4046
Website: http://www.kidshealth
.org
E-mail: info@kidshealth.org

Partnership for a Drug-Free America

405 Lexington Ave., Suite 1601
New York, NY 10174
Phone: 212-922-1560
Fax: 212-922-1570
Website: http://www
.drugfreeamerica.org

SMART Recovery

7304 Mentor Ave., Suite F
Mentor, OH 44060
Toll-Free: 866-951-5357
Phone: 440-951-5357
Fax: 440-951-5358
Website: http://www
.smartrecovery.org

Students Against Destructive Decisions (SADD)

255 Main Street
Marlborough, MA 01752
Toll-Free: 877-SADD-INC
(7233-462)
Fax: 508-481-5759
Website: http://www.sadd.org
E-mail: info@sadd.org

Women for Sobriety, Inc.

P.O. Box 618
Quakertown, PA 18951
Phone: 215-536-8026
Fax: 215-538-9026
Website: http://www
.womenforsobriety.org

World Health Organization

Avenue Appia 20
1211 Geneva 27
Switzerland
Telephone: 41-22-791-21-11
Fax: 41-22-791-31-11
Website: http://www.who.int
E-mail: info@who.int

Index

Index

Page numbers followed by 'n' indicate a footnote. Page numbers in *italics* indicate a table or illustration.

A

AA *see* Alcoholics Anonymous
"The ABCs of BAC" (NHTSA) 178n
abstinence (alcohol), defined 551
abuser, defined 551
acamprosate
  alcohol dependence 372–73
  described 511
acetaldehyde
  alcohol metabolism 78
  described 74, 371–72
  hangover 189
acetylcholine, alcohol addiction 75
acute liver failure, described 208
acute pancreatitis, described 255–56
acute respiratory distress syndrome (ARDS), alcohol use 238–39
A.D.A.M., Inc., publications
  alcoholic neuropathy 231n
  delirium tremens 502n
  Wernicke-Korsakoff syndrome 199n
addiction
  defined 551
  overview 60–67

ADDICTIONSandRECOVERY.org, contact information 574
adolescents
  alcohol-related problems 39
  alcohol use 111–14
  brain changes 65–66, 197–99
  brain development 110, 112–13
  substance abuse disorders 116–27
  substance use prevention messages 158–61
  underage drinking 85–92
  women 45
"Adolescents at Risk for Substance Abuse Disorders" (NIAAA) 116n
"Adopting and Fostering Children with Fetal Alcohol Spectrum Disorders" (SAMHSA) 329n
adoption, fetal alcohol spectrum disorders 329–32
adrenaline, withdrawal 498
Adult Children of Alcoholics, contact information 560, 574
advertising
  alcohol use 100–105
  underage drinking 164–66
African Americans, alcohol use 20–21
age factor
  alcohol dependence 28–29, *86*
  alcohol-related problems 38–41

581

Health Reference Series

Complete Catalog

List price $93 per volume. School and library price $84 per volume.

Adolescent Health Sourcebook, 3rd Edition

Basic Consumer Health Information about Adolescent Growth and Development, Puberty, Sexuality, Reproductive Health, and Physical, Emotional, Social, and Mental Health Concerns of Teens and Their Parents, Including Facts about Nutrition, Physical Activity, Weight Management, Acne, Allergies, Cancer, Diabetes, Growth Disorders, Juvenile Arthritis, Infections, Substance Abuse, and More

Along with Information about Adolescent Safety Concerns, Youth Violence, a Glossary of Related Terms, and a Directory of Resources

Edited by Amy L. Sutton. 600 pages. 2010. 978-0-7808-1140-9.

Adult Health Concerns Sourcebook

Basic Consumer Health Information about Medical and Mental Concerns of Adults, Including Facts about Choosing Healthcare Providers, Navigating Insurance Options, Maintaining Wellness, Preventing Cancer, Heart Disease, Stroke, Diabetes, and Osteoporosis, and Understanding Aging-Related Health Concerns, Including Menopause, Cognitive Changes, and Changes in the Coronary and Vascular Systems

Along with Tips on Caring for Aging Parents and Dealing with Health-Related Work and Travel Issues, a Glossary, and a Directory of Resources for Additional Help and Information

Edited by Sandra J. Judd. 648 pages. 2008. 978-0-7808-0999-4.

"Provides a thorough list of topics that are important to adult health and for caregivers."
—CHOICE, Nov '08

"Written in easy-to-understand language... the content is well-organized and is intended to aid adults in making health care-related decisions."
—AORN Journal, Dec '08

AIDS Sourcebook, 4th Edition

Basic Consumer Health Information about Human Immunodeficiency Virus (HIV) and Acquired Immunodeficiency Syndrome (AIDS), Featuring Updated Statistics and Facts about Risks, Prevention, Screening, Diagnosis, Treatments, Side Effects, and Complications, and Including a Section about the Impact of HIV/AIDS on the Health of Women, Children, and Adolescents

Along with Tips on Managing Life with AIDS, Reports on Current Research Initiatives and Clinical Trials, a Glossary of Related Terms, and Resource Directories for Further Help and Information

Edited by Ivy L. Alexander. 680 pages. 2008. 978-0-7808-0997-0.

SEE ALSO Contagious Diseases Sourcebook, 2nd Edition

Alcoholism Sourcebook, 3rd Edition

Basic Consumer Health Information about Alcohol Use, Abuse, and Dependence, Featuring Facts about the Physical, Mental, and Social Health Effects of Alcohol Addiction, Including Alcoholic Liver Disease, Pancreatic Disease, Cardiovascular Disease, Neurological Disorders, and the Effects of Drinking during Pregnancy

Along with Information about Alcohol Treatment, Medications, and Recovery Programs, in Addition to Tips for Reducing the Prevalence of Underage Drinking, Statistics about Alcohol Use, a Glossary of Related Terms, and Directories of Resources for More Help and Information

Edited by Joyce Brennfleck Shannon. 600 pages. 2010. 978-0-7808-1141-6.

SEE ALSO Drug Abuse Sourcebook, 3rd Edition

Allergies Sourcebook, 3rd Edition

Basic Consumer Health Information about Allergic Disorders, Such as Anaphylaxis, Hives,

Eczema, Rhinitis, Sinusitis, and Conjunctivitis, and Their Triggers, Including Pollen, Mold, Dust Mites, Animal Dander, Insects, Chemicals, Food, Food Additives, and Medications

Along with Advice about the Diagnosis and Treatment of Allergy Symptoms, a Glossary of Related Terms, a Directory of Resources for Help and Information, and Suggestions for Additional Reading

Edited by Amy L. Sutton. 588 pages. 2007. 978-0-7808-0950-5.

SEE ALSO Asthma Sourcebook, 2nd Edition

Alzheimer Disease Sourcebook, 4th Edition

Basic Consumer Health Information about Alzheimer Disease, Other Dementias, and Related Disorders, Including Multi-Infarct Dementia, Dementia with Lewy Bodies, Frontotemporal Dementia (Pick Disease), Wernicke-Korsakoff Syndrome (Alcohol-Related Dementia), AIDS Dementia Complex, Huntington Disease, Creutzfeldt-Jacob Disease, and Delirium

Along with Information about Coping with Memory Loss and Forgetfulness, Maintaining Skills, and Long-Term Planning for People with Dementia, and Suggestions Addressing Common Caregiver Concerns, Updated Information about Current Research Efforts, a Glossary of Related Terms, and Directories of Sources for Additional Help and Information

Edited by Karen Bellenir. 603 pages. 2008. 978-0-7808-1001-3.

"An invaluable resource for persons who have received a diagnosis, for caregivers, and for family members dealing with this insidious disease. It is recommended for public, community college, and ready-reference sections in academic libraries."
—American Reference Books Annual, 2009

SEE ALSO Brain Disorders Sourcebook, 3rd Edition

Arthritis Sourcebook, 3rd Edition

Basic Consumer Health Information about the Risk Factors, Symptoms, Diagnosis, and Treatment of Osteoarthritis, Rheumatoid Arthritis, Juvenile Arthritis, Gout, Infectious Arthritis, and Autoimmune Disorders Associated with Arthritis

Along with Facts about Medications, Surgeries, and Self-Care Techniques to Manage Pain and Disability, Tips on Living with Arthritis, a Glossary of Related Terms, and Resources for Additional Help and Information

Edited by Amy L. Sutton. 600 pages. 2010. 978-0-7808-1077-8.

Asthma Sourcebook, 2nd Edition

Basic Consumer Health Information about the Causes, Symptoms, Diagnosis, and Treatment of Asthma in Infants, Children, Teenagers, and Adults, Including Facts about Different Types of Asthma, Common Co-Occurring Conditions, Asthma Management Plans, Triggers, Medications, and Medication Delivery Devices

Along with Asthma Statistics, Research Updates, a Glossary, a Directory of Asthma-Related Resources, and More

Edited by Karen Bellenir. 581 pages. 2006. 978-0-7808-0866-9.

SEE ALSO Lung Disorders Sourcebook; Respiratory Disorders Sourcebook, 2nd Edition

Attention Deficit Disorder Sourcebook

Basic Consumer Health Information about Attention Deficit/Hyperactivity Disorder in Children and Adults, Including Facts about Causes, Symptoms, Diagnostic Criteria, and Treatment Options Such as Medications, Behavior Therapy, Coaching, and Homeopathy

Along with Reports on Current Research Initiatives, Legal Issues, and Government Regulations, and Featuring a Glossary of Related Terms, Internet Resources, and a List of Additional Reading Material

Edited by Dawn D. Matthews. 447 pages. 2002. 978-0-7808-0624-5.

"Recommended reference source."
—Booklist, Jan '03

SEE ALSO Learning Disabilities Sourcebook, 3rd Edition

Autism and Pervasive Developmental Disorders Sourcebook

Basic Consumer Health Information about Autism Spectrum and Pervasive Developmental Disorders, Such as Classical Autism, Asperger Syndrome, Rett Syndrome, and Childhood Disintegrative Disorder, Including Information about Related Genetic Disorders and Medical Problems and Facts about Causes, Screening Methods, Diagnostic Criteria, Treatments and Interventions, and Family and Education Issues

Along with a Glossary of Related Terms, Tips for Evaluating the Validity of Health Claims, and a Directory of Resources for Additional Help and Information

Edited by Sandra J. Judd. 603 pages. 2007. 978-0-7808-0953-6.

"This book provides a current overview of disorders on the autism spectrum and information about various therapies, educational resources, and help for families with practical issues such as workplace adjustments, living arrangements, and estate planning. It is a useful resource for public and consumer health libraries."
—*American Reference Books Annual, 2009*

SEE ALSO Learning Disabilities Sourcebook, 3rd Edition

Back and Neck Disorders Sourcebook, 2nd Edition

Basic Consumer Health Information about Spinal Pain, Spinal Cord Injuries, and Related Disorders, Such as Degenerative Disk Disease, Osteoarthritis, Scoliosis, Sciatica, Spina Bifida, and Spinal Stenosis, and Featuring Facts about Maintaining Spinal Health, Self-Care, Pain Management, Rehabilitative Care, Chiropractic Care, Spinal Surgeries, and Complementary Therapies

Along with Suggestions for Preventing Back and Neck Pain, a Glossary of Related Terms, and a Directory of Resources

Edited by Amy L. Sutton. 607 pages. 2004. 978-0-7808-0738-9.

"Recommended... An easy to use, comprehensive medical reference book."
—*E-Streams, Sep '05*

"For anyone who has back or neck problems, this book is ideal. Its easy-to-understand language and variety of topics makes this sourcebook a worthwhile read. The price... is reasonable for the amount of information contained in the book"
—*Occupational Therapy in Health Care, 2007*

Blood & Circulatory Disorders Sourcebook, 3rd Edition

Basic Consumer Health Information about Blood and Circulatory System Disorders, Such as Anemia, Leukemia, Lymphoma, Rh Disease, Hemophilia, Thrombophilia, Other Bleeding and Clotting Deficiencies, and Artery, Vascular, and Venous Diseases, Including Facts about Blood Types, Blood Donation, Bone Marrow and Stem Cell Transplants, Tests and Medications, and Tips for Maintaining Circulatory Health

Along with a Glossary of Related Terms and a List of Resources for Additional Help and Information

Edited by Sandra J. Judd. 600 pages. 2010. 978-0-7808-1081-5.

SEE ALSO Leukemia Sourcebook

Brain Disorders Sourcebook, 3rd Edition

Basic Consumer Health Information about Acquired and Traumatic Brain Injuries, Brain Tumors, Cerebral Palsy and Other Genetic and Congenital Brain Disorders, Infections of the Brain, Epilepsy, and Degenerative Neurological Disorders Such as Dementia, Huntington Disease, and Amyotrophic Lateral Sclerosis (ALS)

Along with Information on Brain Structure and Function, Treatment and Rehabilitation Options, a Glossary of Terms Related to Brain Disorders, and a Directory of Resources for More Information

Edited by Joyce Brennfleck Shannon. 600 pages. 2010. 978-0-7808-1083-9.

SEE ALSO Alzheimer Disease Sourcebook, 4th Edition

Breast Cancer Sourcebook, 3rd Edition

Basic Consumer Health Information about Breast Health and Breast Cancer, Including Facts about Environmental, Genetic, and Other Risk Factors, Prevention Efforts, Screening and Diagnostic Methods, Surgical Treatment Options and Other Care Choices, Complementary and Alternative Therapies, and Post-Treatment Concerns

Along with Statistical Data, News about Research Advances, a Glossary of Related Terms, and Directories of Resources for Additional Information and Support

Edited by Karen Bellenir. 606 pages. 2009. 978-0-7808-1030-3.

"A very useful reference for people wanting to learn more about breast cancer and how to negotiate their care or the care of a loved one. The third edition is necessary as information/treatment options continue to evolve."
—*Doody's Review Service, 2009*

SEE ALSO Cancer Sourcebook for Women, 3rd Edition, Women's Health Concerns Sourcebook, 3rd Edition

Breastfeeding Sourcebook

Basic Consumer Health Information about the Benefits of Breastmilk, Preparing to Breastfeed, Breastfeeding as a Baby Grows, Nutrition, and More, Including Information on Special Situations and Concerns Such as Mastitis, Illness, Medications, Allergies, Multiple Births, Prematurity, Special Needs, and Adoption

Along with a Glossary and Resources for Additional Help and Information

Edited by Jenni Lynn Colson. 367 pages. 2002. 978-0-7808-0332-9.

SEE ALSO Pregnancy and Birth Sourcebook, 3rd Edition

Burns Sourcebook

Basic Consumer Health Information about Various Types of Burns and Scalds, Including Flame, Heat, Cold, Electrical, Chemical, and Sun Burns

Along with Information on Short-Term and Long-Term Treatments, Tissue Reconstruction, Plastic Surgery, Prevention Suggestions, and First Aid

Edited by Allan R. Cook. 604 pages. 1999. 978-0-7808-0204-9.

"This is an exceptional addition to the series and is highly recommended for all consumer health collections, hospital libraries, and academic medical centers."
—*E-Streams, Mar '00*

"This key reference guide is an invaluable addition to all health care and public libraries in confronting this ongoing health issue."
—*American Reference Books Annual, 2000*

SEE ALSO Dermatological Disorders Sourcebook, 2nd Edition

Cancer Sourcebook, 5th Edition

Basic Consumer Health Information about Major Forms and Stages of Cancer, Featuring Facts about Head and Neck Cancers, Lung Cancers, Gastrointestinal Cancers, Genitourinary Cancers, Lymphomas, Blood Cell Cancers, Endocrine Cancers, Skin Cancers, Bone Cancers, Metastatic Cancers, and More

Along with Facts about Cancer Treatments, Cancer Risks and Prevention, a Glossary of Related Terms, Statistical Data, and a Directory of Resources for Additional Information

Edited by Karen Bellenir. 1105 pages. 2007. 978-0-7808-0947-5.

"The 5th, updated edition of Cancer Sourcebook should be in every public and health lending library collection... An unparalleled discussion essential for any health collections considering an all-in-one basic general reference."
—*California Bookwatch, Aug '07*

SEE ALSO Breast Cancer Sourcebook, 3rd Edition, Cancer Survivorship Sourcebook, Leukemia Sourcebook

Cancer Sourcebook for Women, 4th Edition

Basic Consumer Health Information about Gynecologic Cancers and Other Cancers of Special Concern to Women, Including Cancers of the Breast, Cervix, Colon, Lung, Ovaries, Thyroid, and Uterus

Along with Facts about Benign Conditions of the Female Reproductive System, Cancer Risk

Factors, Diagnostic and Treatment Procedures, Side Effects of Cancer and Cancer Treatments, Women's Issues in Cancer Survivorship, a Glossary of Related Terms, and a Directory of Resources for Additional Help and Information

Edited by Karen Bellenir. 600 pages. 2010. 978-0-7808-1139-3.

SEE ALSO Breast Cancer Sourcebook, 3rd Edition, Women's Health Concerns Sourcebook, 3rd Edition

Cancer Survivorship Sourcebook

Basic Consumer Health Information about the Physical, Educational, Emotional, Social, and Financial Needs of Cancer Patients from Diagnosis, through Cancer Treatment, and Beyond, Including Facts about Researching Specific Types of Cancer and Learning about Clinical Trials and Treatment Options, and Featuring Tips for Coping with the Side Effects of Cancer Treatments and Adjusting to Life after Cancer Treatment Concludes

Along with Suggestions for Caregivers, Friends, and Family Members of Cancer Patients, a Glossary of Cancer Care Terms, and Directories of Related Resources

Edited by Karen Bellenir. 633 pages. 2007. 978-0-7808-0985-7.

"Well organized and comprehensive in coverage, the book speaks to issues encountered both during and after cancer treatment. Recommended for consumer health and public libraries."
—*Library Journal, Aug 1 '07*

"Cancer Survivorship Sourcebook will be useful to anyone who has a friend or loved one with a cancer diagnosis."
—*American Reference Books Annual, 2008*

SEE ALSO *Cancer Sourcebook, 5th Edition, Disease Management Sourcebook*

Cardiovascular Disorders Sourcebook, 4th Edition

Basic Consumer Health Information about Heart and Blood Vessel Diseases and Disorders, Such as Angina, Heart Attack, Heart Failure, Cardiomyopathy, Arrhythmias, Valve Disease, Atherosclerosis, Aneurysms, and

Congenital Heart Defects, Including Information about Cardiovascular Disease in Women, Men, Children, Adolescents, and Minorities

Along with Facts about Diagnosing, Managing, and Preventing Cardiovascular Disease, a Glossary of Related Medical Terms, and a Directory of Resources for Additional Information

Edited by Amy L. Sutton. 600 pages. 2010. 978-0-7808-1080-8.

Caregiving Sourcebook

Basic Consumer Health Information for Caregivers, Including a Profile of Caregivers, Caregiving Responsibilities and Concerns, Tips for Specific Conditions, Care Environments, and the Effects of Caregiving

Along with Facts about Legal Issues, Financial Information, and Future Planning, a Glossary, and a Listing of Additional Resources

Edited by Joyce Brennfleck Shannon. 583 pages. 2001. 978-0-7808-0331-2.

"Essential for most collections."
—*Library Journal, Apr 1 '02*

"An ideal addition to the reference collection of any public library. Health sciences information professionals may also want to acquire the Caregiving Sourcebook for their hospital or academic library for use as a ready reference tool by health care workers interested in aging and caregiving."
—*E-Streams, Jan '02*

Child Abuse Sourcebook, 2nd Edition

Basic Consumer Health Information about the Physical, Sexual, and Emotional Abuse of Children, Neglect, Münchhausen Syndrome by Proxy (MSBP), and Shaken Baby Syndrome, and Featuring Facts about Withholding Medical Care, Corporal Punishment, Child Maltreatment in Youth Sports, and Parental Substance Abuse

Along with Information about Child Protective Services, Foster Care, Adoption, Parenting Challenges, Abuse Prevention Programs, and Intervention, Treatment, and Recovery Guidelines, a Glossary of Related Terms, and Resources for Additional Help and Information

Edited by Joyce Brennfleck Shannon. 600 pages. 2009. 978-0-7808-1037-2.

SEE ALSO Domestic Violence Sourcebook, 3rd Edition

Childhood Diseases and Disorders Sourcebook, 2nd Edition

Basic Consumer Health Information about the Physical, Mental, and Developmental Health of Pre-Adolescent Children, Including Facts about Infectious Diseases, Asthma, Allergies, Diabetes, and Other Acute and Chronic Conditions Affecting the Gastrointestinal Tract, Ears, Nose, Throat, Liver, Kidneys, Heart, Blood, Brain, Muscles, Bones, and Skin

Along with Reports on Recommended Childhood Vaccinations, Wellness Guidelines, a Glossary of Related Medical Terms, and a List of Resources for Parents

Edited by Sandra J. Judd. 694 pages. 2009. 978-0-7808-1031-0.

"The strength of this source is the wide range of information given about childhood health issues... It is most appropriate for public libraries and academic libraries that field medical questions."
—*American Reference Books Annual, 2009*

SEE ALSO Healthy Children Sourcebook

Colds, Flu and Other Common Ailments Sourcebook

Basic Consumer Health Information about Common Ailments and Injuries, Including Colds, Coughs, the Flu, Sinus Problems, Headaches, Fever, Nausea and Vomiting, Menstrual Cramps, Diarrhea, Constipation, Hemorrhoids, Back Pain, Dandruff, Dry and Itchy Skin, Cuts, Scrapes, Sprains, Bruises, and More

Along with Information about Prevention, Self-Care, Choosing a Doctor, Over-the-Counter Medications, Folk Remedies, and Alternative Therapies, and Including a Glossary of Important Terms and a Directory of Resources for Further Help and Information

Edited by Chad T. Kimball. 622 pages. 2001. 978-0-7808-0435-7.

"A good starting point for research on common illnesses. It will be a useful addition to public and consumer health library collections."
—*American Reference Books Annual, 2002*

"Will prove valuable to any library seeking to maintain a current, comprehensive reference collection of health resources... Excellent reference."
—*The Bookwatch, Aug '01*

SEE ALSO Contagious Diseases Sourcebook, 2nd Edition

Communication Disorders Sourcebook

Basic Information about Deafness and Hearing Loss, Speech and Language Disorders, Voice Disorders, Balance and Vestibular Disorders, and Disorders of Smell, Taste, and Touch

Edited by Linda M. Ross. 533 pages. 1996. 978-0-7808-0077-9.

"This is skillfully edited and is a welcome resource for the layperson. It should be found in every public and medical library."
—*Booklist Health Sciences Supplement, Oct '97*

Complementary & Alternative Medicine Sourcebook, 4th Edition

Basic Consumer Health Information about Ayurveda, Acupuncture, Aromatherapy, Chiropractic Care, Diet-Based Therapies, Guided Imagery, Herbal and Vitamin Supplements, Homeopathy, Hypnosis, Massage, Meditation, Naturopathy, Pilates, Reflexology, Reiki, Shiatsu, Tai Chi, Traditional Chinese Medicine, Yoga, and Other Complementary and Alternative Medical Therapies

Along with Statistics, Tips for Selecting a Practitioner, Treatments for Specific Health Conditions, a Glossary of Related Terms, and a Directory of Resources for Additional Help and Information

Edited by Amy L. Sutton. 600 pages. 2010. 978-0-7808-1082-2.

Congenital Disorders Sourcebook, 2nd Edition

Basic Consumer Health Information about Nonhereditary Birth Defects and Disorders

Related to Prematurity, Gestational Injuries, Congenital Infections, and Birth Complications, Including Heart Defects, Hydrocephalus, Spina Bifida, Cleft Lip and Palate, Cerebral Palsy, and More

Along with Facts about the Prevention of Birth Defects, Fetal Surgery and Other Treatment Options, Research Initiatives, a Glossary of Related Terms, and Resources for Additional Information and Support

Edited by Sandra J. Judd. 619 pages. 2007. 978-0-7808-0945-1.

"Congenital Disorders Sourcebook provides an excellent, non-technical overview of many aspects of pregnancy with the focus on congenital disorders."
— *American Reference Books Annual, 2008*

"An excellent readable reference aimed at the lay public for difficult to understand medical problems. An excellent starting point for the interested parent or family member who may then be motivated to seek more information."
— *Doody's Review Service, 2007*

SEE ALSO *Pregnancy and Birth Sourcebook, 3rd Edition*

Contagious Diseases Sourcebook, 2nd Edition

Basic Consumer Health Information about Diseases Spread from Person to Person through Direct Physical Contact, Airborne Transmissions, Sexual Contact, or Contact with Blood or Other Body Fluids, Including Pneumococcal, Staphylococcal, and Streptococcal Diseases, Colds, Influenza, Lice, Measles, Mumps, Tuberculosis, and Others

Along with Facts about Self-Care and Over-the-Counter Medications, Antibiotics and Drug Resistance, Disease Prevention, Vaccines, and Bioterrorism, a Glossary, and a Directory of Resources for More Information

Edited by Joyce Brennfleck Shannon. 600 pages. 2010. 978-0-7808-1075-4.

SEE ALSO *AIDS Sourcebook, 4th Edition, Hepatitis Sourcebook*

Cosmetic and Reconstructive Surgery Sourcebook, 2nd Edition

Basic Consumer Information about Plastic Surgery and Non-Surgical Appearance-Enhancing Procedures, Including Facts about Botulinum Toxin, Collagen Replacement, Dermabrasion, Chemical Peels, Eyelid Surgery, Nose Reshaping, Lip Augmentation, Liposuction, Breast Enlargement and Reduction, Tummy Tucking, and Other Skin, Hair, Facial, and Body Shaping Procedures

Along with Information about Reconstructive Procedures for Congenital Disorders, Disfiguring Diseases, Burns, and Traumatic Injuries, a Glossary of Related Terms, and a Directory of Additional Resources

Edited by Karen Bellenir. 483 pages. 2007. 978-0-7808-0951-2.

"A comprehensive source for people considering cosmetic surgery... also recommended for medical students who will perform these procedures later in their careers; and public librarians and academic medical librarians who may assist patrons interested in this information."
— *Medical Reference Services Quarterly, Fall '08*

"A practical guide for health care consumers and health care workers... This easy-to-read reference guide would be useful for novice and veteran health care consumers, surgical technology students, nursing students, and perioperative nurses new to plastic and reconstructive surgery. It also may be helpful for medical-surgical nurses as a guide for patient teaching in their practices."
— *AORN Journal, Aug '08*

SEE ALSO *Surgery Sourcebook, 2nd Edition*

Death and Dying Sourcebook, 2nd Edition

Basic Consumer Health Information about End-of-Life Care and Related Perspectives and Ethical Issues, Including End-of-Life Symptoms and Treatments, Pain Management, Quality-of-Life Concerns, the Use of Life Support, Patients' Rights and Privacy Issues, Advance Directives, Physician-Assisted Suicide, Caregiving, Organ and Tissue Donation, Autopsies, Funeral Arrangements, and Grief

Along with Statistical Data, Information about the Leading Causes of Death, a Glossary, and Directories of Support Groups and Other Resources

Edited by Joyce Brennfleck Shannon. 626 pages. 2006. 978-0-7808-0871-3.

Dental Care and Oral Health Sourcebook, 3rd Edition

Basic Consumer Health Information about Dental Care and Oral Health Throughout the Lifespan, Including Facts about Cavities, Bad Breath, Cold and Canker Sores, Dry Mouth, Toothaches, Gum Disease, Malocclusion, Temporomandibular Joint and Muscle Disorders, Oral Cancers, and Dental Emergencies

Along with Information about Mouth Hygiene, Crowns, Bridges, Implants, and Fillings, Surgical, Orthodontic, and Cosmetic Dental Procedures, Pain Management, Health Conditions that Impact Oral Care, a Glossary of Related Terms, and a Directory of Additional Resources

Edited by Amy L. Sutton. 619 pages. 2008. 978-0-7808-1032-7.

"Could serve as turning point in the battle to educate consumers in issues concerning oral health. Tightly written in terms the average person can understand, yet comprehensive in scope and authoritative in tone, it is another excellent sourcebook in the Health Reference Series... Should be in the reference department of all public libraries, and in academic libraries that have a public constituency."
—American Reference Books Annual, 2009

Depression Sourcebook, 2nd Edition

Basic Consumer Health Information about Unipolar Depression, Bipolar Disorder, Dysthymia, Seasonal Affective Disorder, Postpartum Depression, and Other Depressive Disorders, Including Facts about Populations at Special Risk, Coexisting Medical Conditions, Symptoms, Treatment Options, and Suicide Prevention

Along with Statistical Data, a Glossary of Related Terms, and a Directory of Resources for Additional Help and Information

Edited by Sandra J. Judd. 646 pages. 2008. 978-0-7808-1003-7.

"Recommended for public libraries."
—American Reference Books Annual, 2009

SEE ALSO Mental Health Disorders Sourcebook, 4th Edition

Dermatological Disorders Sourcebook, 2nd Edition

Basic Consumer Health Information about Conditions and Disorders Affecting the Skin, Hair, and Nails, Such as Acne, Rosacea, Rashes, Dermatitis, Pigmentation Disorders, Birthmarks, Skin Cancer, Skin Injuries, Psoriasis, Scleroderma, and Hair Loss, Including Facts about Medications and Treatments for Dermatological Disorders and Tips for Maintaining Healthy Skin, Hair, and Nails

Along with Information about How Aging Affects the Skin, a Glossary of Related Terms, and a Directory of Resources for Additional Help and Information

Edited by Amy L. Sutton. 617 pages. 2006. 978-0-7808-0795-2.

"Well organized... presents a plethora of information in a manner that is appropriate in style and readability for the intended audience."
—Physical Therapy, Nov '06

"Helpfully brings together... sources in one convenient place, saving the user hours of research time."
—American Reference Books Annual, 2006

SEE ALSO Burns Sourcebook

Diabetes Sourcebook, 4th Edition

Basic Consumer Health Information about Type 1 and Type 2 Diabetes Mellitus, Gestational Diabetes, Monogenic Forms of Diabetes, and Insulin Resistance, with Guidelines for Lifestyle Modifications and the Medical Management of Diabetes, Including Facts about Insulin, Insulin Delivery Devices, Oral Diabetes Medications, Self-Monitoring of Blood Glucose, Meal Planning, Physical Activity Recommendations, Foot Care, and Treatment Options for People with Kidney Failure

Along with a Section about Diabetes Complications and Co-Occurring Conditions, a Glossary of Related Terms, and Directories of Resources for Additional Help and Information

Edited by Karen Bellenir. 627 pages. 2008. 978-0-7808-1005-1.

"Completely and comprehensively covering almost everything a student or physician would need to know... well worth the investment."

—Internet Bookwatch, Dec '08

SEE ALSO Endocrine and Metabolic Disorders Sourcebook, 2nd Edition

Diet and Nutrition Sourcebook, 3rd Edition

Basic Consumer Health Information about Dietary Guidelines and the Food Guidance System, Recommended Daily Nutrient Intakes, Serving Proportions, Weight Control, Vitamins and Supplements, Nutrition Issues for Different Life Stages and Lifestyles, and the Needs of People with Specific Medical Concerns, Including Cancer, Celiac Disease, Diabetes, Eating Disorders, Food Allergies, and Cardiovascular Disease

Along with Facts about Federal Nutrition Support Programs, a Glossary of Nutrition and Dietary Terms, and Directories of Additional Resources for More Information about Nutrition

Edited by Joyce Brennfleck Shannon. 605 pages. 2006. 978-0-7808-0800-3.

"A valuable resource tool for any individual."

—Journal of Dental Hygiene, Apr '07

"From different recommended eating habits to reduce disease and common ailments to nutrition advice for those with specific conditions, Diet and Nutrition Sourcebook is especially important because so much is changing in this area, and so rapidly."

—California Bookwatch, Jun '06

SEE ALSO Eating Disorders Sourcebook, 2nd Edition, Vegetarian Sourcebook

Digestive Diseases and Disorders Sourcebook

Basic Consumer Health Information about Diseases and Disorders that Impact the Upper and Lower Digestive System, Including Celiac

Disease, Constipation, Crohn's Disease, Cyclic Vomiting Syndrome, Diarrhea, Diverticulosis and Diverticulitis, Gallstones, Heartburn, Hemorrhoids, Hernias, Indigestion (Dyspepsia), Irritable Bowel Syndrome, Lactose Intolerance, Ulcers, and More

Along with Information about Medications and Other Treatments, Tips for Maintaining a Healthy Digestive Tract, a Glossary, and Directory of Digestive Diseases Organizations

Edited by Karen Bellenir. 323 pages. 2000. 978-0-7808-0327-5.

"An excellent addition to all public or patient-research libraries."

—American Reference Books Annual, 2001

"Recommended reference source."

—Booklist, May '00

SEE ALSO Gastrointestinal Diseases and Disorders Sourcebook, 2nd Edition

Disabilities Sourcebook

Basic Consumer Health Information about Physical and Psychiatric Disabilities, Including Descriptions of Major Causes of Disability, Assistive and Adaptive Aids, Workplace Issues, and Accessibility Concerns

Along with Information about the Americans with Disabilities Act, a Glossary, and Resources for Additional Help and Information

Edited by Dawn D. Matthews. 602 pages. 2000. 978-0-7808-0389-3.

"A must for libraries with a consumer health section."

—American Reference Books Annual, 2002

"A much needed addition to the Omnigraphics Health Reference Series. A current reference work to provide people with disabilities, their families, caregivers or those who work with them, a broad range of information in one volume, has not been available until now... It is recommended for all public and academic library reference collections."

—E-Streams, May '01

"An excellent source book in easy-to-read format covering many current topics; highly recommended for all libraries."

—CHOICE, Jan '01

Disease Management Sourcebook

Basic Consumer Health Information about Coping with Chronic and Serious Illnesses, Navigating the Health Care System, Communicating with Health Care Providers, Assessing Health Care Quality, and Making Informed Health Care Decisions, Including Facts about Second Opinions, Hospitalization, Surgery, and Medications

Along with a Section about Children with Chronic Conditions, Information about Legal, Financial, and Insurance Issues, a Glossary of Related Terms, and Directories of Additional Resources

Edited by Joyce Brennfleck Shannon. 621 pages. 2008. 978-0-7808-1002-0.

"Consumers need to know how to manage their health care the same way they manage anything else in their lives. The text is very readable and is written for the layperson and consumer. The cost is not prohibitive. This book should be in all collections of health care libraries and public libraries."
— *American Reference Books Annual, 2009*

"The information is very current, and the selection of font and layout make the book easy to read. A hardback that will stand up to much usage, this is an excellent resource for consumers... Recommended. General readers."
—*CHOICE, Nov '08*

"Intended for lay readers, this resource clarifies the many confusing and overwhelming details associated with chronic disease care. Meticulous and clearly explained, the book even includes diagrams intended to ease comprehension of over-the-counter medication labels. An essential guide to navigating the health-care rapids."
—*Library Journal, Aug '08*

Domestic Violence Sourcebook, 3rd Edition

Basic Consumer Health Information about Warning Signs, Risk Factors, and Health Consequences of Intimate Partner Violence, Sexual Violence and Rape, Stalking, Human Trafficking, Child Maltreatment, Teen Dating Violence, and Elder Abuse

Along with Facts about Victims and Perpetrators, Strategies for Violence Prevention, and Emergency Interventions, Safety Plans, and Financial and Legal Tips for Victims, a Glossary of Related Terms, and Directories of Resources for Additional Information and Support

Edited by Joyce Brennfleck Shannon. 634 pages. 2009. 978-0-7808-1038-9.

"A recommended pick for any library interested in consumer health and social issues... A 'must' for any serious health collection."
—*California Bookwatch, Jul '09*

SEE ALSO *Child Abuse Sourcebook, 2nd Edition*

Drug Abuse Sourcebook, 3rd Edition

Basic Consumer Health Information about the Abuse of Cocaine, Club Drugs, Hallucinogens, Heroin, Inhalants, Marijuana, and Other Illicit Substances, Prescription Medications, and Over-the-Counter Medicines

Along with Facts about Addiction and Related Health Effects, Drug Abuse Treatment and Recovery, Drug Testing, Prevention Programs, Glossaries of Drug-Related Terms, and Directories of Resources for More Information

Edited by Joyce Brennfleck Shannon. 600 pages. 2010. 978-0-7808-1079-2.

SEE ALSO *Alcoholism Sourcebook, 3rd Edition*

Ear, Nose, and Throat Disorders Sourcebook, 2nd Edition

Basic Consumer Health Information about Disorders of the Ears, Hearing Loss, Vestibular Disorders, Nasal and Sinus Problems, Throat and Vocal Cord Disorders, and Otolaryngologic Cancers, Including Facts about Ear Infections and Injuries, Genetic and Congenital Deafness, Sensorineural Hearing Disorders, Tinnitus, Vertigo, Ménière Disease, Rhinitis, Sinusitis, Snoring, Sore Throats, Hoarseness, and More

Along with Reports on Current Research Initiatives, a Glossary of Related Medical Terms, and a Directory of Sources for Further Help and Information

Edited by Sandra J. Judd. 631 pages. 2007. 978-0-7808-0872-0.

"A resource book for the general public that provides comprehensive coverage of basic up-to-date medical information about the causes, symptoms, diagnosis, and treatment of diseases and disorders that affect the ears, nose, sinuses, throat, and voice... The majority of information is presented in question and answer format, much like questions a patient might ask of a health care provider. An extensive index facilitates the reader's ability to easily access information on any specific topic."
—*Journal of Dental Hygiene, Oct '07*

"A handy compilation of information on common and some not so common ailments of the ears, nose, and throat."
—*Doody's Review Service, 2007*

▉

Eating Disorders Sourcebook, 2nd Edition
Basic Consumer Health Information about Anorexia Nervosa, Bulimia, Binge Eating, Compulsive Exercise, Female Athlete Triad, and Other Eating Disorders, Including Facts about Body Image and Other Cultural and Age-Related Risk Factors, Prevention Efforts, Adverse Health Effects, Treatment Options, and the Recovery Process

Along with Guidelines for Healthy Weight Control, a Glossary, and Directories of Additional Resources

Edited by Joyce Brennfleck Shannon. 557 pages. 2007. 978-0-7808-0948-2.

"Recommended for the reference collection of large public libraries."
—*American Reference Books Annual, 2008*

"A basic health reference any health or general library needs."
—*Internet Bookwatch, Jun '07*

SEE ALSO Diet and Nutrition Sourcebook, 3rd Edition, Mental Health Disorders Sourcebook, 4th Edition

▉

Emergency Medical Services Sourcebook
Basic Consumer Health Information about Preventing, Preparing for, and Managing Emergency Situations, When and Who to Call for Help, What to Expect in the Emergency Room, the Emergency Medical Team,

Patient Issues, and Current Topics in Emergency Medicine

Along with Statistical Data, a Glossary, and Sources of Additional Help and Information

Edited by Jenni Lynn Colson. 472 pages. 2002. 978-0-7808-0420-3.

"Handy and convenient for home, public, school, and college libraries. Recommended."
—*CHOICE, Apr '03*

"This reference can provide the consumer with answers to most questions about emergency care in the United States, or it will direct them to a resource where the answer can be found."
—*American Reference Books Annual, 2003*

SEE ALSO Injury and Trauma Sourcebook

▉

Endocrine and Metabolic Disorders Sourcebook, 2nd Edition
Basic Consumer Health Information about Hormonal and Metabolic Disorders that Affect the Body's Growth, Development, and Functioning, Including Disorders of the Pancreas, Ovaries and Testes, and Pituitary, Thyroid, Parathyroid, and Adrenal Glands, with Facts about Growth Disorders, Addison Disease, Cushing Syndrome, Conn Syndrome, Diabetic Disorders, Multiple Endocrine Neoplasia, Inborn Errors of Metabolism, and More

Along with Information about Endocrine Functioning, Diagnostic and Screening Tests, a Glossary of Related Terms, and Directories of Additional Resources

Edited by Joyce Brennfleck Shannon. 597 pages. 2007. 978-0-7808-0952-9.

SEE ALSO Diabetes Sourcebook, 4th Edition

▉

Environmental Health Sourcebook, 3rd Edition
Basic Consumer Health Information about the Environment and Its Effects on Human Health, Including Facts about Air, Water, and Soil Contamination, Hazardous Chemicals, Foodborne Hazards and Illnesses, Household Hazards Such as Radon, Mold, and Carbon Monoxide, Consumer Hazards from Toxic Products and Imported Goods, and Disorders

Linked to Environmental Causes, Including Chemical Sensitivity, Cancer, Allergies, and Asthma

Along with Information about the Impact of Environmental Hazards on Specific Populations, a Glossary of Related Terms, and Resources for Additional Help and Information.

Edited by Laura Larsen. 600 pages. 2010. 978-0-7808-1078-5

Ethnic Diseases Sourcebook

Basic Consumer Health Information for Ethnic and Racial Minority Groups in the United States, Including General Health Indicators and Behaviors, Ethnic Diseases, Genetic Testing, the Impact of Chronic Diseases, Women's Health, Mental Health Issues, and Preventive Health Care Services

Along with a Glossary and a Listing of Additional Resources

Edited by Joyce Brennfleck Shannon. 648 pages. 2001. 978-0-7808-0336-7.

"Not many books have been written on this topic to date, and the Ethnic Diseases Sourcebook is a strong addition to the list. It will be an important introductory resource for health consumers, students, health care personnel, and social scientists. It is recommended for public, academic, and large hospital libraries."

— American Reference Books Annual, 2002

"Will prove valuable to any library seeking to maintain a current, comprehensive reference collection of health resources... An excellent source of health information about genetic disorders which affect particular ethnic and racial minorities in the U.S."

—The Bookwatch, Aug '01

Eye Care Sourcebook, 3rd Edition

Basic Consumer Health Information about Eye Care and Eye Disorders, Including Facts about the Diagnosis, Prevention, and Treatment of Refractive Disorders, Cataracts, Glaucoma, Macular Degeneration, and Problems Affecting the Cornea, Retina, and Lacrimal Glands

Along with Advice about Preventing Eye Injuries and Tips for Living with Low Vision or Blindness, a Glossary of Related Terms, and Directories of Resources for More Help and Information

Edited by Amy L. Sutton. 646 pages. 2008. 978-0-7808-1000-6.

"A solid reference tool for eye care and a valuable addition to a collection."

—American Reference Books Annual, 2009

Family Planning Sourcebook

Basic Consumer Health Information about Planning for Pregnancy and Contraception, Including Traditional Methods, Barrier Methods, Hormonal Methods, Permanent Methods, Future Methods, Emergency Contraception, and Birth Control Choices for Women at Each Stage of Life

Along with Statistics, a Glossary, and Sources of Additional Information

Edited by Amy Marcaccio Keyzer. 503 pages. 2001. 978-0-7808-0379-4.

"Recommended for public, health, and undergraduate libraries as part of the circulating collection."

—E-Streams, Mar '02

"Will prove valuable to any library seeking to maintain a current, comprehensive reference collection of health resources... Excellent reference."

—The Bookwatch, Aug '01

SEE ALSO Pregnancy and Birth Sourcebook, 3rd Edition

Fitness and Exercise Sourcebook, 3rd Edition

Basic Consumer Health Information about the Physical and Mental Benefits of Fitness, Including Cardiorespiratory Endurance, Muscular Strength, Muscular Endurance, and Flexibility, with Facts about Sports Nutrition and Exercise-Related Injuries and Tips about Physical Activity and Exercises for People of All Ages and for People with Health Concerns

Along with Advice on Selecting and Using Exercise Equipment, Maintaining Exercise Motivation, a Glossary of Related Terms, and a Directory of Resources for More Help and Information

Edited by Amy L. Sutton. 635 pages. 2007. 978-0-7808-0946-8.

"Updates the consumer information on the physical and mental benefits of physical activity throughout the lifespan offered in earlier editions... Recommended. All readers; all levels."

—CHOICE, Oct '07

"An exceptionally well-rounded coverage perfect for any concerned about developing and understanding a fitness program."

—California Bookwatch, Jun '07

SEE ALSO Sports Injuries Sourcebook, 3rd Edition

Food Safety Sourcebook

Basic Consumer Health Information about the Safe Handling of Meat, Poultry, Seafood, Eggs, Fruit Juices, and Other Food Items, and Facts about Pesticides, Drinking Water, Food Safety Overseas, and the Onset, Duration, and Symptoms of Foodborne Illnesses, Including Types of Pathogenic Bacteria, Parasitic Protozoa, Worms, Viruses, and Natural Toxins

Along with the Role of the Consumer, the Food Handler, and the Government in Food Safety, a Glossary, and Resources for Additional Help and Information

Edited by Dawn D. Matthews. 327 pages. 1999. 978-0-7808-0326-8.

"Recommended reference source."

—Booklist, May '00

"This book takes the complex issues of food safety and foodborne pathogens and presents them in an easily understood manner. [It does] an excellent job of covering a large and often confusing topic."

— American Reference Books Annual, 2000

Forensic Medicine Sourcebook

Basic Consumer Information for the Layperson about Forensic Medicine, Including Crime Scene Investigation, Evidence Collection and Analysis, Expert Testimony, Computer-Aided Criminal Identification, Digital Imaging in the Courtroom, DNA Profiling, Accident Reconstruction, Autopsies, Ballistics, Drugs and Explosives Detection, Latent Fingerprints,

Product Tampering, and Questioned Document Examination

Along with Statistical Data, a Glossary of Forensics Terminology, and Listings of Sources for Further Help and Information

Edited by Annemarie S. Muth. 574 pages. 1999. 978-0-7808-0232-2.

"Given the expected widespread interest in its content and its easy to read style, this book is recommended for most public and all college and university libraries."

—E-Streams, Feb '01

"A wealth of information, useful statistics, references are up-to-date and extremely complete. This wonderful collection of data will help students who are interested in a career in any type of forensic field. It is a great resource for attorneys who need information about types of expert witnesses needed in a particular case. It also offers useful information for fiction and nonfiction writers whose work involves a crime. A fascinating compilation. All levels."

—CHOICE, Jan '00

"There are several items that make this book attractive to consumers who are seeking certain forensic data... This is a useful current source for those seeking general forensic medical answers."

—American Reference Books Annual, 2000

Gastrointestinal Diseases and Disorders Sourcebook, 2nd Edition

Basic Consumer Health Information about the Upper and Lower Gastrointestinal (GI) Tract, Including the Esophagus, Stomach, Intestines, Rectum, Liver, and Pancreas, with Facts about Gastroesophageal Reflux Disease, Gastritis, Hernias, Ulcers, Celiac Disease, Diverticulitis, Irritable Bowel Syndrome, Hemorrhoids, Gastrointestinal Cancers, and Other Diseases and Disorders Related to the Digestive Process

Along with Information about Commonly Used Diagnostic and Surgical Procedures, Statistics, Reports on Current Research Initiatives and Clinical Trials, a Glossary, and Resources for Additional Help and Information

Edited by Sandra J. Judd. 654 pages. 2006. 978-0-7808-0798-3.

"The text is designed for the general reader seeking information on prevention, disease warning signs, diagnostic and therapeutic questions... It is an excellent resource for the general reader to conveniently locate credible, coordinated and indexed information... The sourcebook will prove very helpful for patients, caregivers and should be available in every physician waiting room."
—*Doody's Review Service, 2006*

SEE ALSO *Diet and Nutrition Sourcebook, 3rd Edition, Digestive Diseases and Disorders Sourcebook*

Genetic Disorders Sourcebook, 4th Edition

Basic Consumer Health Information about Hereditary Diseases and Disorders, Including Facts about the Human Genome, Genetic Inheritance Patterns, Disorders Associated with Specific Genes, Such as Sickle Cell Disease, Hemophilia, and Cystic Fibrosis, Chromosome Disorders, Such as Down Syndrome, Fragile X Syndrome, and Turner Syndrome, and Complex Diseases and Disorders Resulting from the Interaction of Environmental and Genetic Factors, Such as Allergies, Cancer, and Obesity

Along with Facts about Genetic Testing, Suggestions for Parents of Children with Special Needs, Reports on Current Research Initiatives, a Glossary of Genetic Terminology, and Resources for Additional Help and Information

Edited by Sandra J. Judd. 600 pages. 2010. 978-0-7808-1076-1.

Head Trauma Sourcebook

Basic Information for the Layperson about Open-Head and Closed-Head Injuries, Treatment Advances, Recovery, and Rehabilitation

Along with Reports on Current Research Initiatives

Edited by Karen Bellenir. 414 pages. 1997. 978-0-7808-0208-7.

Headache Sourcebook

Basic Consumer Health Information about Migraine, Tension, Cluster, Rebound and Other Types of Headaches, with Facts about the Cause and Prevention of Headaches, the Effects of Stress and the Environment, Headaches during Pregnancy and Menopause, and Childhood Headaches

Along with a Glossary and Other Resources for Additional Help and Information

Edited by Dawn D. Matthews. 342 pages. 2002. 978-0-7808-0337-4.

"Highly recommended for academic and medical reference collections."
—*Library Bookwatch, Sep '02*

SEE ALSO *Pain Sourcebook, 3rd Edition*

Healthy Aging Sourcebook

Basic Consumer Health Information about Maintaining Health through the Aging Process, Including Advice on Nutrition, Exercise, and Sleep, Help in Making Decisions about Midlife Issues and Retirement, and Guidance Concerning Practical and Informed Choices in Health Consumerism

Along with Data Concerning the Theories of Aging, Different Experiences in Aging by Minority Groups, and Facts about Aging Now and Aging in the Future; and Featuring a Glossary, a Guide to Consumer Help, Additional Suggested Reading, and Practical Resource Directory

Edited by Jenifer Swanson. 537 pages. 1999. 978-0-7808-0390-9.

"Recommended reference source."
—*Booklist, Feb '00*

SEE ALSO *Adult Health Sourcebook, Physical and Mental Issues in Aging Sourcebook*

Healthy Children Sourcebook

Basic Consumer Health Information about the Physical and Mental Development of Children between the Ages of 3 and 12, Including Routine Health Care, Preventative Health Services, Safety and First Aid, Healthy Sleep, Dental Care, Nutrition, and Fitness, and Featuring Parenting Tips on Such Topics as Bedwetting, Choosing Day Care, Monitoring TV and Other Media, and Establishing a Foundation for Substance Abuse Prevention

Along with a Glossary of Commonly Used Pediatric Terms and Resources for Additional Help and Information.

Edited by Chad T. Kimball. 624 pages. 2003. 978-0-7808-0247-6.

"Should be required reading for parents and teachers."
—E-Streams, Jun '04

"It is hard to imagine that any other single resource exists that would provide such a comprehensive guide of timely information on health promotion and disease prevention for children aged 3 to 12."
—American Reference Books Annual, 2004

"This easy-to-read volume is a tremendous resource."
—AORN Journal, May '05

SEE ALSO Childhood Diseases and Disorders Sourcebook, 2nd Edition

Healthy Heart Sourcebook for Women

Basic Consumer Health Information about Cardiac Issues Specific to Women, Including Facts about Major Risk Factors and Prevention, Treatment and Control Strategies, and Important Dietary Issues

Along with a Special Section Regarding the Pros and Cons of Hormone Replacement Therapy and Its Impact on Heart Health, and Additional Help, Including Recipes, a Glossary, and a Directory of Resources

Edited by Dawn D. Matthews. 321 pages. 2000. 978-0-7808-0329-9.

"A good reference source and recommended for all public, academic, medical, and hospital libraries."
—Medical Reference Services Quarterly, Summer '01

"Contains very important information about coronary artery disease that all women should know. The information is current and presented in an easy-to-read format. The book will make a good addition to any library."
—American Medical Writers Association Journal, Summer '00

SEE ALSO Cardiovascular Diseases and Disorders Sourcebook, 4th Edition, Women's Health Concerns Sourcebook, 3rd Edition

Hepatitis Sourcebook

Basic Consumer Health Information about Hepatitis A, Hepatitis B, Hepatitis C, and Other Forms of Hepatitis, Including Autoimmune Hepatitis, Alcoholic Hepatitis, Nonalcoholic Steatohepatitis, and Toxic Hepatitis, with Facts about Risk Factors, Screening Methods, Diagnostic Tests, and Treatment Options

Along with Information on Liver Health, Tips for People Living with Chronic Hepatitis, Reports on Current Research Initiatives, a Glossary of Terms Related to Hepatitis, and a Directory of Sources for Further Help and Information

Edited by Sandra J. Judd. 570 pages. 2006. 978-0-7808-0749-5.

"The breadth of information found in this one book would not be readily found in another source. Highly recommended."
—American Reference Books Annual, 2006

SEE ALSO Contagious Diseases Sourcebook, 2nd Edition

Household Safety Sourcebook

Basic Consumer Health Information about Household Safety, Including Information about Poisons, Chemicals, Fire, and Water Hazards in the Home

Along with Advice about the Safe Use of Home Maintenance Equipment, Choosing Toys and Nursery Furniture, Holiday and Recreation Safety, a Glossary, and Resources for Further Help and Information

Edited by Dawn D. Matthews. 587 pages. 2002. 978-0-7808-0338-1.

"As a sourcebook on household safety this book meets its mark. It is encyclopedic in scope and covers a wide range of safety issues that are commonly seen in the home."
—E-Streams, Jul '02

Hypertension Sourcebook

Basic Consumer Health Information about the Causes, Diagnosis, and Treatment of High Blood Pressure, with Facts about Consequences, Complications, and Co-Occurring Disorders, Such as Coronary Heart Disease, Diabetes, Stroke, Kidney Disease, and Hypertensive Retinopathy, and Issues in Blood Pressure

Control, Including Dietary Choices, Stress Management, and Medications

Along with Reports on Current Research Initiatives and Clinical Trials, a Glossary, and Resources for Additional Help and Information

Edited by Dawn D. Matthews and Karen Bellenir. 588 pages. 2004. 978-0-7808-0674-0.

"Academic, public, and medical libraries will want to add the Hypertension Sourcebook to their collections."
—*E-Streams, Aug '05*

"The strength of this source is the wide range of information given about hypertension."
—*American Reference Books Annual, 2005*

***SEE ALSO** Stroke Sourcebook, 2nd Edition*

Immune System Disorders Sourcebook, 2nd Edition

Basic Consumer Health Information about Disorders of the Immune System, Including Immune System Function and Response, Diagnosis of Immune Disorders, Information about Inherited Immune Disease, Acquired Immune Disease, and Autoimmune Diseases, Including Primary Immune Deficiency, Acquired Immunodeficiency Syndrome (AIDS), Lupus, Multiple Sclerosis, Type 1 Diabetes, Rheumatoid Arthritis, and Graves' Disease

Along with Treatments, Tips for Coping with Immune Disorders, a Glossary, and a Directory of Additional Resources

Edited by Joyce Brennfleck Shannon. 643 pages. 2005. 978-0-7808-0748-8.

"Highly recommended for academic and public libraries."
—*American Reference Books Annual, 2006*

"The updated second edition is a 'must' for any consumer health library seeking a solid resource covering the treatments, symptoms, and options for immune disorder sufferers... An excellent guide."
—*MBR Bookwatch, Jan '06*

***SEE ALSO** AIDS Sourcebook, 4th Edition, Arthritis Sourcebook, 3rd Edition*

Infant and Toddler Health Sourcebook

Basic Consumer Health Information about the Physical and Mental Development of Newborns, Infants, and Toddlers, Including Neonatal Concerns, Nutrition Recommendations, Immunization Schedules, Common Pediatric Disorders, Assessments and Milestones, Safety Tips, and Advice for Parents and Other Caregivers

Along with a Glossary of Terms and Resource Listings for Additional Help

Edited by Jenifer Swanson. 570 pages. 2000. 978-0-7808-0246-9.

"As a reference for the general public, this would be useful in any library."
—*E-Streams, May '01*

"Recommended reference source."
—*Booklist, Feb '01*

Infectious Diseases Sourcebook

Basic Consumer Health Information about Non-Contagious Bacterial, Viral, Prion, Fungal, and Parasitic Diseases Spread by Food and Water, Insects and Animals, or Environmental Contact, Including Botulism, E. Coli, Encephalitis, Legionnaires' Disease, Lyme Disease, Malaria, Plague, Rabies, Salmonella, Tetanus, and Others, and Facts about Newly Emerging Diseases, Such as Hantavirus, Mad Cow Disease, Monkeypox, and West Nile Virus

Along with Information about Preventing Disease Transmission, the Threat of Bioterrorism, and Current Research Initiatives, with a Glossary and Directory of Resources for More Information

Edited by Karen Bellenir. 610 pages. 2004. 978-0-7808-0675-7.

"This reference continues the excellent tradition of the Health Reference Series in consolidating a wealth of information on a selected topic into a format that is easy to use and accessible to the general public."
—*American Reference Books Annual, 2005*

"Recommended for public and academic libraries."
—*E-Streams, Jan '05*

***SEE ALSO** Environmental Health Sourcebook, 3rd Edition*

Injury and Trauma Sourcebook

Basic Consumer Health Information about the Impact of Injury, the Diagnosis and Treatment of Common and Traumatic Injuries, Emergency Care, and Specific Injuries Related to Home, Community, Workplace, Transportation, and Recreation

Along with Guidelines for Injury Prevention, a Glossary, and a Directory of Additional Resources

Edited by Joyce Brennfleck Shannon. 675 pages. 2002. 978-0-7808-0421-0.

"Practitioners should be aware of guides such as this in order to facilitate their use by patients and their families."
—Doody's Health Sciences Book Review Journal, Sep-Oct '02

"Recommended reference source."
—Booklist, Sep '02

"Highly recommended for academic and medical reference collections."
—Library Bookwatch, Sep '02

SEE ALSO *Emergency Medical Services Sourcebook, Sports Injuries Sourcebook, 3rd Edition*

Learning Disabilities Sourcebook, 3rd Edition

Basic Consumer Health Information about Dyslexia, Auditory and Visual Processing Disorders, Communication Disorders, Dyscalculia, Dysgraphia, and Other Conditions That Impede Learning, Including Attention Deficit/Hyperactivity Disorder, Autism Spectrum Disorders, Hearing and Visual Impairments, Chromosome-Based Disorders, and Brain Injury

Along with Facts about Brain Function, Assessment, Therapy and Remediation, Accommodations, Assistive Technology, Legal Protections, and Tips about Family Life, School Transitions, and Employment Strategies, a Glossary of Related Terms, and Directories of Additional Resources

Edited by Joyce Brennfleck Shannon. 613 pages. 2009. 978-0-7808-1039-6.

"Intended to be a starting point for people who need to know about learning disabilities. Each chapter on a specific disability includes readable,

well-organized descriptions... The book is well indexed and a glossary is included. Chapters on organizations and helpful websites will aid the reader who needs more information."**
—American Reference Books Annual, 2009

"This book provides the necessary information to better understand learning disabilities and work with children who have them... It would be difficult to find another book that so comprehensively explains learning disabilities without becoming incomprehensible to the average parent who needs this information."
—Doody's Review Service, 2009

SEE ALSO *Attention Deficit Disorder Sourcebook, Autism and Pervasive Developmental Disorders Sourcebook*

Leukemia Sourcebook

Basic Consumer Health Information about Adult and Childhood Leukemias, Including Acute Lymphocytic Leukemia (ALL), Chronic Lymphocytic Leukemia (CLL), Acute Myelogenous Leukemia (AML), Chronic Myelogenous Leukemia (CML), and Hairy Cell Leukemia, and Treatments Such as Chemotherapy, Radiation Therapy, Peripheral Blood Stem Cell and Marrow Transplantation, and Immunotherapy

Along with Tips for Life During and After Treatment, a Glossary, and Directories of Additional Resources

Edited by Joyce Brennfleck Shannon. 564 pages. 2003. 978-0-7808-0627-6.

"Unlike other medical books for the layperson... the language does not talk down to the reader... This volume is highly recommended for all libraries."
—American Reference Books Annual, 2004

"A fine title which ranges from diagnosis to alternative treatments, staging, and tips for life during and after diagnosis."
—The Bookwatch, Dec '03

SEE ALSO *Blood & Circulatory Disorders Sourcebook, 3rd Edition, Cancer Sourcebook, 5th Edition*

Liver Disorders Sourcebook

Basic Consumer Health Information about the Liver and How It Works; Liver Diseases, Including Cancer, Cirrhosis, Hepatitis, and

Toxic and Drug Related Diseases; Tips for Maintaining a Healthy Liver; Laboratory Tests, Radiology Tests, and Facts about Liver Transplantation

Along with a Section on Support Groups, a Glossary, and Resource Listings

Edited by Joyce Brennfleck Shannon. 580 pages. 2000. 978-0-7808-0383-1.

"This title is recommended for health sciences and public libraries with consumer health collections."
—E-Streams, Oct '00

"Recommended reference source."
—Booklist, Jun '00

SEE ALSO Gastrointestinal Diseases and Disorders Sourcebook, 2nd Edition, Hepatitis Sourcebook

Lung Disorders Sourcebook

Basic Consumer Health Information about Emphysema, Pneumonia, Tuberculosis, Asthma, Cystic Fibrosis, and Other Lung Disorders, Including Facts about Diagnostic Procedures, Treatment Strategies, Disease Prevention Efforts, and Such Risk Factors as Smoking, Air Pollution, and Exposure to Asbestos, Radon, and Other Agents

Along with a Glossary and Resources for Additional Help and Information

Edited by Dawn D. Matthews. 657 pages. 2002. 978-0-7808-0339-8.

"Highly recommended for academic and medical reference collections."
—Library Bookwatch, Sep '02

SEE ALSO Asthma Sourcebook, 2nd Edition, Respiratory Disorders Sourcebook, 2nd Edition

Medical Tests Sourcebook, 3rd Edition

Basic Consumer Health Information about X-Rays, Blood Tests, Stool and Urine Tests, Biopsies, Mammography, Endoscopic Procedures, Ultrasound Exams, Computed Tomography, Magnetic Resonance Imaging (MRI), Nuclear Medicine, Genetic Testing, Home-Use Tests, and More

Along with Facts about Preventive Care and Screening Test Guidelines, Screening and

Assessment Tests Associated with Such Specific Concerns as Cancer, Heart Disease, Allergies, Diabetes, Thyroid Disfunction, and Infertility, a Glossary of Related Terms, and a Directory of Resources for Additional Help and Information

Edited by Karen Bellenir. 627 pages. 2008. 978-0-7808-1040-2

"This volume has a wide scope that makes it useful... Can be a valuable reference guide."
—American Reference Books Annual, 2009

"Would be a valuable contribution to any consumer health or public library."
—Doody's Book Review Service, 2009

Men's Health Concerns Sourcebook, 3rd Edition

Basic Consumer Health Information about Wellness in Men and Gender-Related Differences in Health, With Facts about Heart Disease, Cancer, Traumatic Injury, and Other Leading Causes of Death in Men, Reproductive Concerns, Sexual Dysfunction, Disorders of the Prostate, Penis, and Testes, Sex-Linked Genetic Disorders, and Other Medical and Mental Concerns of Men

Along with Statistical Data, a Glossary of Related Terms, and a Directory of Resources for Additional Information

Edited by Sandra J. Judd. 632 pages. 2009. 978-0-7808-1033-4.

"A good addition to any reference shelf in academic, consumer health, or hospital libraries."
—ARBAOnline, Oct '09

SEE ALSO Prostate and Urological Disorders Sourcebook

Mental Health Disorders Sourcebook, 4th Edition

Basic Consumer Health Information about the Causes and Symptoms of Mental Health Problems, Including Depression, Bipolar Disorder, Anxiety Disorders, Posttraumatic Stress Disorder, Obsessive-Compulsive Disorder, Eating Disorders, Addictions, and Personality and Psychotic Disorders

Along with Information about Medications and Treatments, Mental Health Concerns in

Children, Adolescents, and Adults, Tips on Living with Mental Health Disorders, a Glossary of Related Terms, and a Directory of Resources for Additional Help and Information

Edited by Amy L. Sutton. 680 pages. 2009. 978-0-7808-1041-9.

"Mental health concerns are presented in everyday language and intended for patients and their families as well as the general public... This resource is comprehensive and up to date... The easy-to-understand writing style helps to facilitate assimilation of needed facts and specifics on often challenging topics."
—ARBAOnline, Oct '09

"No health collection should be without this resource, which will reach into many a general lending library as well."
—Internet Bookwatch, Oct '09

SEE ALSO Depression Sourcebook, 2nd Edition, Stress-Related Disorders Sourcebook, 2nd Edition

Mental Retardation Sourcebook

Basic Consumer Health Information about Mental Retardation and Its Causes, Including Down Syndrome, Fetal Alcohol Syndrome, Fragile X Syndrome, Genetic Conditions, Injury, and Environmental Sources

Along with Preventive Strategies, Parenting Issues, Educational Implications, Health Care Needs, Employment and Economic Matters, Legal Issues, a Glossary, and a Resource Listing for Additional Help and Information

Edited by Joyce Brennfleck Shannon. 627 pages. 2000. 978-0-7808-0377-0.

"Public libraries will find the book useful for reference and as a beginning research point for students, parents, and caregivers."
—American Reference Books Annual, 2001

"The strength of this work is that it compiles many basic fact sheets and addresses for further information in one volume. It is intended and suitable for the general public."
—E-Streams, Nov '00

"An invaluable overview."
—Reviewer's Bookwatch, Jul '00

Movement Disorders Sourcebook, 2nd Edition

Basic Consumer Health Information about the Symptoms and Causes of Movement Disorders, Including Parkinson Disease, Amyotrophic Lateral Sclerosis, Cerebral Palsy, Muscular Dystrophy, Multiple Sclerosis, Myasthenia, Myoclonus, Spina Bifida, Dystonia, Essential Tremor, Choreatic Disorders, Huntington Disease, Tourette Syndrome, and Other Disorders That Cause Slowed, Absent, or Excessive Movements

Along with Information about Surgical and Nonsurgical Interventions, Physical Therapies, Strategies for Independent Living, a Glossary of Related Terms, and a Directory of Resources for Additional Help and Information

Edited by Amy L. Sutton. 618 pages. 2009. 978-0-7808-1034-1.

"The second updated edition of Movement Disorders Sourcebook is a winner, providing the latest research and health findings on all kinds of movement disorders in children and adults... a top pick for any health or general lending library's health reference collection."
—California Bookwatch, Aug '09

SEE ALSO Muscular Dystrophy Sourcebook

Multiple Sclerosis Sourcebook

Basic Consumer Health Information about Multiple Sclerosis (MS) and Its Effects on Mobility, Vision, Bladder Function, Speech, Swallowing, and Cognition, Including Facts about Risk Factors, Causes, Diagnostic Procedures, Pain Management, Drug Treatments, and Physical and Occupational Therapies

Along with Guidelines for Nutrition and Exercise, Tips on Choosing Assistive Equipment, Information about Disability, Work, Financial, and Legal Issues, a Glossary of Related Terms, and a Directory of Additional Resources

Edited by Joyce Brennfleck Shannon. 553 pages. 2007. 978-0-7808-0998-7.

Muscular Dystrophy Sourcebook

Basic Consumer Health Information about Congenital, Childhood-Onset, and Adult-Onset

Forms of Muscular Dystrophy, Such as Duchenne, Becker, Emery-Dreifuss, Distal, Limb-Girdle, Facioscapulohumeral (FSHD), Myotonic, and Ophthalmoplegic Muscular Dystrophies, Including Facts about Diagnostic Tests, Medical and Physical Therapies, Management of Co-Occurring Conditions, and Parenting Guidelines

Along with Practical Tips for Home Care, a Glossary, and Directories of Additional Resources

Edited by Joyce Brennfleck Shannon. 552 pages. 2004. 978-0-7808-0676-4.

"This book is highly recommended for public and academic libraries as well as health care offices that support the information needs of patients and their families."
—E-Streams, Apr '05

"Excellent reference."
—The Bookwatch, Jan '05

SEE ALSO *Movement Disorders Sourcebook, 2nd Edition*

Obesity Sourcebook

Basic Consumer Health Information about Diseases and Other Problems Associated with Obesity, and Including Facts about Risk Factors, Prevention Issues, and Management Approaches

Along with Statistical and Demographic Data, Information about Special Populations, Research Updates, a Glossary, and Source Listings for Further Help and Information

Edited by Wilma Caldwell and Chad T. Kimball. 360 pages. 2001. 978-0-7808-0333-6.

"The book synthesizes the reliable medical literature on obesity into one easy-to-read and useful resource for the general public."
—American Reference Books Annual, 2002

"Well suited for the health reference collection of a public library or an academic health science library that serves the general population."
—E-Streams, Sep '01

Osteoporosis Sourcebook

Basic Consumer Health Information about Primary and Secondary Osteoporosis and Juvenile Osteoporosis and Related Conditions, Including Fibrous Dysplasia, Gaucher Disease, Hyperthyroidism, Hypophosphatasia,

Myeloma, Osteopetrosis, Osteogenesis Imperfecta, and Paget's Disease

Along with Information about Risk Factors, Treatments, Traditional and Non-Traditional Pain Management, a Glossary of Related Terms, and a Directory of Resources

Edited by Allan R. Cook. 568 pages. 2001. 978-0-7808-0239-1.

"This resource is recommended as a great reference source for public, health, and academic libraries, and is another triumph for the editors of Omnigraphics."
—American Reference Books Annual, 2002

"Will prove valuable to any library seeking to maintain a current, comprehensive reference collection of health resources... From prevention to treatment and associated conditions, this provides an excellent survey."
—The Bookwatch, Aug '01

SEE ALSO *Healthy Aging Sourcebook, Women's Health Concerns Sourcebook, 3rd Edition*

Pain Sourcebook, 3rd Edition

Basic Consumer Health Information about Acute and Chronic Pain, Including Nerve Pain, Bone Pain, Muscle Pain, Cancer Pain, and Disorders Characterized by Pain, Such as Arthritis, Temporomandibular Muscle and Joint (TMJ) Disorder, Carpal Tunnel Syndrome, Headaches, Heartburn, Sciatica, and Shingles, and Facts about Diagnostic Tests and Treatment Options for Pain, Including Over-the-Counter and Prescription Drugs, Physical Rehabilitation, Injection and Infusion Therapies, Implantable Technologies, and Complementary Medicine

Along with Tips for Living with Pain, a Glossary of Related Terms, and a Directory of Additional Resources

Edited by Joyce Brennfleck Shannon. 644 pages. 2008. 978-0-7808-1006-8.

"Excellent for ready-reference users and can be used for beginning students in health fields... appropriate for the consumer health collection in both public and academic libraries."
—American Reference Books Annual, 2009

SEE ALSO Arthritis Sourcebook, 3rd Edition; Back and Neck Sourcebook, 2nd Edition;

Headache Sourcebook; Sports Injuries Source-book, 3rd Edition

Pediatric Cancer Sourcebook

Basic Consumer Health Information about Leukemias, Brain Tumors, Sarcomas, Lymphomas, and Other Cancers in Infants, Children, and Adolescents, Including Descriptions of Cancers, Treatments, and Coping Strategies

Along with Suggestions for Parents, Caregivers, and Concerned Relatives, a Glossary of Cancer Terms, and Resource Listings

Edited by Edward J. Prucha. 575 pages. 1999. 978-0-7808-0245-2.

"An excellent source of information. Recommended for public, hospital, and health science libraries with consumer health collections."
—*E-Streams, Jun '00*

"A valuable addition to all libraries specializing in health services and many public libraries."
—*American Reference Books Annual, 2000*

SEE ALSO *Childhood Diseases and Disorders Sourcebook, 2nd Edition, Healthy Children Sourcebook*

Physical and Mental Issues in Aging Sourcebook

Basic Consumer Health Information on Physical and Mental Disorders Associated with the Aging Process, Including Concerns about Cardiovascular Disease, Pulmonary Disease, Oral Health, Digestive Disorders, Musculoskeletal and Skin Disorders, Metabolic Changes, Sexual and Reproductive Issues, and Changes in Vision, Hearing, and Other Senses

Along with Data about Longevity and Causes of Death, Information on Acute and Chronic Pain, Descriptions of Mental Concerns, a Glossary of Terms, and Resource Listings for Additional Help

Edited by Jenifer Swanson. 660 pages. 1999. 978-0-7808-0233-9.

"This is a treasure of health information for the layperson."
—*CHOICE Health Sciences Supplement, May '00*

"Recommended for public libraries."
—*American Reference Books Annual, 2000*

SEE ALSO *Healthy Aging Sourcebook*

Podiatry Sourcebook, 2nd Edition

Basic Consumer Health Information about Disorders, Diseases, and Deformities that Affect the Foot and Ankle, Including Sprains, Corns, Calluses, Bunions, Plantar Warts, Plantar Fasciitis, Neuromas, Clubfoot, Flat Feet, Achilles Tendonitis, and Much More

Along with Information about Selecting a Foot Care Specialist, Foot Fitness, Shoes and Socks, Diagnostic Tests and Corrective Procedures, Financial Assistance for Corrective Devices, a Glossary of Related Terms, and a Directory of Resources for Additional Help and Information

Edited by Ivy L. Alexander. 516 pages. 2007. 978-0-7808-0944-4.

"An excellent resource... Although there have been various types of 'foot books' published in the past, none are as comprehensive as this one. 5 Stars (out of 5)!"
—*Doody's Review Service, 2007*

"Perfect for both health libraries and general-interest lending collections."
—*Internet Bookwatch, Jul '07*

Pregnancy and Birth Sourcebook, 3rd Edition

Basic Consumer Health Information about Pregnancy and Fetal Development, Including Facts about Fertility and Conception, Physical and Emotional Changes during Pregnancy, Prenatal Care and Diagnostic Tests, High-Risk Pregnancies and Complications, Labor, Delivery, and the Postpartum Period

Along with Tips on Maintaining Health and Wellness during Pregnancy and Caring for Newborn Infants, a Glossary of Related Terms, and Directories of Resources for Additional Help and Information

Edited by Amy L. Sutton. 645 pages. 2009. 978-0-7808-1074-7.

SEE ALSO *Breastfeeding Sourcebook, Congenital Disorders Sourcebook, 2nd Edition, Family Planning Sourcebook, Women's Health Concerns Sourcebook, 3rd Edition*

Prostate and Urological Disorders Sourcebook

Basic Consumer Health Information about Urogenital and Sexual Disorders in Men, Including Prostate and Other Andrological Cancers, Prostatitis, Benign Prostatic Hyperplasia, Testicular and Penile Trauma, Cryptorchidism, Peyronie Disease, Erectile Dysfunction, and Male Factor Infertility, and Facts about Commonly Used Tests and Procedures, Such as Prostatectomy, Vasectomy, Vasectomy Reversal, Penile Implants, and Semen Analysis

Along with a Glossary of Andrological Terms and a Directory of Resources for Additional Information

Edited by Karen Bellenir. 604 pages. 2006. 978-0-7808-0797-6.

"Certain to be a popular pick among library reference holdings... No prior knowledge is assumed for any of the conditions or terms herein, making it a most accessible general-interest reference."
— *California Bookwatch, Apr '06*

SEE ALSO *Men's Health Concerns Sourcebook, 3rd Edition, Urinary Tract and Kidney Diseases and Disorders Sourcebook, 2nd Edition*

Prostate Cancer Sourcebook

Basic Consumer Health Information about Prostate Cancer, Including Information about the Associated Risk Factors, Detection, Diagnosis, and Treatment of Prostate Cancer

Along with Information on Non-Malignant Prostate Conditions, and Featuring a Section Listing Support and Treatment Centers and a Glossary of Related Terms

Edited by Dawn D. Matthews. 340 pages. 2001. 978-0-7808-0324-4.

"Recommended reference source."
— *Booklist, Jan '02*

"A valuable resource for health care consumers seeking information on the subject... All text is written in a clear, easy-to-understand language that avoids technical jargon. Any library that collects consumer health resources would strengthen their collection with the addition of the Prostate Cancer Sourcebook."
— *American Reference Books Annual, 2002*

SEE ALSO *Cancer Sourcebook, 5th Edition, Men's Health Concerns Sourcebook, 3rd Edition*

Rehabilitation Sourcebook

Basic Consumer Health Information about Rehabilitation for People Recovering from Heart Surgery, Spinal Cord Injury, Stroke, Orthopedic Impairments, Amputation, Pulmonary Impairments, Traumatic Injury, and More, Including Physical Therapy, Occupational Therapy, Speech/Language Therapy, Massage Therapy, Dance Therapy, Art Therapy, and Recreational Therapy

Along with Information on Assistive and Adaptive Devices, a Glossary, and Resources for Additional Help and Information

Edited by Dawn D. Matthews. 519 pages. 2000. 978-0-7808-0236-0.

"This is an excellent resource for public library reference and health collections."
— *American Reference Books Annual, 2001*

"Recommended reference source."
— *Booklist, May '00*

Respiratory Disorders Sourcebook, 2nd Edition

Basic Consumer Health Information about Infectious, Inflammatory, and Chronic Conditions Affecting the Lungs and Respiratory System, Including Pneumonia, Bronchitis, Influenza, Tuberculosis, Sarcoidosis, Asthma, Cystic Fibrosis, Chronic Obstructive Pulmonary Disease, Lung Abscesses, Pulmonary Embolism, Occupational Lung Diseases, and Other Bacterial, Viral, and Fungal Infections

Along with Facts about the Structure and Function of the Lungs and Airways, Methods of Diagnosing Respiratory Disorders, and Treatment and Rehabilitation Options, a Glossary of Related Terms, and a Directory of Resources for Additional Help and Information

Edited by Sandra L. Judd. 638 pages. 2008. 978-0-7808-1007-5.

"An excellent book for patients, their families, or for those who are just curious about respiratory disease. Public libraries and physician offices would find this a valuable resource as well. 4 Stars! (out of 5)"
— *Doody's Review Service, 2009*

"A great addition for public and school libraries because it provides concise health information... readers can start with this reference source and get satisfactory answers before proceeding to other medical reference tools for

more in depth information... A good guide for health education on lung disorders."
—*American Reference Books Annual, 2009*

SEE ALSO *Asthma Sourcebook, 2nd Edition, Lung Disorders Sourcebook*

Sexually Transmitted Diseases Sourcebook, 4th Edition

Basic Consumer Health Information about Chlamydial Infections, Gonorrhea, Hepatitis, Herpes, HIV/AIDS, Human Papillomavirus, Pubic Lice, Scabies, Syphilis, Trichomoniasis, Vaginal Infections, and Other Sexually Transmitted Diseases, Including Facts about Risk Factors, Symptoms, Diagnosis, Treatment, and the Prevention of Sexually Transmitted Infections

Along with Updates on Current Research Initiatives, a Glossary of Related Terms, and Resources for Additional Help and Information

Edited by Laura Larsen. 623 pages. 2009. 978-0-7808-1073-0.

"Extremely beneficial... The question-and-answer format along with the index and table of contents make this well-organized resource extremely easy to reference, read, and comprehend... an invaluable medical reference source for lay readers, and a highly appropriate addition for public library collections, health clinics, and any library with a consumer health collection"
—*ARBAOnline, Oct '09*

SEE ALSO *AIDS Sourcebook, 4th Edition, Contagious Diseases Sourcebook, 2nd Edition, Men's Health Concerns Sourcebook, 3rd Edition, Women's Health Concerns Sourcebook, 3rd Edition*

Sleep Disorders Sourcebook, 3rd Edition

Basic Consumer Health Information about Sleep Disorders, Including Insomnia, Sleep Apnea and Snoring, Jet Lag and Other Circadian Rhythm Disorders, Narcolepsy, and Parasomnias, Such as Sleep Walking and Sleep Talking, and Featuring Facts about Other Health Problems that Affect Sleep, Why Sleep Is Necessary, How Much Sleep Is Needed, the Physical and Mental Effects of Sleep Deprivation, and Pediatric Sleep Issues

Along with Tips for Diagnosing and Treating Sleep Disorders, a Glossary of Related Terms, and a List of Resources for Additional Help and Information

Edited by Sandra J. Judd. 600 pages. 2010. 978-0-7808-1084-6.

Smoking Concerns Sourcebook

Basic Consumer Health Information about Nicotine Addiction and Smoking Cessation, Featuring Facts about the Health Effects of Tobacco Use, Including Lung and Other Cancers, Heart Disease, Stroke, and Respiratory Disorders, Such as Emphysema and Chronic Bronchitis

Along with Information about Smoking Prevention Programs, Suggestions for Achieving and Maintaining a Smoke-Free Lifestyle, Statistics about Tobacco Use, Reports on Current Research Initiatives, a Glossary of Related Terms, and Directories of Resources for Additional Help and Information

Edited by Karen Bellenir. 595 pages. 2004. 978-0-7808-0323-7.

"Provides everything needed for the student or general reader seeking practical details on the effects of tobacco use."
—*The Bookwatch, Mar '05*

"Public libraries and consumer health care libraries will find this work useful."
—*American Reference Books Annual, 2005*

SEE ALSO *Respiratory Disorders Sourcebook, 2nd Edition*

Sports Injuries Sourcebook, 3rd Edition

Basic Consumer Health Information about Sprains and Strains, Fractures, Growth Plate Injuries, Overtraining Injuries, and Injuries to the Head, Face, Shoulders, Elbows, Hands, Spinal Column, Knees, Ankles, and Feet, and with Facts about Heat-Related Illness, Steroids and Sport Supplements, Protective Equipment, Diagnostic Procedures, Treatment Options, and Rehabilitation

Along with a Glossary of Related Terms and a Directory of Resources for Additional Help and Information

Edited by Sandra J. Judd. 623 pages. 2007. 978-0-7808-0949-9.

SEE ALSO Fitness and Exercise Sourcebook, 3rd Edition, Podiatry Sourcebook, 2nd Edition

Stress-Related Disorders Sourcebook, 2nd Edition

Basic Consumer Health Information about Stress and Stress-Related Disorders, Including Types of Stress, Sources of Acute and Chronic Stress, the Impact of Stress on the Body's Systems, and Mental and Emotional Health Problems Associated with Stress, Such as Depression, Anxiety Disorders, Substance Abuse, Posttraumatic Stress Disorder, and Suicide

Along with Advice about Getting Help for Stress-Related Disorders, Information about Stress Management Techniques, a Glossary of Stress-Related Terms, and a Directory of Resources for Additional Help and Information

Edited by Amy L. Sutton. 608 pages. 2007. 978-0-7808-0996-3.

"Accessible to the lay reader. Highly recommended for medical and psychiatric collections."
—*Library Journal, Mar '08*

"Well-written for a general readership, the 2nd Edition of Stress-Related Disorders Sourcebook is a useful addition to the health reference literature."
—*American Reference Books Annual, 2008*

SEE ALSO Mental Health Disorders Sourcebook, 4th Edition

Stroke Sourcebook, 2nd Edition

Basic Consumer Health Information about Stroke, Including Ischemic, Hemorrhagic, and Mini Strokes, as Well as Risk Factors, Prevention Guidelines, Diagnostic Tests, Medications and Surgical Treatments, and Complications of Stroke

Along with Rehabilitation Techniques and Innovations, Tips on Staying Healthy and Maintaining Independence after Stroke, a Glossary of Related Terms, and a Directory of Resources for Stroke Survivors and Their Families

Edited by Amy L. Sutton. 626 pages. 2008. 978-0-7808-1035-8.

"An encyclopedic handbook on stroke that is written in a language the layperson can understand... This is one of the most helpful, readable books on stroke. This volume is highly recommended and should be in every medical, hospital and public library; in addition, every family practitioner should have a copy in his or her office."
—*American Reference Books Annual, 2009*

SEE ALSO Brain Disorders Sourcebook, 3rd Edition, Hypertension Sourcebook

Surgery Sourcebook, 2nd Edition

Basic Consumer Health Information about Common Inpatient and Outpatient Surgeries, Including Critical Care and Trauma, Gastrointestinal, Gynecologic and Obstetric, Cardiac and Vascular, Neurologic, Ophthalmologic, Orthopedic, Reconstructive and Cosmetic, and Other Major and Minor Surgeries

Along with Information about Anesthesia and Pain Relief Options, Risks and Complications, Postoperative Recovery Concerns, and Innovative Surgical Techniques and Tools, a Glossary of Related Terms, and a Directory of Additional Resources

Edited by Amy L. Sutton. 645 pages. 2008. 978-0-7808-1004-4.

"Large public libraries and medical libraries would benefit from this material in their reference collections."
—*American Reference Books Annual, 2009*

SEE ALSO Cosmetic and Reconstructive Surgery Sourcebook, 2nd Edition

Thyroid Disorders Sourcebook

Basic Consumer Health Information about Disorders of the Thyroid and Parathyroid Glands, Including Hypothyroidism, Hyperthyroidism, Graves Disease, Hashimoto Thyroiditis, Thyroid Cancer, and Parathyroid Disorders, Featuring Facts about Symptoms, Risk Factors, Tests, and Treatments

Along with Information about the Effects of Thyroid Imbalance on Other Body Systems, Environmental Factors That Affect the Thyroid Gland, a Glossary, and a Directory of Additional Resources

Edited by Joyce Brennfleck Shannon. 573 pages. 2005. 978-0-7808-0745-7.

"Recommended for consumer health collections."
—*American Reference Books Annual*, 2006

"Highly recommended pick for Basic Consumer health reference holdings at all levels."
—*The Bookwatch*, Aug '05

SEE ALSO *Endocrine and Metabolic Disorders Sourcebook, 2nd Edition*

Transplantation Sourcebook

Basic Consumer Health Information about Organ and Tissue Transplantation, Including Physical and Financial Preparations, Procedures and Issues Relating to Specific Solid Organ and Tissue Transplants, Rehabilitation, Pediatric Transplant Information, the Future of Transplantation, and Organ and Tissue Donation

Along with a Glossary and Listings of Additional Resources

Edited by Joyce Brennfleck Shannon. 610 pages. 2002. 978-0-7808-0322-0.

"Recommended for libraries with an interest in offering consumer health information."
—*E-Streams*, Jul '02

"This is a unique and valuable resource for patients facing transplantation and their families."
—*Doody's Review Service*, Jun '02

Traveler's Health Sourcebook

Basic Consumer Health Information for Travelers, Including Physical and Medical Preparations, Transportation Health and Safety, Essential Information about Food and Water, Sun Exposure, Insect and Snake Bites, Camping and Wilderness Medicine, and Travel with Physical or Medical Disabilities

Along with International Travel Tips, Vaccination Recommendations, Geographical Health Issues, Disease Risks, a Glossary, and a Listing of Additional Resources

Edited by Joyce Brennfleck Shannon. 619 pages. 2000. 978-0-7808-0384-8.

"Recommended reference source."
—*Booklist*, Feb '01

"This book is recommended for any public library, any travel collection, and especially any collection for the physically disabled."
—*American Reference Books Annual*, 2001

SEE ALSO *Worldwide Health Sourcebook*

Urinary Tract and Kidney Diseases and Disorders Sourcebook, 2nd Edition

Basic Consumer Health Information about the Urinary System, Including the Bladder, Urethra, Ureters, and Kidneys, with Facts about Urinary Tract Infections, Incontinence, Congenital Disorders, Kidney Stones, Cancers of the Urinary Tract and Kidneys, Kidney Failure, Dialysis, and Kidney Transplantation

Along with Statistical and Demographic Information, Reports on Current Research in Kidney and Urologic Health, a Summary of Commonly Used Diagnostic Tests, a Glossary of Related Terms, and a Directory of Resources for Additional Help and Information

Edited by Ivy L. Alexander. 621 pages. 2005. 978-0-7808-0750-1.

"A good choice for a consumer health information library or for a medical library needing information to refer to their patients."
—*American Reference Books Annual*, 2006

SEE ALSO *Prostate and Urological Disorders Sourcebook*

Vegetarian Sourcebook

Basic Consumer Health Information about Vegetarian Diets, Lifestyle, and Philosophy, Including Definitions of Vegetarianism and Veganism, Tips about Adopting Vegetarianism, Creating a Vegetarian Pantry, and Meeting Nutritional Needs of Vegetarians, with Facts Regarding Vegetarianism's Effect on Pregnant and Lactating Women, Children, Athletes, and Senior Citizens

Along with a Glossary of Commonly Used Vegetarian Terms and Resources for Additional Help and Information

Edited by Chad T. Kimball. 337 pages. 2002. 978-0-7808-0439-5.

"Organizes into one concise volume the answers to the most common questions concerning vegetarian diets and lifestyles. This title is recommended for public and secondary school libraries."

—*E-Streams, Apr '03*

"Invaluable reference for public and school library collections alike."
—*Library Bookwatch, Apr '03*

"The articles in this volume are easy to read and come from authoritative sources. The book does not necessarily support the vegetarian diet but instead provides the pros and cons of this important decision... Recommended for public libraries and consumer health libraries."
—*American Reference Books Annual, 2003*

SEE ALSO *Diet and Nutrition Sourcebook, 3rd Edition*

▪

Women's Health Concerns Sourcebook, 3rd Edition
Basic Consumer Health Information about Issues and Trends in Women's Health and Health Conditions of Special Concern to Women, Including Endometriosis, Uterine Fibroids, Menstrual Irregularities, Menopause, Sexual Dysfunction, Infertility, Cancer in Women, and Other Such Chronic Disorders as Lupus, Fibromyalgia, and Thyroid Disease

Along with Statistical Data, Tips for Maintaining Wellness, a Glossary, and a Directory of Resources for Further Help and Information

Edited by Sandra J. Judd. 679 pages. 2009. 978-0-7808-1036-5.

"This useful resource provides information about a wide range of topics that will help women understand their bodies, prevent or treat disease, and maintain health... A detailed index helps readers locate information. This is a useful addition to public and consumer health library collections"
—*ARBAOnline, Jun '09*

SEE ALSO *Breast Cancer Sourcebook, 3rd Edition, Cancer Sourcebook for Women, 4th Edition, Healthy Heart Sourcebook for Women*

▪

Workplace Health and Safety Sourcebook
Basic Consumer Health Information about Workplace Health and Safety, Including the Effect of Workplace Hazards on the Lungs,

Skin, Heart, Ears, Eyes, Brain, Reproductive Organs, Musculoskeletal System, and Other Organs and Body Parts

Along with Information about Occupational Cancer, Personal Protective Equipment, Toxic and Hazardous Chemicals, Child Labor, Stress, and Workplace Violence

Edited by Chad T. Kimball. 610 pages. 2000. 978-0-7808-0231-5.

"As a reference for the general public, this would be useful in any library."
—*E-Streams, Jun '01*

"Provides helpful information for primary care physicians and other caregivers interested in occupational medicine... General readers; professionals."
—*CHOICE, May '01*

▪

Worldwide Health Sourcebook
Basic Information about Global Health Issues, Including Malnutrition, Reproductive Health, Disease Dispersion and Prevention, Emerging Diseases, Risky Health Behaviors, and the Leading Causes of Death

Along with Global Health Concerns for Children, Women, and the Elderly, Mental Health Issues, Research and Technology Advancements, and Economic, Environmental, and Political Health Implications, a Glossary, and a Resource Listing for Additional Help and Information

Edited by Joyce Brennfleck Shannon. 597 pages. 2001. 978-0-7808-0330-5.

"Named an Outstanding Academic Title."
—*CHOICE, Jan '02*

"Yet another handy but also unique compilation in the extensive Health Reference Series, this is a useful work because many of the international publications reprinted or excerpted are not readily available. Highly recommended."
—*CHOICE, Nov '01*

SEE ALSO *Traveler's Health Sourcebook*

Teen Health Series
Complete Catalog
List price $69 per volume. School and library price $62 per volume.

Abuse and Violence Information for Teens
Health Tips about the Causes and Consequences of Abusive and Violent Behavior
Including Facts about the Types of Abuse and Violence, the Warning Signs of Abusive and Violent Behavior, Health Concerns of Victims, and Getting Help and Staying Safe

Edited by Sandra Augustyn Lawton. 411 pages. 2008. 978-0-7808-1008-2.

"A useful resource for schools and organizations providing services to teens and may also be a starting point in research projects."
— *Reference and Research Book News, Aug '08*

"Violence is a serious problem for teens... This resource gives teens the information they need to face potential threats and get help—either for themselves or for their friends."
— *American Reference Books Annual, 2009*

Accident and Safety Information for Teens
Health Tips about Medical Emergencies, Traumatic Injuries, and Disaster Preparedness
Including Facts about Motor Vehicle Accidents, Burns, Poisoning, Firearms, Natural Disasters, National Security Threats, and More

Edited by Karen Bellenir. 420 pages. 2008. 978-0-7808-1046-4.

"Aimed at teenage audiences, this guide provides practical information for handling a comprehensive list of emergencies, from sport injuries and auto accidents to alcohol poisoning and natural disasters."
— *Library Journal, Apr 1, '09*

"Useful in the young adult collections of public libraries as well as high school libraries."
— *American Reference Books Annual, 2009*

SEE ALSO *Sports Injuries Information for Teens, 2nd Edition*

Alcohol Information for Teens, 2nd Edition
Health Tips about Alcohol and Alcoholism
Including Facts about Alcohol's Effects on the Body, Brain, and Behavior, the Consequences of Underage Drinking, Alcohol Abuse Prevention and Treatment, and Coping with Alcoholic Parents

Edited by Lisa Bakewell. 410 pages. 2009. 978-0-7808-1043-3.

"This handbook, written for a teenage audience, provides information on the causes, effects, and preventive measures related to alcohol abuse among teens... The chapters are quick to make a connection to their teenage reading audience. The prose is straightforward and the book lends itself to spot reading. It should be useful both for practical information and for research, and it is suitable for public and school libraries."
— *ARBAOnline, Jun '09*

SEE ALSO *Drug Information for Teens, 2nd Edition*

Allergy Information for Teens
Health Tips about Allergic Reactions Such as Anaphylaxis, Respiratory Problems, and Rashes
Including Facts about Identifying and Managing Allergies to Food, Pollen, Mold, Animals, Chemicals, Drugs, and Other Substances

Edited by Karen Bellenir. 410 pages. 2006. 978-0-7808-0799-0.

"This is a comprehensive, readable text on the subject of allergic diseases in teenagers. 5 Stars (out of 5)!"
— *Doody's Review Service, Jun '06*

"This authoritative and useful self-help title is a solid addition to YA collections, whether for personal interest or reports."
— *School Library Journal, Jul '06*

Asthma Information for Teens, 2nd Ed.
Health Tips about Managing Asthma and Related Concerns

Including Facts about Asthma Causes, Triggers and Symptoms, Diagnosis, and Treatment

Edited by Kim Wohlenhaus. 400 pages. 2010. 978-0-7808-1086-0.

Body Information for Teens
Health Tips about Maintaining Well-Being for a Lifetime
Including Facts about the Development and Functioning of the Body's Systems, Organs, and Structures and the Health Impact of Lifestyle Choices

Edited by Sandra Augustyn Lawton. 458 pages. 2007. 978-0-7808-0443-2.

Cancer Information for Teens, 2nd Edition
Health Tips about Cancer Awareness, Symptoms, Prevention, Diagnosis, and Treatment
Including Facts about Common Cancers Affecting Teens, Causes, Detection, Coping Strategies, Clinical Trials, Nutrition and Exercise, Cancer in Friends or Family, and More

Edited by Karen Bellenir and Lisa Bakewell. 445 pages. 2010. 978-0-7808-1085-3.

Complementary and Alternative Medicine Information for Teens
Health Tips about Non-Traditional and Non-Western Medical Practices
Including Information about Acupuncture, Chiropractic Medicine, Dietary and Herbal Supplements, Hypnosis, Massage Therapy, Prayer and Spirituality, Reflexology, Yoga, and More

Edited by Sandra Augustyn Lawton. 407 pages. 2007. 978-0-7808-0966-6.

"This volume covers CAM specifically for teenagers but of general use also. It should be a welcome addition to both public and academic libraries."
—American Reference Books Annual, 2008

"This volume provides a solid foundation for further investigation of the subject, making it useful for both public and high school libraries."
—VOYA: Voice of Youth Advocates, Jun '07

Diabetes Information for Teens
Health Tips about Managing Diabetes and Preventing Related Complications
Including Information about Insulin, Glucose Control, Healthy Eating, Physical Activity, and Learning to Live with Diabetes

Edited by Sandra Augustyn Lawton. 410 pages. 2006. 978-0-7808-0811-9.

"A comprehensive instructional guide for teens... some of the material may also be directed towards parents or teachers. 5 stars (out of 5)!"
—Doody's Review Service, 2006

"Students dealing with their own diabetes or that of a friend or family member or those writing reports on the topic will find this a valuable resource."
—School Library Journal, Aug '06

"This text is directed to the teen population and would be an excellent library resource for a health class or for the teacher as a reference for class preparation. It can, however, serve a much wider audience. The clinical educator on diabetes may find it valuable to educate the newly diagnosed client regardless of age. It also would be an excellent reference and education tool for a preventive medicine seminar on diabetes."
—Physical Therapy, Mar '07

Diet Information for Teens, 2nd Edition
Health Tips about Diet and Nutrition
Including Facts about Dietary Guidelines, Food Groups, Nutrients, Healthy Meals, Snacks, Weight Control, Medical Concerns Related to Diet, and More

Edited by Karen Bellenir. 432 pages. 2006. 978-0-7808-0820-1.

"A very quick and pleasant read in spite of the fact that it is very detailed in the information it gives... A book for anyone concerned about diet and nutrition."
—American Reference Books Annual, 2007

SEE ALSO Eating Disorders Information for Teens, 2nd Edition

Drug Information for Teens, 2nd Edition

Health Tips about the Physical and Mental Effects of Substance Abuse

Including Information about Marijuana, Inhalants, Club Drugs, Stimulants, Hallucinogens, Opiates, Prescription and Over-the-Counter Drugs, Herbal Products, Tobacco, Alcohol, and More

Edited by Sandra Augustyn Lawton. 468 pages. 2006. 978-0-7808-0862-1.

"As with earlier installments in Omnigraphics' Teen Health Series, Drug Information for Teens is designed specifically to meet the needs and interests of middle and high school students... Strongly recommended for both academic and public libraries."
—*American Reference Books Annual, 2007*

"Solid thoughtful advice is given about how to handle peer pressure, drug-related health concerns, and treatment strategies."
—*School Library Journal, Dec '06*

SEE ALSO *Alcohol Information for Teens, 2nd Edition, Tobacco Information for Teens, 2nd Edition*

Eating Disorders Information for Teens, 2nd Edition

Health Tips about Anorexia, Bulimia, Binge Eating, And Other Eating Disorders

Including Information about Risk Factors, Diagnosis and Treatment, Prevention, Related Health Concerns, and Other Issues

Edited by Sandra Augustyn Lawton. 377 pages. 2009. 978-0-7808-1044-0.

"This handy reference offers basic information and addresses specific disorders, consequences, prevention, diagnosis and treatment, healthy eating, and more. It is written in a conversational style that is easy to understand... Will provide plenty of facts for reports as well as browsing potential for students with an interest in the topic."
—*School Library Journal, Jun '09*

"Written in a straightforward style that will appeal to its teenage audience. The author does not play down the danger of living with an eating disorder and urges those struggling with this problem to seek professional help.

This work, as well as others in this series, will be a welcome addition to high school and undergraduate libraries."
—*American Reference Books Annual, 2009*

SEE ALSO *Diet Information for Teens, 2nd Edition*

Fitness Information for Teens, 2nd Edition

Health Tips about Exercise, Physical Well-Being, and Health Maintenance

Including Facts about Conditioning, Stretching, Strength Training, Body Shape and Body Image, Sports Nutrition, and Specific Activities for Athletes and Non-Athletes

Edited by Lisa Bakewell. 432 pages. 2009. 978-0-7808-1045-7.

"This no-nonsense guide packs a great deal into its pages... This is a helpful reference for basic diet and exercise information for health reports or personal use."
—*School Library Journal, April 2009*

"An excellent source for general information on why teens should be active, making time to exercise, the equipment people might need, various types of activities to try, how to maintain health and wellness, and how to avoid barriers to becoming healthier... This would still be an excellent addition to a public library ready-reference collection or a high school health library collection."
—*American Reference Books Annual, 2009*

"This easy to read, well-written, up-to-date overview of fitness for teenagers provides excellent wellness and exercise tips, information, and directions... It is a useful tool for them to obtain a base knowledge in fitness topics and different sports."
—*Doody's Review Service, 2009*

SEE ALSO *Diet Information for Teens, 2nd Edition, Sports Injuries Information for Teens, 2nd Edition*

Learning Disabilities Information for Teens

Health Tips about Academic Skills Disorders and Other Disabilities That Affect Learning

Including Information about Common Signs of Learning Disabilities, School Issues, Learning to Live with a Learning Disability, and Other Related Issues

Edited by Sandra Augustyn Lawton. 400 pages. 2006. 978-0-7808-0796-9.

"This book provides a wealth of information for any reader interested in the signs, causes, and consequences of learning disabilities, as well as related legal rights and educational interventions... Public and academic libraries should want this title for both students and general readers."

—American Reference Books Annual, 2006

Mental Health Information for Teens, 3rd Edition
Health Tips about Mental Wellness and Mental Illness
Including Facts about Mental and Emotional Health, Depression and Other Mood Disorders, Anxiety Disorders, Behavior Disorders, Self-Injury, Psychosis, Schizophrenia, and More

Edited by Karen Bellenir. 400 pages. 2010. 978-0-7808-1087-7.

SEE ALSO *Stress Information for Teens, Suicide Information for Teens, 2nd Edition*

Pregnancy Information for Teens
Health Tips about Teen Pregnancy and Teen Parenting
Including Facts about Prenatal Care, Pregnancy Complications, Labor and Delivery, Postpartum Care, Pregnancy-Related Lifestyle Concerns, and More

Edited by Sandra Augustyn Lawton. 434 pages. 2007. 978-0-7808-0984-0.

Sexual Health Information for Teens, 2nd Edition
Health Tips about Sexual Development, Reproduction, Contraception, and Sexually Transmitted Infections
Including Facts about Puberty, Sexuality, Birth Control, Chlamydia, Gonorrhea, Herpes, Human Papillomavirus, Syphilis, and More

Edited by Sandra Augustyn Lawton. 430 pages. 2008. 978-0-7808-1010-5.

"This offering represents the most up-to-date information available on an array of topics including abstinence-only sexual education and pregnancy-prevention methods... The range of coverage—from puberty and anatomy to sexually transmitted diseases—is thorough and extensive. Each chapter includes a bibliographic citation, and the three back sections containing additional resources, further reading, and the index are all first-rate... This volume will be well used by students in need of the facts, whether for educational or personal reasons."

—School Library Journal, Nov '08

"Presents information related to the emotional, physical, and biological development of both males and females that occurs during puberty. It also strives to address some of the issues and questions that may arise... The text is easy to read and understand for young readers, with satisfactory definitions within the text to explain new terms."

—American Reference Books Annual, 2009

Skin Health Information for Teens, 2nd Edition
Health Tips about Dermatological Concerns and Skin Cancer Risks
Including Facts about Acne, Warts, Hives, and Other Conditions and Lifestyle Choices, Such as Tanning, Tattooing, and Piercing, That Affect the Skin, Nails, Scalp, and Hair

Edited by Edited by Kim Wohlenhaus. 418 pages. 2009. 978-0-7808-1042-6.

"The material in this work will be easily understood by teenagers and young adults. The publisher has liberally used bulleted lists and sidebars to keep the reader's attention... A useful addition to school and public library collections."

—ARBAOnline, Oct '09

Sleep Information for Teens
Health Tips about Adolescent Sleep Requirements, Sleep Disorders, and the Effects of Sleep Deprivation
Including Facts about Why People Need Sleep, Sleep Patterns, Circadian Rhythms, Dreaming, Insomnia, Sleep Apnea, Narcolepsy, and More

Edited by Karen Bellenir. 355 pages. 2008. 978-0-7808-1009-9.

"Clear, concise, and very readable and would be a good source of sleep information for anyone—not just teenagers. This work is highly recommended for medical libraries, public school libraries, and public libraries."
—*American Reference Books Annual, 2009*

SEE ALSO Body Information for Teens

Sports Injuries Information for Teens, 2nd Edition
Health Tips about Acute, Traumatic, and Chronic Injuries in Adolescent Athletes
Including Facts about Sprains, Fractures, and Overuse Injuries, Treatment, Rehabilitation, Sport-Specific Safety Guidelines, Fitness Suggestions, and More

Edited by Karen Bellenir. 429 pages. 2008. 978-0-7808-1011-2.

"An engaging selection of informative articles about the prevention and treatment of sports injuries... The value of this book is that the articles have been vetted and are often augmented with inserts of useful facts, definitions of technical terms, and quick tips. Sensitive topics like injuries to genitalia are discussed openly and responsibly. This revised edition contains updated articles and defines sport more broadly than the first edition."
—*School Library Journal, Nov '08*

"This work will be useful in the young adult collections of public libraries as well as high school libraries... A useful resource for student research."
—*American Reference Books Annual, 2009*

SEE ALSO Accident and Safety Information for Teens

Stress Information for Teens
Health Tips about the Mental and Physical Consequences of Stress
Including Information about the Different Kinds of Stress, Symptoms of Stress, Frequent Causes of Stress, Stress Management Techniques, and More

Edited by Sandra Augustyn Lawton. 392 pages. 2008. 978-0-7808-1012-9.

"Understanding what stress is, what causes it, how the body and the mind are impacted by it, and what teens can do are the general categories addressed here... The chapters are brief but informative, and the list of community-help organizations is exhaustive. Report writers will find information quickly and easily, as will those who have personal concerns. The print is clear and the format is readable, making this an accessible resource for struggling readers and researchers."
—*School Library Journal, Dec '08*

"The articles selected will specifically appeal to young adults and are designed to answer their most common questions."
— *American Reference Books Annual, 2009*

SEE ALSO Mental Health Information for Teens, 3rd Edition

Suicide Information for Teens, 2nd Edition
Health Tips about Suicide Causes and Prevention
Including Facts about Depression, Risk Factors, Getting Help, Survivor Support, and More

Edited by Kim Wohlenhaus. 400 pages. 2010. 978-0-7808-1088-4.

SEE ALSO Mental Health Information for Teens, 3rd Edition

Tobacco Information for Teens, 2nd Edition
Health Tips about the Hazards of Using Cigarettes, Smokeless Tobacco, and Other Nicotine Products
Including Facts about Nicotine Addiction, Nicotine Delivery Systems, Secondhand Smoke, Health Consequences of Tobacco Use, Related Cancers, Smoking Cessation, and Tobacco Use Statistics

Edited by Karen Bellenir. 400 pages. 2010. 978-0-7808-1153-9.

SEE ALSO Drug Information for Teens, 2nd Edition

Health Reference Series

Adolescent Health Sourcebook, 3rd Edition

Adult Health Concerns Sourcebook

AIDS Sourcebook, 4th Edition

Alcoholism Sourcebook, 3rd Edition

Allergies Sourcebook, 3rd Edition

Alzheimer Disease Sourcebook, 4th Edition

Arthritis Sourcebook, 3rd Edition

Asthma Sourcebook, 2nd Edition

Attention Deficit Disorder Sourcebook

Autism & Pervasive Developmental Disorders Sourcebook

Back & Neck Sourcebook, 2nd Edition

Blood & Circulatory Disorders Sourcebook, 3rd Edition

Brain Disorders Sourcebook, 3rd Edition

Breast Cancer Sourcebook, 3rd Edition

Breastfeeding Sourcebook

Burns Sourcebook

Cancer Sourcebook for Women, 4th Edition

Cancer Sourcebook, 5th Edition

Cancer Survivorship Sourcebook

Cardiovascular Disorders Sourcebook, 4th Edition

Caregiving Sourcebook

Child Abuse Sourcebook

Childhood Diseases & Disorders Sourcebook, 2nd Edition

Colds, Flu & Other Common Ailments Sourcebook

Communication Disorders Sourcebook

Complementary & Alternative Medicine Sourcebook, 4th Edition

Congenital Disorders Sourcebook, 2nd Edition

Contagious Diseases Sourcebook

Cosmetic & Reconstructive Surgery Sourcebook, 2nd Edition

Death & Dying Sourcebook, 2nd Edition

Dental Care & Oral Health Sourcebook, 3rd Edition

Depression Sourcebook, 2nd Edition

Dermatological Disorders Sourcebook, 2nd Edition

Diabetes Sourcebook, 4th Edition

Diet & Nutrition Sourcebook, 3rd Edition

Digestive Diseases & Disorder Sourcebook

Disabilities Sourcebook

Disease Management Sourcebook

Domestic Violence Sourcebook, 3rd Edition

Drug Abuse Sourcebook, 3rd Edition

Ear, Nose & Throat Disorders Sourcebook, 2nd Edition

Eating Disorders Sourcebook, 3rd Edition

Emergency Medical Services Sourcebook

Endocrine & Metabolic Disorders Sourcebook, 2nd Edition

Environmental Health Sourcebook, 3rd Edition

Ethnic Diseases Sourcebook

Eye Care Sourcebook, 3rd Edition

Family Planning Sourcebook

Fitness & Exercise Sourcebook, 4th Edition

Food Safety Sourcebook

Forensic Medicine Sourcebook

Gastrointestinal Diseases & Disorders Sourcebook, 2nd Edition

Genetic Disorders Sourcebook, 3rd Edition

Head Trauma Sourcebook

Headache Sourcebook

Health Insurance Sourcebook

Healthy Aging Sourcebook

Healthy Children Sourcebook

Healthy Heart Sourcebook for Women

Hepatitis Sourcebook

Household Safety Sourcebook

Hypertension Sourcebook

Immune System Disorders Sourcebook, 2nd Edition

Infant & Toddler Health Sourcebook

Infectious Diseases Sourcebook

Injury & Trauma Sourcebook